Nutritional Management of Equine Diseases and Special Cases

Nutritional Management of Equine Diseases and Special Cases

Bryan M. Waldridge

Park Equine Hospital at Woodford,
Versailles, KY, USA

WILEY Blackwell

Dedication

This book is dedicated to my wife, Sonja; my parents; and family who never complain and always understand when I have to go see a sick horse.

Contents

Contributors

Iveta Becvarova, DVM, MS, DACVN
Hill's Pet Nutrition,
Prague, Czech Republic

Ramesh C. Gupta, DVM, MVSc, PhD, DABT, FACT,
FACN, FATS
Toxicology Department,
Breathitt Veterinary Center,
Murray State University,
Hopkinsville, KY, USA

Peter Huntington, BVSc (Hons), MANZCVS
Kentucky Equine Research,
Mulgrave, Victoria, Australia

Anthony P. Knight, BVSc, MS, DACVIM
Professor Emeritus,
Colorado State University,
Fort Collins, CO, USA

Amelia Munsterman, DVM, MS, DACVS, DACVECC
Department of Surgical Sciences,
University of Wisconsin,
Madison WI, USA

Nicole Passler, DVM, MS
Equine Source Plasma Project,
College of Veterinary Medicine,
Auburn University,
Auburn, AL, USA

DG Pugh, DVM, MS, MAg, DACT, DACVN, DACVM
Alabama Veterinary Diagnostic Laboratory System,
Auburn, AL, USA

Stephanie J. Valberg, DVM, PhD, Diplomate ACVIM,
ACVSMR
Mary Anne McPhail Equine Performance Center,
Michigan State University,
East Lansing, MI, USA

Bryan M. Waldridge, DVM, MS, DABVP, DACVIM
Park Equine Hospital at Woodford,
Versailles, KY, USA

Sara Ziska, DVM, PhD
College of Veterinary Medicine,
Auburn University,
Auburn, AL, USA

Preface

Water, hay, and oats are all that a horse needs.

Anonymous

Even in modern times, this is often said from the race-track to the farm. However, from a nutritional perspective it does not hold true for all horses. Depending on hay quality and type: energy, protein, and calcium may be deficient, especially for working horses and mares in late gestation. Working horses may require such a large amount of oats to meet energy requirements that they would be at risk for hindgut acidosis and subsequent laminitis. A horse may not be physically able to eat enough hay to meet increased energy requirements, depending on the hay's energy content and quality.

We are fortunate to have a plethora of horse feeds that are formulated by knowledgeable equine nutritionists and tested to ensure that they meet horses' requirements. Most commercial feeds are fortified with vitamins and minerals to meet requirements if the horse is fed as directed on the bag. Modern feeding and overfeeding practices, as well as the horse's transition from a working to a companion animal, have created problems such as Equine Metabolic Syndrome. Horses are both living longer and becoming fatter with our help.

Like most equine practices, feeding horses can become as infinitely complicated as we make it to be. Many horses receive multiple supplements and many contain the same ingredients. At least, this is expensive and unnecessary and at worst, it can result in toxicity. Unfortunately, supplementation and feeding decisions are often based on the advice of a self-proclaimed authority or because someone else does it with apparent success.

The purpose of this book is to guide decision making and clarify the sometimes-confusing subject of equine nutrition. Thank you to my coauthors for their contributions, including my former major professor Dr. David Pugh, whose guidance and education have been a tremendous gift.

Bryan M. Waldridge

1 Miniature horses and ponies

DG Pugh, DVM, MS, MAg, DACT, DACVN, DACVM; Nicole Passler, DVM, MS; and Sara Ziska, DVM, PhD

This chapter will discuss feeding of miniature horses and ponies, two of the smallest members of the genus, species, and subspecies *Equus ferus caballus*. Both miniature horses and ponies should be fed in a similar fashion as light breeds, with the obvious exception that they are smaller and therefore require less total nutrients on a body weight basis. Many of the common feeding and husbandry practices applicable for other breeds may be applicable to both miniature and pony breeds.[1]

1.1 Miniature Horses

Although the American Miniature horse was declared a single breed in the late 1970s by the American Horse Association, many miniature horse breeders consider several distinct breeds to exist (e.g., Australian Miniature Pony, Dartmoor Pony, Falabella, Micro Mini, Miniature Toy Horse, etc.). These breeds can be traced back to royal families in Europe of the seventeenth century. Presently, these equids are used as pets, show, and service animals. Miniature horses usually live 25–35 years and are described as being less than 97 cm (38 in) in height at the withers (probably all carry some genes for dwarfism). Many non-guide miniature horses may weigh up to 90 kg, while the minis used as service animals should be less than 66 cm (26 in) in height and weigh between 24–45 kg (55–100 lb).

1.2 General Feeding of Miniature Horses

Unlike ponies, there are few controlled scientific studies on nutritional requirements of miniature horses.[1–3] Minis are considered an "easy keeper" breed and should not be overfed to prevent obesity. As with other horse breeds, energy requirements for maintenance usually can be met by feeding 1.0–1.8% of their body weight daily in dry matter derived from good quality forages or 1–2 kg of good quality dry forage daily. Miniature horses can be fed small amounts of grass or hay and concentrates or used to graze or "mow" lawns. Supplemental grain should be fed only as needed and added to the diet based upon body condition score (BCS). The principles of body condition scoring are the same for miniatures as for other breeds of horses. Miniature horses should be maintained at an ideal BCS of 5–6/9 (ribs can easily be palpated, but not seen, and there are no obvious fat deposits on the neck, shoulders, withers, or tail base). Body condition scoring should be used to determine energy intake adequacy or lack thereof.[1] When BCS falls below 5/9, caretakers should consider increasing either the quality and/or quantity of forages or slowly introducing a small amount (0.25–0.5 lb/day) of concentrate. Common mistakes made with concentrate feeding include overestimation of body weight and underestimation of concentrate offered. Both mistakes can result in obesity and possibly one of many metabolic disorders (e.g., equine metabolic syndrome, laminitis, hyperlipemia, etc.) seen in overweight miniature horses. Owners of miniature horses should be encouraged to purchase scales to actually weigh feed to avoid overfeeding. Scales used by fishermen to weigh fish are inexpensive and can be readily purchased. As for other horses, access to fresh clean water is critical to ensure adequate feed intake, minimize colic risk, and maintain overall health. The general guidelines for water, energy, protein, mineral, and vitamin requirements as a percent of diet are based upon age, growth, production status (e.g. early, mid, late gestation, or lactation), and use of miniature horses, and are similar to other breeds.[1]

Miniature horses are susceptible to many of the nutritionally related conditions seen in other breeds, but may be more prone to enteroliths[4] and hyperlipemia.[5,6]

Nutritional Management of Equine Diseases and Special Cases, First Edition. Edited by Bryan M. Waldridge.

Caregivers should be cognizant of normal horse feeding practices and adopt well-conceived, basic feeding programs as discussed in other chapters of this text.

1.3 Pony Feeding

Ponies are horses less than 147 cm (14.2 hands or 58 in) in height at the withers. Pony breeds typically have shorter heads with broader foreheads, thicker necks, wider barrels, and shorter legs compared to other horses. Pony breeds are used as pets, show, riding, and working animals. There are many distinct breeds of ponies with varying uses that help determine proper feeding programs (e.g., carriage ponies vs hunter/jumper ponies).

Because of their size and availability, ponies have been utilized in many equine nutrition research projects. Therefore, much information is available specifically discussing pony nutrition.[7–11] Feeding practices for other light breeds are usually applicable to ponies.[1] Many pony breeds will reach 75% of their mature weight by 12 months of age, while Thoroughbred horses only reach approximately 69% of mature weight at the same age.[1] Therefore, feeding practices should be adjusted for ponies compared to other breeds because of their faster growth rate. Because most pony breeds were selected and evolved under conditions of sparse or poor quality pasture and rugged terrain, they tend to be easier to maintain than other horse breeds. With the possible exception of working, lactating, and growing ponies, most ponies will rarely require concentrates and easily become obese. Ponies are predisposed to many metabolic conditions, such as hyperlipemia and equine metabolic syndrome.[1,12,13] Increased fat supplementation with soybean oil at 10% of dry matter intake was associated with glucose intolerance in Shetland ponies.[14] Ponies appear to have a higher voluntary intake than other horse breeds.[1,11,15] In one study, ponies consumed 3.9 kg of alfalfa hay per 100 kg of body weight (3.9% of body weight in dry matter intake).[11] Caretakers should be cautious and utilize high energy feedstuffs only when necessary. When providing a concentrate or concentrates, the BCS should be continuously monitored to minimize obesity.

As for miniature horses, ponies should be fed good quality forages at 1.0–1.8% of their body weight in dry matter daily. Body condition scores should be estimated for ponies as for other breeds, with diet modifications implemented to maintain ideal body condition near 5–6/9. Ponies at maintenance (neither gaining nor losing weight) usually can survive on hay only or grass pastures, while those used for light work may require 20% of their dietary intake in the form of a concentrate. Feed should be withheld from ponies only when medically indicated and with strict observation. Prolonged periods of inadequate energy intake result in hyperlipemia, which is exacerbated by preexisting conditions such as illness, pregnancy, and/or obesity.[1]

References

1. National Research Council. Nutrient Requirements of Horses, 6th ed. National Research Council, The National Academies Press, 2007.
2. Hoyt JK, Potter GD, Greene LW, et al. Mineral balance in resting and exercised miniature horses. J Equine Vet Sci 1995;15(7):310–314.
3. Hoyt JK, Potter GD, Greene LW, et al. Copper balance in miniature horses fed varying amounts of zinc. J Equine Vet Sci 1995;15(8):357–359.
4. Cohen ND, Vontur CA, Rakestraw PC. Risk factors for enterolithiasis among horses in Texas. J Am Vet Med Assoc 2000;216:1787–1794.
5. Moore BR, Abood SK, Hinchcliff KW. Hyperlipemia in 9 miniature horses and miniature donkeys. J Vet Intern Med 1994;8(5):376–381.
6. Golenz MR, Knight DA, Yvorchuk-St Jean KE. Use of a human enteral feeding preparation for treatment of hyperlipemia and nutritional support during healing of an esophageal laceration in a miniature horse. J Am Vet Med Assoc 1992;200(7):951–953.
7. Vermorel, M; J Vernet; W Martin-Rosset. Digestive and energy utilisation of two diets by ponies and horses. Livest Prod Sci 1997;51:13–19.
8. Kane E, Baker JP, Bull LS. Utilization of corn oil supplemented diet by the pony. J Anim Sci 1979;48:1379–1384.
9. Goodson J, Tyznik WJ, Cline JH, et al. Effects of an abrupt diet change from hay to concentrate on microbial numbers and physical environment in the cecum of the pony. Appl Environ Microb 1988;54(8):1946–1950.
10. Cuddeford D, Pearson RA, Archibald RF, et al. Digestibility and gastro-intestinal transit time of diets containing different proportions of alfalfa and oat straw given to thoroughbreds, Shetland ponies, highland ponies, and donkeys. 1995; Anim Sci 61:407–417.
11. Pearson RA, Archibald RF, Muirhead RH. The effect of forage quality and level of feeding on digestibility and gastrointestinal transit time of oat straw and alfalfa given to ponies and donkeys. Brit J Nutr 2001;85:599–606.
12. Treiber K, Carter R, Gay L, et al. Inflammatory and redox status of ponies with a history of pasture-associated laminitis. Vet Immunol Immunopathol 2009;129(3–4):216–20.

13. Hughes KJ, Hodgson DR, Dart AJ. Hyperlipaemia in a 7-week-old miniature pony foal. Aust Vet J 2002;80(6):350–1.

14. Schmidt O, Deegen E, Fuhrmann H, et al. Effects of fat feeding and energy level on plasma metabolites and hormones in Shetland ponies. J Vet Med 2001;48A:39–49.

15. Argo C McG, Cox JE, Lockyear C, et al. Adaptive changes in the appetite, growth, and feeding behaviour of pony mares offered ad libitum access to a complete diet in either a pelleted or chaffbased form. Anim Scis 2002; 74:517–528.

2 Draft horses, mules, and donkeys

DG Pugh, DVM, MS, MAg, DACT, DACVN, DACVM; Sara Ziska, DVM, PhD; and Nicole Passler, DVM, MS

Draft horses, donkeys, and their hybrid crosses are discussed together in this chapter, as all three are traditionally thought of as working animals or "beasts of burden." Draft horses, mules, and donkeys still are used as working animals, but also as pets, for trail riding, cart pulling, showing, and other recreational uses. As all three are of the genus *Equus*, this chapter will review some of the differences between them and other horse breeds with respect to feeding.

2.1 Draft Horses

There are approximately 30 breeds of draft or draught horses found in the world today. These large horses (550–1180 kg or 1400–2600 lb) are utilized in farming and logging industries, blood or plasma donation, biological and pharmaceutical production, advertising campaigns, as carriage horses, show horses, and pets. The most popular breeds of draft horses in the United States, Belgians, Clydesdales, Percherons, and Shires, all originated in Western Europe. These breeds were selected for their tall stature, heavy bone and frame structure, muscular hindquarters, and patience to haul large loads.

Traditionally, these large working animals were thought to have a similar nutrient metabolism as pony breeds. Historically, draft breeds have been fed slightly less feed per kg of body weight than light breeds. The most recent National Research Council feeding guidelines for horses[1] suggested that idle, mature, healthy draft horses could subsist on 30.3 kcal of digestible energy (DE)/kg of body weight daily. This energy requirement is slightly lower than 33.3 kcal/kg of body weight daily recommended for light horse breeds. Obviously, during work, growth, lactation, or other periods of increased energy expenditure, the energy requirements are greater. The total energy requirement is higher for draft horses (700 kg or greater) than light horse breeds (Thoroughbred, Quarter Horse, etc.), as these breeds may weigh substantially less (425–480 kg). Mature draft horses should be fed a minimum of 1.5% of their body weight in roughage daily, with a total dry matter intake between 1.5–3.0% of their body weight daily. Still, these breeds can be fed using many of the general guidelines applicable to light breeds.

Good quality grass-legume mixed pastures or hay will usually suffice for draft horses at maintenance (neither gaining nor losing weight). The caregiver should always be cognizant of carbohydrate concentrations in the forage and pastures, as with any breed of horse, to minimize the risk of colic and laminitis.

Feeding to maintain a body condition score (BCS) of 5–6/9 is optimal in most circumstances. The energy density of the diet and/or use of supplemental high energy feedstuffs (e.g., concentrates) should be adjusted to support growth, production, lactation, late gestation, work, and needs for increased energy use with the goal of maintaining a BCS between 5–6/9. Total dietary energy required will depend on the type of work, duration of work, weight of loads, or the amount of force exerted to perform work. Again, body condition should be used to adjust energy intake to meet demands and maintain BCS in the 5–6/9 range. Unfortunately, draft horses may be prone to Polysaccharide Storage Myopathy, Exertional Rhabdomyolysis, Equine Metabolic Syndrome, and other diet-related conditions.[1-3] Thus, feeding diets high in carbohydrates should be done with extreme caution, and then only when necessary. Nutritional myopathies are discussed in Chapter 4.

Overall, these breeds seem less prone to developmental orthopedic disease.[1,4,5] Of the draft horses, Clydesdales and Percherons appear to be the breeds most affected with metabolic bone diseases.[5] The caregiver is cautioned to follow feeding practices that minimize developmental orthopedic disease in growing animals.

Nutritional Management of Equine Diseases and Special Cases, First Edition. Edited by Bryan M. Waldridge.
© 2017 John Wiley & Sons, Inc. Published 2017 by John Wiley & Sons, Inc.

Unfortunately, the large size of draft horses presents other management issues that directly affect feeding. The authors have observed more catastrophic outcomes when draft breeds develop laminitis and increased heat stress with obesity, as compared to lighter breeds. The caregiver should strive to maintain a BCS of 5–6/9 and carefully monitor obese animals, particularly in times of warm weather or when laminitis is a concern.

Due to their impressive body weight, it is not uncommon for draft horses to require 24 gallons (91 L) of fresh, clean water daily. Dehydration may result if caregivers are unable to meet these extreme demands, which increases the risk of developing intestinal impactions and other potentially life-threatening conditions.

2.2 Donkeys

Donkeys or asses (*Equus africanus asinus* or *Equus asinus*) are traditionally thought of as working animals, and in many parts of the world are depended upon in this manner. In modern-day North America, donkeys or "burros" are used for work, show, cart and/or carriage pulling, competitive riding, drug smuggling, guard animals, training animals, and pets. There are 15–20 breeds of donkeys, including miniature, standard, large standard, and mammoth stock, which vary greatly in height (81–157 cm or 32–62 in). The female is commonly referred to as a jenny or jennet. Intact males are commonly called a jack or jackass. These animals characteristically have longer ears and make loud vocal noises ("bray"), as compared to horses. Their reproductive cycle has similarities to that of the horse and has been described.[6]

Donkeys are believed to have evolved in arid to semi-arid climates and show extraordinary tolerance for heat and dehydration. They seem able to continue eating for several days in the absence of drinkable water. This is in contrast to horses, which decrease forage and feed consumption in the face of dehydration. In modern agricultural husbandry practices, as with other equids, clean, fresh water should be offered to donkeys free choice, despite their relative hardiness.

Donkeys appear to readily adapt to new environments and feedstuffs, which is not common in other equids.[1] It is an accepted husbandry practice to feed donkeys less than horses on a body weight basis, as they are not simply small horses.[1] Donkeys have a narrow muzzle and mobile lips, which allow for greater feed selection in comparison to most horses. Therefore, they can selectively consume higher quality portions of available forages. Donkeys will subsist on more mature forages than are willingly consumed by most horses (e.g., bark on trees and shrubs), but can and will consume traditional feedstuffs.[1,7,8] On poor quality forage diets, donkeys appear to have a lower dry matter intake requirement than ponies.[9,10] Reported voluntary dry matter intake ranges for donkeys have been between 0.83–2.6% of body weight, depending on the type and quality of the feed stuff, along with physiologic requirements.[11,12] However, dry matter intake between 1.75–2.25% of body weight of moderate to good quality forage will routinely meet maintenance requirements in mature donkeys.[1] When offered moderate to good quality forages, donkeys will readily adapt to consume complete diets and employ their selective grazing habits only when offered mixed forage diets of differing quality.[13]

Traditional donkey feeding practices infer that donkeys are more efficient in digestion than horses. Donkeys appear to have higher apparent digestibility for dietary dry matter and fiber than ponies and horses, particularly when fed poor quality forages (e.g., oat straw).[11,14] The higher digestibility ability of donkeys could be attributed to longer gut retention time or greater microbial cellulolytic activity in the cecum, compared to other equids.[15,16]

Some reports have shown that donkeys may require only 3.8–7.4% protein in their diet, due to efficient dietary protein utilization.[17,18] Despite these findings, the authors recommend that dietary protein intake in donkey diets should be fed similar to recommendations for horses. Consequently, feeding as for horses should meet requirements for donkeys, with respect to protein intake.

In parts of the world where high quality feedstuffs are plentiful, obesity in donkeys is a major concern. Caregivers should be mindful to feed donkeys only to a desired body condition and avoiding over-conditioning. Energy-protein malnutrition, mineral deficiencies, and emaciation are of most concern in many tropical areas of the world where donkeys are used as work animals.

Donkeys fed to obesity will develop a fat roll over the neck (pones) and fat on the barrel and hips, which are quite unsightly. Donkeys, much like pony breeds, may be prone to hyperlipemia during stress and feed deprivation.[1]

Caregivers should closely monitor donkeys for feed intake in times of stress (e.g., changes in weather, illness, etc.). Because of the stoic disposition of donkeys, close attention to dietary intake and body condition is imperative. Body condition scoring systems for donkeys have been described.[19,20] The Vall system assigns a score from 1 (emaciated) to 4 (good), with emphasis placed on the appearance of the flank and back.[19]

Diets appropriate and practical for horses can typically be fed to donkeys, with caregivers mindful to avoid obesity. Diets should include 6–10% protein intake for maintenance needs, free access to fresh clean water, and a good quality mineral mixture designed for horses.

2.3 Mules

Mules are the offspring of a male donkey (jack or jackass) and a female horse (mare). Their size, shape, and use are often determined by the breed characteristics of both the sire and dam. Thus, mules can be found in all statures, colors, and types of conformations. Mules were used primarily for riding, packing, and/or working animals. Today, mules are still used for these purposes, as well as guard animals for small ruminants, showing, recreation, and pets. The female mule is traditionally referred to as a female, mare mule, molly, or molly mule, whereas the male mule is traditionally referred to as a male, gelded/stud mule, or john mule. Mules are considered more sure-footed, patient, hardier, and slower than horses, and less obstinate than donkeys. As donkeys have 62 chromosomes and horses have 64 chromosomes, mule hybrids are rarely fertile. The cross between a stallion and a jenny is called a hinney; hinnies tend to be more donkey-like and much less common than mules.

Mules are routinely fed less than horses but more than donkeys on a body weight basis. Regrettably, there are few controlled studies on nutritional requirements for mules.[20] Mules are physiologically more similar to horses than donkeys and feeding practices should take this into account. Accordingly, mules from Quarter Horse mares and used for Quarter Horse-like purposes should be fed in a similar manner for the mare. However, caregivers must remain cognizant that these mules are also part donkey and therefore may require less total dietary intake than Quarter Horses of similar size. This principle is applicable across lines of mules; that is mules

should be fed in a similar fashion to that of the dam. As with donkeys, obesity can be a major problem in mules, so caution should be exercised when feeding high energy diets. Overall, energy, protein, and mineral requirements in mules appear to be very similar to horses, with the exception that mules may digest feedstuffs more efficiently than horses.

References

1. National Research Council, Nutrient requirements of horses, 6th ed. National Research Council: The National Academies Press, 2007.
2. Valentine BA, Credille KM, Lavoie JP, et al. Severe polysaccharide storage myopathy in Belgian and Percheron draft horse. *Equine Vet J* 1997;29:220–225.
3. Valentine BA, Habecker PL, Patterson JS, et al. Incidence of polysaccharide storage myopathy in draft horse-related breeds: a necropsy study of 37 horses and a mule. *J Vet Diagn Invest* 2001;13:63–68.
4. Stromberg B. A review of the salient features of osteochondrosis in the horse. *Equine Vet J* 1979;11:211–214.
5. Riley CB, Scott WM, Caron JP, et al. Osteochondritis dessicans and subchondral cystic lesions in draft horses: a retrospective study. *Can Vet J* 1998;39:627–633.
6. Wilborn RR, Pugh DG. Donkey reproduction. In: McKinnon AO, Squires EL, Vaala WE, et al., eds, *Equine reproduction*. 2nd ed. Ames: Wiley-Blackwell, 2011;2835–2838.
7. Mueller PJ, Protos P, Houpt KA, et al. Chewing behavior in the domestic donkey (*Equus asimus*) fed fibrous forage. *Appl Anim Behav Sci* 1998;60:241–251.
8. Suhartanto B, Tisserand JL. 1996. A comparison of the utilization of hay and straw by ponies and donkeys. 47th EAAP meeting, Lillehammer.
9. Pearson RA, Merritt JB. Intake, digestion and gastrointestinal transit time in resting donkeys and ponies and exercised donkeys given *ad libitum* hay and straw diets. *Equine Vet J* 1991;23:339–343.
10. Tisserand JL, Pearson RA. Nutritional requirements, feed intake and digestion in working donkeys: a comparison with other work animals. In: Pearson RA, Lhoste P, Saastamoinen M, and Martin-Rosset W, eds, *Working animals in agriculture and transport. a collection of some current research and development observations*. EAAP Technical Series No 6. Wageningen, Netherlands: Wageningen Academic Publishers, 2003;63–73.
11. Pearson RA, Archibald RF, Muirhead RH. The effect of forage quality and level of feeding on digestibility and gastrointestinal transit time of oat straw and alfalfa given to ponies and donkeys. *Br J Nutr* 2001;85:599–606.
12. Pearson RA. Effects of exercise on digestive efficiency in donkeys given *ad libitum* hay and straw diets. In: Pearson AA,

Fielding D, eds, *Donkeys, mules and horses in tropical agricultural development*. Edinburgh: University of Edinburgh Press, 1991;79–85.

13. Maloiy GMO. The effect of dehydration and heat stress on intake and digestion of food in the Somali donkey. *Environ Physio Biochem* 1973;3:36–39.

14. Araujo LOD, Goncalves LC, Rezende ASC, et al. Digistibilidade aparente em equideos submetidos a dieta composta de concentrado e volumosos, fornecido com diferentes intervalos de tempo (Apparent digestibility in equids of diets differing in concerntration and volume when fed over different time periods). *Arquivo Brasileiro de Medicina Veterinaria Zootecnia* 1997;49: 225–237.

15. Cuddeford D, Pearson RA, Archibald RF, et al. Digestibility and gastro-intestinal transit time of diets containing different proportions of alfalfa and oat straw given to thoroughbreds, shetland ponies, highland ponies, and donkeys. *Animal Science* 1995;61:407–417.

16. Suhartanto B, Julliand V, Faurie F, et al. Comparison of digestion in donkeys and ponies. In: Proceedings of the 1st European Conference on Equine Nutrition. *Pferdeheilkunde Sondergabe* 1992;158–161.

17. Muller PJ, Protos P, Houpt KA, et al. Voluntary intake of roughage diets by donkeys. In: Bakkoury M, Prentis A, eds. *Working equines*. Rabat, Morocco: Aetes Editions, 1994 137–148.

18. Schlegal ML, Miller M, Crawshaw G, et al. Practical diets and blood mineral and vitamin concentrations of captive exotic equids housed at Disney's Animal Kingdom and the Toronto Zoo. Second Annual Crissey Zoological Nutrition Symposium, December 10–11, Raleigh, North Carolina, 2004; 39–46.

19. Vall E, Ebangi AL, Abakar O. A method of estimating body condition score (BCS) in donkeys. In: Pearson RA, Lhoste P, Saastamoinen M, Martin-Rosset W, eds. *Working animals in agriculture and transport. A collection of some current research and development observations*. EAAP Technical Series No 6. Wageningen, Netherlands: Wageningen Academic Publishers, 2003;93–102.

20. Pearson RA, Quassat M. *A guide to live weight estimation and body condition scoring of donkeys*. Edinburgh: University of Edinburgh Press, 2000.

3 Gastrointestinal system

Amelia Munsterman, DVM, MS, DACVS, DACVECC

Nutritional support of the critically ill patient is no longer seen only as an adjunct therapy. Recent studies in humans support that early and adequate nutritional support can reduce complications, shorten the duration and severity of disease, and improve patient outcomes. However, it is important to note that, even in human medicine, recommendations for nutritional support are limited by the heterogeneity of patient populations, their illnesses, and statistical power. In the veterinary literature, these limitations are even more restrictive. This chapter offers basic guidelines for nutritional support of adult horses with colic, based on a review of available literature and expert opinion.

3.1 The Association between Nutrition and Colic

The horse was designed to be a continuously grazing animal, with hindgut fermentation supporting the digestion of high fiber, low carbohydrate feeds. Modern horse keeping either neglects this fact or is unable to provide a lifestyle for the needs of the horse's digestive system, which was evolutionarily refined for fiber digestion. Intermittent feedings, large boluses of cereal based feeds, and stall confinement are the norm for most modern horses. While the horse is able to adapt to some extent, it is not unexpected that the adaptations that allow horses to live among us periodically fail. Nutrition is often implicated as the cause of gastrointestinal pain, however, the multifactorial nature of the problem, including types of feed, quality of feedstuffs, and variations in feeding practices, make it difficult to pinpoint epidemiologically the true role of diet in colic.

In veterinary medicine, the search for the cause and effect of a condition is often hampered by financial limitations, small group sizes, and limited record keeping. It is important, however, to take an unbiased and critical view of all the information provided, since the knowledge we gain will be used to directly influence the treatments provided. Evidence based medicine is the practice of integrating unbiased research and clinical expertise, and applies a grading scheme to the published literature. It acknowledges that all evidence is not created equal and requires careful consideration when applying research to the clinical patient. In this chapter, only studies with a level of evidence of grade 2 or higher were included to provide statistical evidence linking colic and nutrition (see Table 3.1). When assessing the evidence, the veterinary practitioner is cautioned to keep in mind the strengths and weaknesses of the published literature in order to make decisions based only on the most valuable information available. The first step in linking feeds to colic is to analyze the evidence related to the most common feeds provided to horses, including grasses, dried forages, and concentrates.

3.1.1 Feeds and Colic: Pastures

The horse was evolutionarily designed to graze grasses. The large colon, specifically, developed to ferment these grasses into short chain fatty acids (acetate, propionate, and butyrate) for energy.[1] While grasses have the capability of storing large quantities of carbohydrates, as starches and fructans, which could upset the delicate microbial populations, continuous grazing should allow the bacteria to respond to any changes in carbohydrate content gradually.[2–5] However, access to pastures with high levels of fermentable carbohydrates has been implicated as a cause of colic and laminitis and may relate to the apparent seasonality of colic events.[6–8] While grazing on pasture has been regarded as protective against colic, its effect may be tempered by other factors, including water supply, weather, rate of feed intake, stocking density, quality of pasture, and supplements provided.

Pasture access was found to reduce the likelihood of colic in a case control observational study of 364 horses,

Nutritional Management of Equine Diseases and Special Cases, First Edition. Edited by Bryan M. Waldridge.
© 2017 John Wiley & Sons, Inc. Published 2017 by John Wiley & Sons, Inc.

Table 3.1 Classification levels for evidence based medicine applied to veterinary publications (Source: Bedenice, 2007, Reproduced with permission of Elsevier).[330]

Level of Evidence	Veterinary Literature Classification	Grade of Recommendation
1a	Systematic review of randomized controlled trials	A
1b	Individual randomized controlled trial (clinical patients or disease models in the horse)	A
2	Retrospective, non-randomized cohort study or case control study	B
3	Case series	B
4	Research model in the horse or a similar species	C
5	*In vitro* testing or expert opinion based on physiologic justification	D

which noted a three-fold increase in the risk of colic for horses with no pasture turnout or that had a recent reduction in paddock size or time at pasture (95% CI 1.4–6.6, P=0.007).[9] A separate case control study in the UK noted that stall confinement tended to increase the risk of colic (OR=9.30, 95% CI 1.68–51.40, P=0.011). Stabling for 24 hours per day was associated with the greatest risk for colic (OR=35.2).[10] Lack of grazing activities may also predispose to specific types of colic, including enterolithiasis, which was noted to occur 2.8 (95% CI 1.06–7.59, P=0.04)[11] to 4.0 (95% CI 1.3–12.2, P=0.02)[12] times more frequently in horses that spent less than 50% of their time outdoors. Access to pasture did not reduce the risk of colic in a report by Reeves et al.,[13] but if water was not available in the paddock, it more than doubled the risk of colic (OR=2.2, 95% CI 1.2–4.3). Despite this published evidence, it is difficult to separate any beneficial effect of grazing activities from the patterns and timing of ingestion, the horse's activity levels, and the effects of exercise on intestinal motility.

3.1.2 Feeds and Colic: Dried Forages

Hay often provides a large portion of the modern horse's diet due to the confines of space and resources. While dried forages provide some consistency to the horse's diet, there is still variability that can occur between batches due to changes in source, the type of hay fed, and even the preservation process that produced the hay. Poor quality forages with high concentrations of hemicellulose, cellulose, and lignin increase the risk of impaction-related colic.[9,14–16] Feeding hay from round bales may also increase the risk by 2.5 times (95% CI 1.1–5.6, P=0.028), likely due to the methods of preservation, exposure to the elements before and during feeding, and the unchecked quantities available to the horse.[9]

Abrupt changes in the type or batch of hay have been noted to be a common cause of colic. In a case control study of horses experiencing colic in Texas, it was noted that while a feed change in the previous two weeks was significantly associated with colic (OR=5.0, 95% CI 2.6–9.7, P<0.001), a change of hay increased the risk even further (OR=9.8, 95% 1.2–81.5, P=0.035).[6] This was confirmed in an additional study in 2001 (OR=4.9 95% 2.1–11.4, P<0.001).[9] On the eastern seaboard of the United States, a change in diet was again linked to colic, specifically with a change in hay resulting in a 2.1 times increase in colic incidence (95% CI 1.2–3.8, P=0.01).[17]

The specific type of hay also may play an important role in the risk of colic. Coastal Bermudagrass hay has been implicated in one cohort study as a cause of colic (OR=1.65, 95% CI 1.01–2.7, P=0.045),[14] and has been suggested in numerous retrospective case series to cause ileal impactions.[18–20] Coastal Bermudagrass hay was confirmed as a risk factor for ileal impactions in a retrospective case control study by Little and Blikslager,[15] who found that horses fed Coastal Bermudagrass had a 4.4 times higher risk for ileal impaction (95% CI 2.1–9.1) versus non-colic controls; a 5.7 times higher risk (95% CI 2.4–13.6) for medical colic, and a 2.7 times higher risk (95% CI 1.2–6.5) for surgical colic. However, this study also noted that feeding Coastal Bermudagrass alone did not increase the risk of colic in general and diluting it with other hays did not reduce the risk of ileal impactions.

Alfalfa hay has been associated with an alkalinizing effect on the colonic ingesta, resulting in alterations in microflora and a reduction in volatile fatty acid production, which produces an environment suited to the formation of enteroliths.[21] In one study, the odds of enterolithiasis were increased if the diet was comprised of >50% alfalfa (OR = 4.2, 95% CI 1.3–12.9, P = 0.01).[12] Two additional studies confirmed this finding, supporting the restriction of alfalfa hay from the diet of horses at risk for enterolithiasis.[11,22] One possible explanation is that the high magnesium content of alfalfa contributes to its alkalinizing effect on colon contents.[22,23] In addition, the high protein content may decrease magnesium absorption and increase ammonia to precipitate minerals and form enteroliths.[24] Conversely, grass hays may be useful for prevention of enteroliths and were noted to have a protective effect if fed at greater than 50% of the diet.[11]

3.1.3 Feeds and Colic: Concentrates

Carbohydrate rich feeds, including grains, are the most commonly implicated dietary cause of colic in the horse, likely due to the well-documented influences of this substrate on the flora of the equine gastrointestinal tract.[4,25] While carbohydrates are much more abundant in grains, there is also a significant difference in the type of carbohydrate present versus forages. In general, carbohydrates can be grouped into two groups: rapidly hydrolyzable carbohydrates (starches, hexoses, disaccharides, and some oligosaccharides), which are primarily degraded in the small intestine and fermentable carbohydrates degraded by bacterial populations to short chain fatty acids (acetate, propionate, and butyrate) in the large intestine and cecum.[7] Grains contain larger quantities of rapidly hydrolysable carbohydrates.

Hydrolysable carbohydrates in the small intestine are normally degraded by pancreatic α-amylase to oligosaccharides, which are further digested by brush-border enzymes to glucose for absorption.[26–28] While glucose transport by enterocytes can be improved with adaptation to high starch feeds, this adaptation relies on the presence of monosaccharides produced by amylase to stimulate this adaptive process.[29] However, the overall activity of amylase in the horse is low compared to other species[30] and highly variable between horses.[27,29] The lack of sufficient amylase has been proposed as the rate limiting step of carbohydrate digestion in the horse.[31]

Research supports this conclusion by documenting starch intake exceeding 0.4% of body weight in one meal can allow hydrolyzable carbohydrates to pass into the hindgut of the horse.[32] In the cecum and colon, carbohydrates are fermented to lactic acid by saccharolytic bacteria, reducing colonic pH and therefore the

survival of bacteria required for fiber fermentation (Clostridiaceae, Spirochaetaceae, and *Fibrobacter* spp.).[33–35] Changes in the microbial environment can alter fermentable carbohydrate digestion,[36] reduce the production of volatile fatty acids,[34,35,37,38] dehydrate the ingesta,[39,40] increase transit times,[40] and result in gas distention of the large intestine,[28] predisposing the horse to colic.

In clinical patients, the association of concentrates with colic was variable, having a significant effect in one study (OR = 2.6, 95% CI 0.9–7.2, P = 0.064),[9] but no effect in a second study.[12] While feeding more than 2.7 kg of oats per day increased the risk of colic in the study by Hudson et al. (OR = 5.9, 95% CI 1.6–22, P = 0.009),[9] previous work noted that any whole grain (oats, barley, etc.) was associated with an increased risk of colic if fed in amounts greater than 2.5 kg per meal (OR = 4.8, 95% CI 1.4–16.6, P = 0.01).[17] Another study found that only whole corn was a risk factor.[13] Pelleting grain may increase the risk of colic, but studies were not as clear.[15,17,41] However, changes in the concentrate fed was shown statistically to increase the risk of colic (OR = 3.6, 95% CI 1.6–5.4, P < 0.001).[17] Current recommendations regarding concentrates advise feeding less than 0.2% of body weight per meal to prevent adverse effects on digestion.[42.]

3.1.4 General Practices to Prevent Colic

Prevention of colic should be centered on providing a consistent diet, since dietary change is the factor most commonly associated with colic in the horse.[6,9,14,17,43,44.] Variations in the type of feed (forages, concentrates, as well as pasture turnout), quantity provided, and frequency that feed is offered all may play a role in altering the pH of ingesta and the bacterial populations that are relied upon for effective digestion.[6,9,17] Therefore, the horse should be provided at least 60% of its diet from forage sources, at a minimum of 1–1.5% of body weight.[45] Concentrates should be kept to a minimum and provided in three or more feedings per day to reduce acid production in the stomach and colon.[42,45] If additional energy sources are required, vegetable oil, strained sugar beet pulp, or soy hulls are good alternatives to starch-based feeds. Finally, any change in the horse's diet should occur over 7–10 days, to allow adjustment of the microbial population, small intestinal enzymes, and glucose transporters required for carbohydrate digestion.[46]

3.2 Nutritional Plans for Horses with Colic

3.2.1 Identifying Nutritional Status

The first step in selecting a nutrition plan for a horse with colic is to evaluate the animal's existing nutritional status and body condition score (BCS). Horses in good BCS are believed to be able to withstand fasting for 2–3 days with no adverse effects. However, horses with emaciated BCS or with comorbidities that affect their ability to gain and maintain weight are candidates for immediate nutritional support. Concurrent conditions that may indicate the need for supplementation include growth, sepsis, endotoxemia, lactation, gestation in the third trimester, abdominal or thoracic abscesses, diarrhea, bowel resection, intestinal ischemia, or malabsorptive diseases.[47,48] While underweight horses are easy to identify as in need of support, overconditioned horses may have a similar need for early nutritional intervention due to their intolerance of feed deprivation and the risk of hyperlipemia.[49]

It can be difficult to assess overall nutritional status at initial examination, often due to lack of a reliable history of dietary intake, recent weight loss, duration of illness, and recent changes in diet. Several scales have been proposed for humans to determine baseline nutritional deficiencies, including weight, height, protein markers, historical observations of dietary changes and nutrient intake, gastrointestinal function, and comorbid conditions.[50] However, these tools were designed for accuracy based upon specific populations of patients, therefore, their results cannot be extrapolated between groups and especially between species.[51–54]

In addition, these scales force the clinician to choose an outcome, either recognizing established malnutrition or identifying the risk of malnutrition. Unfortunately, veterinarians usually would like to identify both risks in horses. There is currently no validated tool for use in equine patients, but a good history, physical examination, laboratory data, and feed analysis can provide information into the patient's nutritional needs. Adequate investigation should allow the veterinarian to identify horses who are already malnourished, as well as those that may require additional nutritional support to prevent inadequacies.

Initially, the veterinarian should obtain a complete history, including signalment, training regimen, and current housing. Changes in body condition can be derived from medical records, but more commonly this requires a careful interview of the owner to reduce bias. Any pertinent medical history, including previous colic surgery and current medications, should be noted. It is important to record not only prescribed medications, but alternative therapies including enzyme supplements, probiotics, vitamins, minerals, and herbal remedies. Any changes in diet, housing, performance, appetite, attitude, and fecal production should be discussed.

The patient should then be thoroughly examined to further the clinician's understanding of the patient's current nutritional status. If possible, body weight should be objectively measured with a scale to obtain an admission baseline for assessment of changes during hospitalization. Body weight is also useful to determine nutrient requirements and doses of medications, as well as to make adjustments in the feeding management. Repeated measurement of body weight should be obtained at a consistent time, ideally before feeding in the morning, to prevent acute alterations due to water intake and gastrointestinal fill. It is also important to consider hydration status, body cavity effusions, and feed intake at the time of weighing when assessing changes in body weight. For example, body weight can change between 5–12% based on level of hydration and procedures such as large colon lavage can remove 50–70 l of ingesta at one time.[55] When a scale is not available, body weight can be estimated from measurement of the heart girth and the length of the horse using the following formula.[56]

$$\text{Weight in pounds} = \left(\text{heart girth} \left[\text{inches} \right] \right)^2 \\ \times \text{body length} \left[\text{inches} \right] / 330$$

or

$$\text{Weight in kilograms} = \left(\text{heart girth} \left[\text{cm} \right] \right)^2 \\ \times \text{body length} \left[\text{cm} \right] / 11{,}877$$

The heart girth is the circumference of the thorax of the horse, just behind the triceps at the highest point of the withers. Measurement of heart girth should be obtained at exhalation. The length of the horse is obtained by measuring from the point of the shoulder to the tuber ischii. It is important to use an inelastic tape for best accuracy. The tape should not be pulled too tightly and the horse should be standing square and level.

Table 3.2 Equine Body Condition Scoring System (adapted from Henneke et al., 1983).[58]

1 Poor/Severe emaciation	Spinous processes, ribs, tailhead, tuber coxae, and tuber ischii are prominent. Scapula and cervical vertebrae are easily palpable. No fatty tissue can be felt.
2 Very thin/ Emaciated	Slight fat covers the base of the spinous processes. Transverse processes of lumbar vertebrae are rounded. Spinous processes, ribs, tailhead, tuber coxae, and tuber ischii are prominent. Scapula and cervical vertebrae are faintly palpable.
3 Thin	Transverse processes cannot be palpated. Slight fat cover on ribs and spinous processes. Tailhead prominent, but individual vertebrae not distinguishable. Tuber ischii rounded, but noticeable. Greater trochanter not distinguishable. Withers, shoulders, and neck accentuated.
4 Moderately thin	Slight ridge along back, faint outline of ribs noted, tailhead has some fat, point of hip not distinguishable.
5 Moderate	Back flat, ribs not visible, but palpable. Fat on tailhead is slightly spongy, withers rounded over spinous processes, shoulders and neck blend smoothly.
6 Moderately fleshy	Slight crease down back. Fat over ribs is spongy, fat over tailhead is soft. Fat deposits along sides of withers, behind shoulders, and along sides of neck.
7 Fleshy	May have crease down back. Individual ribs can be felt, but fat is noted between ribs. Fat around tailhead soft. Fat along withers, behind shoulder, and along neck.
8 Fat	Crease down back. Difficult to feel ribs. Fat around tailhead very soft. Area along withers and behind shoulder filled with fat. Neck thickened. Fat along inner thighs.
9 Extremely fat	Obvious crease down back. Fat over ribs, bulging over tailhead, along withers, behind shoulders, and along neck. Fat inside inner thighs may rub. Flank filled with fat.

This formula estimates the mature body weight and this calculation is unaffected by hydration status or ingestion of feed. While the calculation has been shown to be accurate in smaller horses, it should be used with some caution in horses over 15 hands high.[57] For the best estimate of weight, the heart girth and body length should be obtained three times and averaged to reduce error.

While body weight is an objective measure of nutritional status, it does not provide insight into the nutritional history of the horse in terms of chronic catabolic conditions, as well as evaluating states of over-conditioning. Use of a BCS system is recommended to provide a subjective assessment of the horse's adipose reserves and lean muscle mass. A nine-point system has been developed that is useful in light breeds,[58] and it has been applied with modifications in warm-blood horses (see Table 3.2).[59,60] This scale provides a BCS for the amount of fat noted at six discreet areas (neck, withers, behind the shoulders, over the ribs, along the spine, and around the tail head) and is helpful to determine if the weight of a horse is appropriate for its frame. Body condition score has been shown to be positively correlated with body fat percentage[58,61] and has been verified by ultrasonography, which noted a good correlation between BCS and the amount of fat deposited at the tailhead, thirteenth rib, and withers.[62]

Plasma protein biochemical markers, including albumin, transferrin, and retinol binding protein, have been used in humans to determine nutritional status, assuming that a decrease in plasma protein is due to reduced hepatic synthesis.[63] However, most of these traditional protein markers are acute phase proteins and are not validated for critical patients.[64–66] Albumin, in particular, is affected by a number of changes related to disease status. Blood albumin concentration is reduced by overhydration, dilution, increased renal, vascular, or gastrointestinal permeability, and decreased production by the liver due to disease or a negative acute phase response. The half-life of albumin in the horse is 19–21 days, therefore, changes in serum concentration will not be immediately noted.[67] In horses, albumin has not been shown to be sensitive to nutritional status or supplemental feeding, in agreement with findings in critically ill humans. Albumin significantly increased in horses that were not fed after small intestinal resections, versus those that were supported with parenteral nutrition, likely due to a dilutional effect (P=0.044).[68] Therefore, physical examination and historical information remain the best predictors of nutritional status.

3.2.2 Nutritional Requirements of Horses with Colic

The dietary requirements of healthy horses based on mature body weight have been established through feeding trials and have been published by the National

Research Council (NRC) and others.[69] While daily requirements have been determined for a number of life stages and activities, it is important to recognize that each patient with colic will deviate from these published requirements due to individual variations in nutrient absorption, losses, and metabolism. In addition, these guidelines provide only the minimum requirements for each nutrient; therefore, horses with impaired absorption, digestion, and metabolism may fall short of meeting their need if fed to standard. While helpful, it is difficult to extrapolate these guidelines to horses with colic and additional factors including history, physical exam, and assessment of BCS are essential to determine nutritional needs.

It is thought that well-conditioned horses can withstand a short period of fasting. Donkeys and mules have been kept off feed for 10 days without deleterious effect on the major body organs.[70] The actual length of time that a horse can go without feed may be even longer, based on historical evidence in humans that noted a lack of adverse effects on organ systems during starvation up to 30 days.[71] There are three factors that affect the metabolism and energy requirements of the colic patient: (1) stall rest, which reduces energy needs, (2) disease processes such as surgery or sepsis that may increase needs, and (3) starvation, which can reduce energy requirements due to reductions in energy lost through fermentation and digestive processes.[72] The effects of starvation and disease are difficult to quantify.

The goal for the equine clinician treating horses with colic is to estimate energy needs using the requirements of the stalled patient in a thermoneutral environment, called the resting energy requirements (RER) or resting energy expenditure. The ideal method for determining RER in critical human patients is through indirect calorimetry, which avoids the inaccuracies of metabolic formulas based on individual patient populations.[73–75] This method calculates the individual patient's caloric requirements from measurements of oxygen uptake and carbon dioxide excretion using closed circuit spirometry.[74,76] Measurements may have inaccuracies due to pain or anxiety,[76–78] changes in ventilation,[79–82] acute changes in pH,[63] sympathomemetic medications,[82–85] leaks or resistance in the spirometry system,[76,78] and the inspired oxygen concentration administered to the patient.[86,87] These variables and the lack of availability of spirometers in veterinary practice make accurate measurements difficult.

The RER of normal, stall rested horses using indirect calorimetry can be estimated by the following calculation:[88]

$$RER = 21.28\,kcal \times body\ weight\,(kg) + 975$$

For a 500-kg horse, the calculated RER using this equation is 11,615 kcal. This number would be an ideal starting point for calculation of feeding plans for horses hospitalized with severe colic. However, most horses affected with colic recover quickly, with little disruption in their activities or routine. Therefore, a second equation, called the daily digestible energy requirement (DER), may be more appropriate.[69] It factors in the additional energy required to maintain normothermia in varied environments as well as minimal activity levels (i.e., walking, grazing).

$$DER\ horses < 600\,kg\,(Mcal) = 1.4 + (0.03 \times BW\,[kg])$$
$$DER\ horses > 600\,kg\,(Mcal) = 1.82 + (BW\,[kg] \times 0.0383)$$
$$- (0.000015 \times BW\,[kg])$$

For a 500-kg horse, DER equates to 16,400 kcal per day. The clinician should consider the severity of illness when calculating the diet for refeeding, to decide if RER or DDE is more appropriate.

Stress factors or multipliers that estimate the increase or decrease in basal metabolic rate have been developed to assess the impact of illness and disease on the energy expenditure of the critically ill.[89] It is important to consider that these factors were developed using subjectively defined study groups, therefore the relevance of these multipliers has recently come into question.[75] There are numerous factors that can influence the metabolic rate of a critical patient (see Table 3.3) and these influences as well as the fact that these multipliers were developed in humans must be considered when extrapolating to the equine patient.

Energy expenditure multipliers for equine patients are lacking, specifically following gastrointestinal surgery, but in humans undergoing surgical procedures, energy expenditure is estimated to be 23–31 kcal/kg/day,[90,91] which is approximately 1.24–1.4 times higher than resting energy expenditure. In horses, the RER of post-operative colic patients has been estimated based on human studies to be 1.3 times the RER.[92] More recently, closed circuit spirometry has been used

Table 3.3 Factors that can influence the resting energy expenditure of the critically ill horse (Source: Reid et al., 2004).[328]

Factors increasing energy expenditure	Factors decreasing energy expenditure
Absorptive abnormalities	Anesthesia
Burns	Hypothermia
Diarrhea	Recumbency
Disease state	Sedation
Gastrointestinal reflux	Stall rest
Hyperthermia	Starvation
Pyrexia	
Surgery	
Trauma/wounds	

to provide a more accurate estimate. A standardized abdominal exploratory via ventral midline incision under general anesthesia resulted in an increase of 1.0 Mcal/kg/day, equating to a 1.1 times increase in RER.[76] Based on this study, adjustments using energy expenditure multipliers are probably not required.

3.3 Routes for Feeding Horses Recovering from Colic

Colic in the horse is often a short-term disease process, such as gas colic or mild impaction.[93] These conditions resolve quickly with minimal medical therapy and allow for rapid reintroduction to oral feedings. However, severe impactions and some surgical conditions, such as small intestinal resections, may require a period of feed withholding during the acute recovery period. Ideally, veterinarians would provide nutritional support by enteral or parenteral methods for any horse held off feed for longer than 4–5 days. In reality, clinicians are often placed in situations based on finances or the unexpected course of the disease that results in a lack of supplementation for longer than expected.

The method for providing nutrition to horses that have experienced colic will vary depending on a number of factors, including the cause of the colic, appetite, surgical procedures performed, duration of illness, and finances of the owner. Most importantly with gastrointestinal disease, the primary problem must be addressed before enteral nutrition is permitted. The overall goal is to gradually reintroduce voluntary intake and there are

strengths and weaknesses to any program. However, there are three basic feeding methods for horses recovering from colic: (1) voluntary intake, (2) supportive enteral nutrition, and (3) supportive parenteral nutrition.

3.3.1 Voluntary Intake

Clinical cases have supported the idea that horses may withstand brief periods of fasting without ill effects.[45] Once feed is provided, if >85% of the calculated RER can be achieved after a gradual reintroduction, then no other form of supportive nutrition is required.[94] In horses with an extended period of anorexia, feed should be reintroduced at 25% of the RER and increased by 25% each day if tolerated, until the amount provided is greater than 85% of the calculated energy requirements.[45] In horses with a shorter course of disease, reintroduction can occur much quicker.

Feeds should be reintroduced once signs of colic have resolved, transit time returns to normal with no evidence of positive nasogastric reflux, and gastrointestinal borborygmi are adequate. Most commonly, horses are first challenged with water provided in small amounts to ensure adequate progressive motility. If oral fluids are tolerated without colic, then feed is introduced. The veterinarian should provide a feed that the owners can readily obtain and will provide the energy needed for work to ensure compliance and prevent feed changes during early convalescence. If dietary factors, such as the type of hay fed, were a predisposing factor for colic, then these feeds should be avoided during the refeeding process. It is also recommended to avoid feeding grains or other concentrates for the first 2 weeks after the colic episode in order to reduce further disturbances in gastrointestinal microflora.[95] If concentrates are required to maintain the horse's level of athletic performance, grains should be reintroduced at a rate of 0.1% of body weight (or 0.5 kg per 500 kg of body weight) per feeding, increasing slowly each day.

Horses recovering from colic rarely refuse voluntary intake of feeds and often will continue to try to eat despite severe abdominal discomfort. There are instances when feeds may be rejected, either due to the novelty of the feed item, consistency, palatability, or boredom. In these horses, a variety of feeds should be provided in a buffet-type setting, to determine which food the horse prefers.[96] While some feedstuffs may not be ideal (i.e., sweet feed), the items that a horse selects may allow the clinician to add small amounts of less palatable, but more wholesome feeds to improve intake. Other methods to improve feed palatability include adding molasses or pancake syrup to sweeten the feed. While pharmaceuticals are controversial as appetite stimulants in horses, there is a report of improvement using diazepam (0.02–0.03 mg/kg, IV).[97] In this study, acepromazine (0.5 mg/kg, IV) also had an effect, although less marked. Cyproheptadine (0.6–1.2 mg/kg, PO, q24 h) and anabolic steroids are also useful to stimulate appetite.

The ideal feed for reintroduction is grass, based on the natural physiology of the horse. Grazing the horse for 20–30 min at a time will provide a slow reintroduction of feeding and allow the clinician to monitor for any unresolved gastrointestinal complications. In addition, the exercise it provides will stimulate gastrointestinal motility. Based on research on digestible energy obtained during grazing over time, this amount of grazing will provide approximately 1.2–1.8 kcal/kg per feeding.[98] Therefore, a 500-kg horse can be grazed initially 3–5 times per day to provide approximately 25% of the RER. Grazing should be increased as tolerated and full feeding should be attained within 2–3 days.

Pastures are often limited, so hay can be provided as an alternative forage. Small quantities of hay should be offered at first. Most sources recommend starting at 0.5 kg (1.1 lb) of good quality hay offered 4–6 times per day.[45] The quality of hay can vary significantly, so when feed analysis is not available, first cutting hays are preferred. This conservative rate of feeding will supply approximately half of the RER when fed 6 times a day to a 500-kg horse. However, concerns about strictures or edema reducing lumen size may reduce the size of these meals initially, to ensure adequate passage of ingesta. Feeding 0.25 kg of hay will provide approximately 25% of the daily needs for a 500-kg horse. This slow introduction of feed is advisable for any horse that has been anorexic for more than 4 days. Weighing the hay will help in monitoring intake, since different grasses, growing climates, and baling techniques can radically affect the weight of the hay per volume, bale weight, and amount of hay per flake.

In general, forages are similar in that they are high in fiber and will stimulate the production of volatile fatty acids in the hindgut. The protein content can vary significantly between types of hay. Therefore, protein supplements may be required for horses fed low protein hay (i.e., Coastal Bermudagrass), especially if the horse is in a state of malnutrition. In addition, calcium and potassium are often deficient in horses held off feed and serum concentrations should be monitored closely when refeeding colicky horses.

Cubed or pelleted forages can be a forage alternative for horses with dental disease, metabolic or respiratory issues, restricted gastrointestinal luminal size, or in areas with reduced availability of suitable feedstuffs (see Table 3.4). These feeds can replace hay or pasture in the diet and soaking can be helpful to reduce dust and decrease the chance of esophageal obstruction. Alfalfa cubes or chopped hay are preferable to pelleted forages, due to the positive effects of long stem fiber on the gastrointestinal flora. A minimum of 1–1.5% of body weight of hay is required for maintenance.[99]

Table 3.4 Nutritional composition of commonly fed forage alternatives that can provide adequate fiber length to horses with dental problems or those who cannot chew and swallow hay.

	DE kcal/ kg DM*	Crude Protein % (min)	Fat % (min)	Crude Fiber % (max)	DM* % (min)	Ca % DM* (min)	P % DM*	Mg % DM*	K % DM*
Alfalfa pellets[a]	2380	17	1.0	28	90	1.40	0.26	0.34	2.41
Chopped alfalfa hay[b]	2112	15	2.5	30	88.2	1.10	0.28	0.19	2.96
Chopped grass forage[b]	2024	8	2.5	30	90.3	0.50	0.21	0.16	1.97
Alfalfa cubes[b]	2156	15	1.5	30	88.0	1.10	0.25	0.28	1.60
Alfalfa-timothy cubes[b]	2112	12	1.8	32	88.0	0.89	0.30	0.25	1.60

* Dry matter
[a] Minnesota Valley Alfalfa Producers, Raymond, MN
[b] Triple Crown Nutrition, Wayzata, MN

Another alternative to forages for horses recovering from colic is complete pelleted rations. Complete feeds are often preferred during recuperation from more complicated causes of colic, such as an anastomosis with questionable lumen size or in cases where large colon fiber digestibility has been compromised by resection or ischemia. There are many complete feeds on the market, but all can be fed as the sole ration if required (see Table 3.5). Complete feeds are nutritionally balanced for maintenance and provide adequate fiber to stimulate mucosal recovery. However, once the horse has fully recovered from the colic episode, a source of long stem fiber, such as hay, chopped hay, or hay cubes, is recommended to ensure healthy hindgut microbial populations.

Pelleted feeds can be introduced at a rate of 25–50% of the total daily ration digestible energy (DE), divided into meals fed every 3–6 h, and increasing by 25% each day until a full ration is reached. For example, a 500-kg horse would require 6.1 kg (13.4 lb) of a complete senior feed per day for maintenance. Starting at 25% of the total daily energy requirements would equate to 1.5 kg (3.3 lb) of feed per day, which would be split into feedings of 0.2 kg (0.5 lb) every 3 h. Pelleted rations can be soaked in water to improve motility through the intestinal lumen, and to provide additional water intake. However, some horses may refuse wet feed due to its texture or temperature. It is imperative to tailor the diet to each horse's individual needs and preferences. Additional dietary adjustments for preexisting malnutrition, performance, and maintenance can be addressed after the horse is re-established on its full ration.

While forages and complete manufactured feeds are ideal based on their nutrient profiles, some horses may refuse to eat these feeds. Additional feed choices may be selected based on availability or clinician preference. Commonly used feedstuffs for horses recovering from colic include beet pulp, vegetable oils, rice bran, and soy hulls (see Table 3.6).

Beet pulp is commonly used as an alternative fiber source, although it should not be used as a sole source of forage since it lacks some necessary vitamins and minerals. The maximum amount that can be fed is unknown, but estimated to be close to 1% of body weight per day.[100] While none of these feeds are complete nutritionally by themselves, they can provide the horse with the variety it is seeking to stimulate appetite and interest. They can also be used in conjunction with complete forage and pelleted diets to increase energy, protein, or improve palatability.

It is important to consider the function of the digestive system when returning the horse to feed. In particular, fats are absorbed after lipolysis in the small intestine. Therefore, small intestinal disease may reduce the ability to convert dietary fats to energy. There should also be concern over providing feeds that could increase the glycemic index in horses with metabolic disorders. Sweet feeds, corn, oats, and other grains should be avoided, whereas beet pulp, alfalfa, rice bran, and soy hulls are relatively safe.[101] However, the preparation of certain feeds must be considered, since beet pulp with molasses has a glycemic index close to oats.[99]

Some clinicians have expressed concern over the energy content of wheat bran, purported to have a laxative effect by drawing water into the intestinal lumen. Wheat bran's glycemic index is intermediate and large amounts in the diet may be of concern in horses with metabolic disease or disruptions in the colonic flora, which may exacerbate diarrhea. In addition, both wheat and rice bran have inverted calcium phosphorus rations, which can lead to nutritional secondary hyperparathyroidism when fed in excess and without supplemental calcium. It is currently recommended to limit these feeds to less than one pound per day in a 500-kg horse.[101]

3.3.2 Supportive Enteral Nutrition

Voluntary intake is the preferred route to provide nutrition in horses recovering from colic. It is rare for a horse to refuse to eat, as long as it is provided with palatable feeds. However, there are instances where oral intake cannot and should not be allowed. Most commonly, this occurs with injury or diseases affecting the oral cavity or esophagus, such as pharyngeal trauma and esophageal strictures, resulting in dysphagia or the inability to swallow. In these instances, enteral nutrition can be provided via an esophagostomy or nasogastric tube to provide nutrients.

Enteral nutrition is preferred over parenteral routes due to the positive effect it provides for mucosal recovery and maintenance of the gastrointestinal barrier to enteric pathogens and endotoxin.[102–104,] Based on work in other species, a complete and balanced oral diet provides nutrients that are selected by different enterocytes along the gastrointestinal tract to maintain this barrier.[105,106] It is especially important in the horse to

Table 3.5 A partial list of commercial complete rations available for horses, including pelleted, powdered, and forage based diets. The feeds listed in this table are provided as representative examples only and are not the only complete feeds available for horses. Nutrient analysis is provided to allow for dietary formulation, as well as weight calculations for initial reintroduction after colic. Initial ration weight is based on a digestible energy requirement (DER) of 16,400 kcal/day for a 500-kg horse and should increase gradually to the full DER over 2–4 days. After recovery from colic, the feed type and amount should be reevaluated based on each individual horse's needs and long stem forages should be added to the diet if possible.

Brand Name	Crude Protein % (min)	Crude Fat % (min)	Crude Fiber % (max)	DE (kcal/kg)	NSC % (min)	Total daily ration for 500 kg horse (based on DER of 16,400 kcal)	Initial daily ration for conservative reintroduction to feed 25% of DE (divided into 4–8 feedings/day)
Purina Equine Senior Horse Feed®[a]	14	5.5	17	2695	20 (18–22)	6.1 kg (13.4 lb)	1.5 kg (3.3 lb)
Purina WellSolve Well-Gel®*[a]	36	6	14	2860	NA	1.5 kg (3.3 lb) per label	0.5 kg (1.1 lb) three times daily per label
Triple Crown Senior Horse Feed™[b]	14	10	17	3400	11.7	4.8 kg (10.6 lb)	1.2 kg (2.7 lb)
Triple Crown Complete Formula™[b]	12	12	15	3900	20.6	4.2 kg (9.3 lb)	1.1 kg (2.3 lb)
Triple Crown Low Starch Formula®[b]	12	6	18	3140	13.5	5.2 kg (11.5 lb)	1.3 kg (2.9 lb)
Triple Crown Safe Starch Forage®[b]	11	6	28	2423	8.7	6.8 kg (14.9 lb)	1.7 kg (3.7 lb)
Nutrena Life Design Senior Horse Feed®[c]	14	5	16	2800–3100	20	5.3–5.9 kg (11.6–13.0 lb)	1.3–1.5 kg (2.9–3.2 lb)
Nutrena Triumph Complete Horse Feed®[c]	12	3.5	25	2800–3000	22	5.4–5.9 kg (12.0–13.0 lb)	1.4–1.5 kg (3.0–3.2 lb)
Seminole Feed Senior Formula®[d]	14	7	16	3086	19	5.3 kg/ 11.7 pounds	1.3 kg (2.9 lb)
Seminole Wellness Senior Mix®[d]	12.0	10.0	18.0	3230	17	5.1 kg (11.1 lb)	1.3 kg (2.8 lb)
Seminole Wellness Equi-Safe®[d]	8.0	4.0	25.0	1984	12	8.3 kg (18.2 lb)	2.1 kg (4.5 lb)

* WellSolve Well-Gel® is a complete feed that can be administered enterally after mixing with 2–3 parts water or fed as a slurry. Diet should not exceed 0.3% of bodyweight per day, for more than 5 days. Additional feed will be required long-term to meet caloric needs, or Well-Gel may be used as a protein, vitamin and mineral supplement if top dressed onto other feeds at a rate of 0.11–0.22 kg/day.

[a] Purina Mills, Gray Summit, MO
[b] Triple Crown Nutrition, Wayzata, MN
[c] Nutrena, Minneapolis, MN
[d] Seminole Feed, Ocala, FL

Table 3.6 Alternative feed supplements for feeding horses after colic to provide additional energy, protein, and fiber to correct dietary deficiencies. (Adapted from National Research Council, Committee on Nutrient Requirements of Horses, 2007)

	DE (kcal/kg DM)	Crude Protein (% DM)	Fat (% DM)	Neutral detergent fiber (% DM)	Calcium (% DM)	Phosphorus (% DM)	Magnesium (% DM)	Potassium (% DM)	Sodium (% DM)
Beet pulp with molasses 3%	2,840	10.0	0.42	44.4	0.89	0.09	0.23	1.11	0.35
Beet pulp without molasses	2,800	10.0	0.44	45.8	0.91	0.09	0.23	0.96	0.31
Wheat bran	3,220	17.3	4.30	42.5	0.13	1.18	0.53	1.32	0.04
Soybean meal (44% crude protein)	3,520	49.9	1.60	14.9	0.40	0.71	0.31	2.22	0.04
Rice bran	3,350	15.5	15.2	26.1	0.07	1.78	0.81	1.57	0.03
Molasses, sugarcane	4,060	5.8	0.20	0.40	1.00	0.10	0.42	4.01	0.22
Vegetable oils	9,190	0	99.9	0	0	0	0	0	0

DM = Dry matter

provide a source of fiber in enteral diets, which is essential for gastrointestinal activity, mucosal blood flow, cell growth, and absorption of nutrients.[107] Enteral nutrition should be provided as early as possible, based on its positive effects on mortality, length of hospitalization, infection, and metabolic response to illness in critically ill human patients.[105,108,109]

In horses, supplemental enteral nutrition can be provided using a nasogastric tube placed into the stomach (approximately at the 12th rib). A 14 French nasogastric tube is preferred for blenderized component diets, but for liquid diets a smaller 18 F feeding tube can be placed. Feeding tubes may be placed by nasogastric intubation or through an esophagostomy aboral to the site of injury or obstruction. While accurate placement can be determined by palpation or aspiration of gastrointestinal contents with larger tubes, smaller tubes will require endoscopy or radiography to ensure proper position. Once inserted, the tube is capped when not in use, secured to the halter with tape, and flushed with warm water before and after each feeding to maintain patency.

There are three types of diets that have been administered by feeding tubes to the horse. First is a blenderized diet of commercially available complete pellets, which can be administered through a 14 F nasogastric tube.[110] Any of the pelleted diets listed in Table 3.6 are nutritionally balanced and can be administered in this fashion. However, it is advisable to avoid any feed that contains whole grains, such as oats, to avoid clogging the tube. It is also helpful to purchase a blender to further reduce particle size. Approximately 0.5 kg (1 lb) of pellets can be mixed with 2–4 l of water to form a slurry meal. If additional calories are needed, vegetable oil can be added and one cup (240 ml) will provide an additional 1.9 Mcal. While time consuming, these blenderized diets are a cost-effective alternative to other enteral diets.

An alternative is to feed a powdered commercial diet (Welsolve Wel-Gel®, Purina Mills, St. Louis, MO) to reduce problems with particle size caused by grinding pellets. This is a complete formula, providing 100% of the NRC requirements for protein, vitamins and minerals, as well as fiber for hindgut fermentation.[46] This diet can be administered through a nasogastric tube at a rate of 0.3% of bodyweight per day for up to 5 days. For horses requiring extended enteral feeding, additional calories may be needed to meet energy requirements, and vegetable oil, dextrose, or molasses can be added to the formula.

Table 3.7 The Naylor Component Diet. This diet is thick and usually fed as-is, rather than via nasogastric tube. Total DE supplied is 2,770 kcal/5 l. (Adapted from Naylor et al., 1992.)[329]

Alfalfa pellets	454 g
Casein/cottage cheese	204 g
Dextrose	204 g
Electrolytes*	52 g
Water	5 l
Electrolyte mixture (approximately meets daily requirements)*	
KCl	75 g
CaCl$_2$	45 g
MgO	25 g
Bicarbonate	15 g
NaCl	10 g

Component diets are a second choice for enteral feeding in the horse. In this case, the dietary requirements are met by selecting whole feeds that will provide the essential nutrients. Often these diets are alfalfa pellet-based, therefore they will still require a larger nasogastric tube for administration. The most commonly cited formula was published by Naylor[49] (see Table 3.7) and is composed of alfalfa, casein, dextrose, and electrolytes. While it is possible for the clinician to more closely tailor the diet to the needs of the specific patient, component diets are more complicated to mix and are often deficient in key vitamins and minerals that preclude long term use.

A more complete equine commercial enteral diet is also available (Critical Care Meals™, MD's Choice, Louisville, TN). The advantages of this diet are the known quantities of essential nutrients and the ability to adjust its composition to meet the needs of an individual patient. Additional ingredients include lactase, glutamine, L-arginine, vitamins, trace minerals, and antioxidants.

A low residue elemental liquid feed (Vital® HN and Osmolite®; Abbott Nutrition, Columbus, OH) is the third type of enteral diet that has been used in adult horses.[110–113] These diets are low fat and composed of soy and whey or casein proteins, individual peptides, sucrose and/or maltodextrin for carbohydrates, and fats from safflower oil, canola, medium chain triglycerides, and lecithin. These diets were designed as a complete enteral feed for human gastrointestinal patients to be administered through an 8 F feeding tube. The nutrient profiles are probably not complete for herbivores and neither diet contains a source of fiber. As a result, low volume diarrhea is common with these diets.[110–113] An additional disadvantage is the higher cost.

Enteral diets are typically introduced starting at 25% of the target on day one, then increasing by 25% each day until the dietary goal is met. If the horse is handling these small feedings well, then the number of feedings per day can be reduced to make it more manageable for caretakers. However, an individual feeding should never exceed 8 liters, based on the stomach volume of a 500-kg horse. Horses on enteral feed should be checked for gastric reflux at each feeding and the diet adjusted accordingly.

Complications of enteral feedings are often the result of diet formulations containing high carbohydrates and low fiber. This is commonly seen with low residue, elemental diets that can cause diarrhea in the horse.[45,110–113] Additional problems include colic, ileus, gastrointestinal stasis, and laminitis. Direct complications of nasogastric intubation include rhinitis, pharyngitis, aspiration, and esophageal or pharyngeal perforation.[114] With esophagostomy, mediastinitis, laryngeal hemiplegia, diverticula, and local infection may result.[115,116] Enteral nutrition is contraindicated in horses with gastrointestinal obstruction, hypovolemia, or cardiovascular shock, when gastrointestinal tract functional is impaired. In these patients, parenteral nutrition is advisable.

When administering enteral nutrition, especially elemental diets, the horse should be monitored carefully with regular physical examinations. The feeding tube should be flushed regularly and the horse weighed daily to determine if the volume of feed is adequate. Once the horse has recovered, it should be gradually weaned from enteral feedings. Reducing the number of feedings and removing the tube in between will allow the horse to start voluntary feedings. It is important to remember that an esophagostomy tube must remain in place for 10–14 days until healing has occurred to prevent mediastinitis.[116]

3.3.3 Parenteral Nutrition

Parenteral nutrition is recommended for horses that are unable to receive enteral feedings. In horses suffering from colic, this is commonly due to gastrointestinal obstructions, sustained anorexia, ileus, or infectious causes. Parenteral feeding should be considered in any horse that is not expected to eat for more than 5 days.[117,118] However, initiation of parenteral nutrition should not be delayed in horses with poor BCS (<3/9),

or in cases with increased metabolic demands, including pregnancy and lactation, which may reduce the body's ability to compensate for even short-term feed withholding. Horses in circulatory shock are also candidates for parenteral nutrition due to reduced gastrointestinal perfusion preventing normal digestion and absorption.

There is currently no evidence from human retrospective studies for early institution of IV nutritional support and there is some evidence that suggests use of parenteral nutrition may even increase infection and mortality rates.[119–121] However, in malnourished patients (<90% of ideal body weight), parenteral nutrition improved survival; therefore, it is advised that supplementation should not be delayed in these cases. In fact, when directly compared to enteral nutrition, parenteral nutrition made no significant difference in the clinical outcome.[122,123] Current recommendations for patients in adequate body condition by the Society of Critical Care Medicine and the American Society for Parenteral and Enteral Nutrition state that parenteral nutrition should be provided only if enteral nutrition is not available and only if the problem persists for more than 7 days.[65] The European Society for Parenteral and Enteral Nutrition however, recommends immediate supplementation if the person is not expected to take food enterally within 3 days, based on aggressive guidelines to prevent malnutrition.[124]

Research in veterinary medicine is more limited, but appears to agree with the more conservative human practice guidelines. In horses receiving parenteral nutrition immediately post-operatively, there has been no evidence of any benefit in terms of duration of hospitalization, survival, or cost of treatment.[125] One study reported increased mortality rates in horses receiving parenteral nutrition, however, the report may have been hampered by the biased selection of more severe cases for administration of parenteral nutrition.[47] Despite this evidence, there have been some benefits reported in horses, including significant improvements in triglyceride concentration and reduced hyperbilirubinemia in post-operative intestinal resections that were administered parenteral nutrition, which may point to an improved plane of nutrition in these horses.[68] Intravenous nutrition may also be used as an adjunct to enteral nutrition, if enteral intake is less than 75% of total caloric need.

Components of parenteral nutrition provide energy via supplementation of carbohydrates and/or lipids, amino acids for protein synthesis, and reduced catabolic muscle scavenging. Additional vitamins, minerals, and electrolytes may also be included, based on the needs of the individual patient. The optimum nutrient composition for parenteral nutrition in the horse is not known. It is important, however, to provide the proper ratio and levels of these ingredients to prevent complications including hepatic lipidosis, hyperglycemia, and sepsis.

The first component of parenteral nutrition is an energy source, typically 50% dextrose. Each gram of dextrose provides 3.4 kcal, but its high osmolality and low caloric density make it difficult to provide sufficient energy to the patient with dextrose solutions alone. Typically, 40–60% of the non-protein calories in parenteral nutrition is supplied by dextrose and this rate appears to be well tolerated by equine patients.[47,118]

It is important to remember that carbohydrates are not an essential nutrient.[119] Glucose synthesis can occur from a number of sources, including lactate, glycerol, and amino acids in the liver, kidneys, muscle, and the gastrointestinal organs.[122,122] In humans, basal glucose requirements have been set at 2 g/kg/day[125] to supply readily available energy to tissues without mitochondrial metabolism (red blood cells, leukocytes, renal medulla) and tissues strongly reliant on glucose such as the brain.[126] While muscle protein catabolism can be reduced with exogenous glucose supplementation, excessive concentrations in parenteral diets may result in inflammation and oxidative injury. In humans, tight glucose control has been advocated as a treatment for oversupplementation or glucose intolerance, but it often leads to hypoglycemia, which may increase mortality.[128] Current recommendations are to simply prevent hyperglycemia with judicious parenteral supplementation.[129]

Lipids are an alternative to carbohydrates that can be used to supply a portion of the metabolic energy needs. They also may be beneficial to temper serum glucose fluctuations. Each gram of lipid provides 9 kcal/g and a 20% lipid solution will provide 2 kcal/ml. A lipid solution of long chain fatty acids is usually comprised of either soy or safflower oils and is iso-osmolar due to the addition of glycerol. Lipids can be used to provide up to 30–40% of the non-protein calories initially, increasing to up to 60% of the total calories supplied.[130] Advantages of incorporating lipids include a reduction in dextrose in the solution, which will significantly lower the tonicity and reduce the risk of thrombophlebitis. In addition, decreased dextrose concentrations

reduce the risk of hepatic lipidosis, osmotic diuresis, and hypokalemia.[118,131,132]

However, lipids increase cost significantly and the long chain fatty acids it provides may inhibit neutrophils, T-cell function, and the reticuloendothelial system, increasing the risk of infection.[121,133,134] It is important to monitor patients closely for lipemia and hypertriglyceridemia, due to endotoxin's inhibitory effect on lipoprotein lipase production and activity that can reduce clearance of lipids.[135] Lipids should be avoided in any patient at risk for hyperlipemia or with increased serum triglycerides.

Precursors for protein synthesis are the final ingredient commonly included in parenteral nutrition for horses. These are provided by amino acid solutions of varying concentrations, ranging from 8.5–10.0%. The goal of amino acid supplementation is to spare the breakdown of lean muscle, used for energy when carbohydrates and fats are scarce, and allow for the production of new proteins. The optimal protein requirements for horses are difficult to quantify, since whole body nitrogen balance is not a reliable measure of adequate protein synthesis in the face of critical illness.[127]

In the healthy horse, enteral protein requirements have been determined to be approximately 40 times the DER in Mcal per day. If the efficiency of digestion and absorption is 70% of total intake, this level of protein supplementation provides approximately 0.9 g protein/kg body weight/day.[69] Since parenteral proteins bypass the digestive process, they are closer to 100% available, giving a parenteral nutrition protein requirement of 0.6–0.8 g/kg/day.[68,125] In critically ill humans, the current recommendations are to increase protein supplementation to 0.8–1.5 g/kg/day to improve nitrogen balance in severely stressed patients, without increasing metabolic demands.[126,136,137] In horses, protein supplementation supplied parenterally has ranged from 0.68–2.0 g/kg/day and since the protein requirements of a horse with colic are not currently known, the clinician is still left with making an educated guess.[47,68,125,139,]

In critically ill patients, the anabolic effects of protein supplementation are hampered further by a number of factors which reduce the ability to replace or increase lean muscle. Physical activity is one factor that is positively correlated with muscle protein synthesis. Inactivity is an unavoidable consequence of convalescence and will reduce the anabolic effect normally produced with amino acid supplementation.[140,141]

Catecholamines and inflammatory mediators also inhibit insulin activity and increase catabolism despite adequate nutritional support.[142] These metabolic factors further complicate calculation of protein requirements for parenteral nutrition.

The level of protein supplementation must also be balanced against the energy supplied by carbohydrates and lipids to prevent the use of protein for energy or storage as fat. The ratio of non-protein energy (kcal) to nitrogen (g) should be between 1:100 to 1:200 kcal/g.[47,134] Protein is 16% nitrogen; therefore, grams of nitrogen are obtained by multiplying 0.16 times the total amount of protein. In general, lower amounts of protein are required in animals with hepatic insufficiency, but nitrogen requirements will increase by 25–30% in permissive hypoalimentation (described in the next Section 3.3.3.1) and may also be higher in malnourished patients.[137]

It is essential to remember that a complete parenteral nutrition formula also includes micronutrients, including trace elements, vitamins, and minerals. While the nutrient requirements for healthy horses have been established by the NRC,[69] it is difficult to extrapolate these guidelines to the requirements of critically ill patients. Pre-existing nutrient deficiencies may complicate the issue. While energy and protein requirements can be monitored through indirect calorimetry, it is not possible to measure micronutrient needs. Supplementation should be provided for any horse on parenteral nutrition for more than 3 days.

3.3.3.1 Calculation of Parenteral Nutrition

The composition of parenteral nutrition administered to a horse with colic can be determined based on the resting energy requirement previously discussed, multiplied by a factor for surgery (optional), and with additional calories added for previous malnutrition. The goal for the nutrition formulation is to prevent muscle wasting and maintain body weight until enteral feeding is resumed. Often, calculations overestimate energy expenditure, which can lead to hyperlipemia, hypercapnea, and hyperglycemia.[144–146] However, hypoalimentation also has negative effects including increased risk of infection and increased mortality.[147,148]

To avoid complications of over or under feeding patients, the current recommendation in human medicine is permissive hypoalimentation for critically ill patients, providing 33–65% of targeted calories

(9–18 kcal/kg/day). This strategy avoids excess calories while providing necessary energy and protein and has been shown to improve survival and reduce sepsis.[147,149] Based on these principles of permissive hypoalimentation when calculating equine parenteral nutrition, the total resting energy requirement should be multiplied by 33–65%, giving an initial rate between 7.7–15.0 kcal/kg/day. Based on the horses' recovery, it can either be weaned from parenteral nutrition onto oral feeds or the rate can be increased up to RER, and then DER or higher based on the needs of the individual patient.[139] When calculating parenteral nutrition for horses, it is important to monitor changes in body weight and disease status to determine if the parenteral nutrition provided is adequate.

Practitioners with access to a compounding pharmacy can calculate exact prescriptions for their patients in terms of calories supplied, protein provided, and components to provide energy requirements. An algorithm is provided to allow for step by step prescriptions of total parenteral nutrition (TPN; see Figure 3.1). In practice, most clinicians use products readily available to mix their own. These include 50% dextrose solutions, 8.5–10.0% amino acid solutions, and 10–20% lipid solutions. There are currently three forms of parenteral nutrition commonly used in the horse.

Dextrose Solutions

First is a parenteral solution composed of dextrose only (see Table 3.8). While dextrose can provide energy in the short term to critical patients, it is not nutritionally complete and will not prevent continued muscle wasting. However, dextrose solutions are commonly used in the horse for one advantage; its reduced cost. If selected, dextrose infusions should be diluted to 5% or less concentration, due to the increased risk of complications when higher (hypertonic: 600 mOsm/L) concentrations are infused into a peripheral vein. One option is to add a hypertonic dextrose solution to a balanced electrolyte solution to obtain the desired concentration. Rates from 0.5–2.0 mg/kg/min have been described, but 1.7 mg/kg/min is commonly used and well tolerated by horses.[150] However, this rate provides only 35% of the RER, the minimum rate for permissive hypoalimentation, and may be inadequate for some horses. Excessive rates of dextrose administration may result in hyperosmolality, hypovolemia and hyperglycemia. In addition, large volumes of isotonic fluids can have a significant

Step 1: Calculate total daily energy expenditure, equivalent to resting energy requirement (RER)

RER = 21.28 kcal × body weight (kg) + 975
or
RER = 23 kcal/kg/day

Example: RER = (21.28 kcal) × (500 kg) + 975 = 11,615 kcal

Step 2:
Calculate non-protein energy requirements and composition

Dextrose solutions only

Energy from dextrose = RER

Example: ml of 50% dextrose required
11,615kcal/(1.7kcal/ml)[a]
= 6,832 ml

Dextrose + Lipid

Range of composition:
Dextrose: 40–100% of RER
Lipid: 40–60% of RER

Example: using 50% dextrose and 20% lipid solutions for each to meet 50% of RER (50:50 kcal basis)

Supply 50% of RER with 50% dextrose solution
0.5 x 11,615 = 5,807 kcal
5,807/(1.7 kcal/ml)[a] = 3,416 ml of dextrose

Supply 50% of RER with 20% lipid solution
0.5 x 11,615 = 5,807 kcal
5,807/(2.0 kcal/ml)[b] = 2,904 ml of lipids

Step 3:
Calculate crude protein (CP) requirements
(Range: 0.6–2.0 g/kg/day)

Total daily CP =
BW (kg) x rate (g/kg/day)

Total volume of 8.5% amino acid solution (AA) required =
CP (g)/(0.085 g/ml)

Total DE provided by CP =
(0.34 kcal/ml) x AA (ml)

Example: using 1.2 g/kg/day
Total daily CP (g) =
500kg x 1.2 g/kg/day = 600 g

Total volume of 8.5% AA = 600 g/(0.085 g/ml) = 7,059 ml

Total DE provided by CP =
(0.34 kcal/ml) × (7,059 ml) = 2,400 kcal

Step 4:
Determine non-protein energy to nitrogen ratio
(Goal: 100–150:1)

Non-protein energy to nitrogen ratio =
total non-protein energy
RER/total nitrogen

CP = 16% nitrogen
Therefore, total nitrogen = 0.16 × CP (g)

Example:
Non-protein energy to nitrogen ratio =
11,615 kcal/(600 g x 0.16) = 121
if < 100, increase RER
if > 150, decrease CP

Step 5: Calculate total daily DE and infusion rate

Total Daily DE =
non-protein energy + energy from protein

Maximum infusion rate =
total volume/24h

Initial infusion rate =
60% of maximum infusion rate

1. **Dextrose (50%) and amino acids (8.5%) only:**
DE = 11,615 kcal + 2,400 kcal = 14,015 kcal
Total volume = 6,832 ml dextrose + 7,059 ml AA = 13,891 ml
kcal/ml = 14,015 kcal/13,891 ml = 1.0 kcal/ml
Maximum infusion rate = 13,891 ml/24 h = 579 ml/h
Initial infusion rate = 0.6 x 579 ml/h = 347 ml/h

2. **Dextrose (50%), amino acid (8.5%), and lipid (20%) infusion:**
DE = 11,615 + 2,400 kcal = 14,015 kcal
Total volume = 3,416 ml dextrose + 7,059 ml AA + 2,904 ml lipid
= 13,379 ml
kcal/ml = 14,014 kcal/13,379 ml = 1.05 kcal/ml
Maximum infusion rate = 13,379 ml/24 h = 557 ml/h
Initial infusion rate = 0.6 x 557 ml/h = 334 ml/h

a. 50% dextrose supplies 1.7 kcal/ml
b. 20% lipid supplies 2.0 kcal/ml

Figure 3.1 Algorithm for calculation of parenteral nutrition in a horse weighing 500 kg.

Table 3.8 Commercially available dextrose solutions for partial parenteral nutrition.

Solution	Concentration dextrose (mg/ml)	Osmolarity (mOsm/L)	kcal/L	Maximum rate for 500-kg horse (ml/h)
2.5% dextrose in water	25	126	85	non-physiologic
5% dextrose in water	50	253	170	non-physiologic
10% dextrose in water	100	505	340	non-physiologic
2.5% dextrose in Plasmalyte® 56	25	236	85	2,040
2.5% dextrose in Plasmalyte® 148	25	420	105	2,040
2.5% dextrose in Normosol® R	25	420	100	2,040
2.5% dextrose in lactated Ringers	25	398	95	2,040
5% dextrose in Plasmalyte® 56	50	363	170	1,020
5% dextrose in Plasmalyte® 148	50	547	190	1,020
5% dextrose in Normosol® R	50	547	185	1,020
5% dextrose in lactated Ringers	50	525	180	1,020

ᵃ Baxter Healthcare Corp, Deerfield, IL
ᵇ Abbott Animal Health, Abbott Park, IL

dilutional affect. Dextrose solutions should be used to provide only short term parenteral nutrition, for less than 3 days total.

Amino Acid and Dextrose Solutions

A combination of protein and carbohydrate solutions is a more physiologic solution for parenteral nutrition in the horse. This method combines provision of the daily RER using 50% dextrose with an amino acid solution that reduces the catabolism of lean muscle. Amino acid solutions vary widely in concentration, but the most common concentrations used in horses are 8.5–10.0% amino acids. The goal for protein supplementation is between 0.6–2.0 g/kg/day. If liver disease or renal failure is diagnosed, then protein supplementation should be lower; conversely, with severe sepsis or burns, higher levels may be required. After calculating the total protein required, it is important to ensure adequate calories are provided to prevent use of the amino acids for energy. Calculation of the non-protein energy to nitrogen ratio

(see algorithm in Figure 3.1) should ensure a ratio between 100–150:1 to provide a balanced formula.

To simplify parenteral nutrition, these solutions are often provided in a dual chamber bag, allowing mixture of the dextrose and amino acids after breaking an internal membrane. The most common solution used in equine medicine is composed of a 1:1 ratio of 50% dextrose and 8.5% amino acids. After mixing, the combined solution provides 1l of a 25% dextrose solution in a 4.25% amino acid mixture, with a total of 1.02 kcal/ml. The non-protein energy to nitrogen ratio is 200:1 and the osmolality of the solution is 780 mOsm/L. Starting at 60% of the resting energy requirement for a 500-kg horse, initial target infusion rates are approximately 343 ml/h. However, it is recommended to start at approximately 25% of this rate (85 ml/h), increasing as tolerated over the first 24 h.

Advantages of lipid free formulations include a lower cost as well as a reduction in infection-related complications by eliminating immunosuppressive long chain fatty acids.[122,133,134] However, the high concentration of dextrose may increase the risk of hyperglycemia, known to increase mortality in human and equine patients.[151,152] In addition, the osmolarity of the solution requires that the formula be diluted before administration, or mixed concurrently with infusion of a crystalloid solution.

Amino Acid, Dextrose, and Lipid Solutions

The combination of nutrients commonly used for equine TPN is a mixture of amino acids, carbohydrates, and lipids. At least 8% of the total energy requirements should be provided by lipids to ensure adequate fatty acid supplementation. While more complicated to calculate, as well as more expensive, it has several advantages. First is the improved osmolarity of the final solution. Undiluted 20% lipid solutions are iso-osmotic with an osmolarity of 260 mOsm/L. This reduces the osmolarity of the final solution, possibly reducing the risk of thrombophlebitis. Also, lipid solutions contain the essential fatty acid linoleic acid, which may become depleted over time in horses held off feed.

Contraindications include any horse at risk, or with evidence of, hyperlipemia which would worsen with administration of additional lipids. The daily dose of lipid should not exceed 2.5 g/kg. It is important to remember that lipids are destabilized by sunlight, pH, storage conditions, and some electrolytes (calcium and magnesium). However, amino acid solutions exert some protection for the lipids. When mixing TPN, the amino acid and dextrose solutions must be combined first, followed by the lipid solution. Any signs of stearation (yellow streaks or droplets) indicate destabilization of the mixture and it should be discarded.

3.3.3.2 Administration of Parenteral Nutrition

In horses, parenteral nutrition can be supplied through a peripheral vein, including the jugular and lateral thoracic. A dedicated silicone or polypropylene multilumen catheter with separate injection ports for medications and fluids is preferred. However, delivery through a single lumen catheter, while not ideal, has been successful, provided a Y port is used to supply medications and fluids separately. It is important to maintain sterility of the lines at all times: gloves should be worn when handling all connections, all ports should be cleaned before use, and triple antibiotic ointment can be applied over all connections to reduce the risk of infection. In addition, all lines should be changed every

24–48 h to reduce the risk of bacterial colonization, especially when using lipids.

Solutions should always be mixed under sterile conditions in a laminar flow hood, however, newer products provide both amino acids and glucose in separate chambers contained inside one bag, which allows for mixing without contamination after breaking the internal seal. Lipids, if needed, will still need to be added under sterile conditions. Additional additives, including vitamins and minerals, must be ensured by the manufacturer to be compatible with the solution, since lipids are destabilized by pH and a number of electrolytes. Lipids, amino acids, and some vitamins are light sensitive; therefore, it is important to protect the solution from direct sunlight before and during administration. Oxidation of fatty acids can result in formation of large droplets that cannot be cleared by the endothelium and could result in lipid embolization.[135] Once mixed, the solution can be stored in the refrigerator at 2–8 °C for up to 24 h prior to use, but should be used within 24 h after removal from refrigeration.

An infusion pump is ideal for administration of parenteral nutrition to ensure accurate and continuous infusions. Parenteral nutrition is typically administered as 60–85% of the calculated total daily resting energy requirements for the horse, due to cost and to avoid complications of overalimentation. In general, parenteral nutrition should be initiated at 25% of this reduced rate, increasing by 25% every 3–6 h if the patient is handling the solution well. Once the patient is at the full infusion rate, serum chemistries, body weight, and changes in disease status will indicate if further increases are needed. Parenteral nutrition should be discontinued in a similar stepwise manner once enteral feeding has started.

Intensive monitoring is required, both during introduction and after the full rate is reached to ensure acceptable serum glucose, triglycerides, electrolytes, and organ function. Blood glucose concentration should be measured at least every 4 h initially, then every 4–6 h once at the full rate of parenteral nutrition. While strict glycemic control has been advocated, it is reasonable to expect to maintain blood glucose between 110–150 g/dl while on parenteral infusions.[65,128] Urine glucose is also effective in determining the horse's glucose tolerance. If the renal threshold is exceeded (serum glucose of 200–220 mg/dl), glucose may be noted in the urine. If hyperglycemia occurs, then the infusion rate should be reduced and rate increases performed more slowly. If hyperglycemia persists, an insulin infusion may be started or the concentration of dextrose in the solution can be reduced.

Serum triglycerides should also be monitored at least once a day, since hyperlipemia is known to occur without gross changes in serum clarity.[135] Blood urea nitrogen (BUN) and serum creatinine should be checked daily to ensure adequate hydration and renal function in the face of protein supplementation. Serum creatinine and BUN concentrations may also be helpful in determining if amino acid supplementation is sufficient. If protein is inadequate, BUN may decrease; conversely, it may increase if supplementation is excessive.[144] Increased BUN with normal creatinine concentration can indicate muscle catabolism and deamination of protein for energy. Finally, liver function should be assessed daily.

3.3.3.3 Complications

The most common complication of parenteral nutrition in the horse is hyperglycemia,[47,68,153] which may be exacerbated by catecholamines, cortisol, endotoxin, and the concentration of the glucose solution itself.[154–157] While high rates of glucose administration (1.91–7.41 mg/kg/min) require gradual introduction and withdrawal due to glucose intolerance and rebound hypoglycemia, slower rates (1.39 mg/kg/min) can be administered and discontinued more abruptly.[47,68] If needed, a continuous rate infusion of regular insulin at 0.04–0.1 IU/kg/h can be added to maintain normoglycemia. Sepsis and severe disease can exacerbate glucose intolerance, requiring frequent monitoring of serum glucose.[68,153,155] Inability to maintain normal serum glucose levels may be the first sign of deterioration in the patient's condition.[68,118,158]

Hyperglycemia may also cause hyperinsulinemia.[68] While parentally administered glucose is known to increase insulin levels, it causes less of an effect than enteral glucose.[159,160] While glucose intolerance may result,[159] hyperinsulinemia may provide some benefit the horse through anabolic effects on skeletal muscle and improvement in glucose and triglyceride uptake.[118]

Intravenous catheter related complications are common in humans, but this seems to be a relatively uncommon occurrence in veterinary patients.[47,118,125,139,161] Catheters should still be monitored closely for signs of infection or thrombosis, including heat, swelling, and lack of patency. While catheters are traditionally left exposed in adult horses, a bandage should be considered due to the increased risk of catheter-related sepsis with parenteral nutrition.

Hyperlipidemia and hypertriglyceridemia are also potential complications of TPN. Ponies, donkeys, and miniature horses are at the highest risk and should be closely monitored with serum biochemistries and triglyceride concentrations.[162] In addition, horses with sepsis or endotoxemia are at an increased risk for hyperlipidemia, due to suppression of lipoprotein lipase activity by inflammatory mediators, enhanced adipose tissue catabolism by catacholamines, and inhibition of hepatic metabolism of chylomicrons.[163]

Hypermagnesemia resulting in seizures has been reported in one horse receiving parenteral nutrition.[47] However, other studies have not noted any significant changes in electrolytes.[68,125] Hypermagnesemia has also been reported in humans with symptoms including loss of muscle tone, apnea, hypotension, and bradycardia.[164] Electrolytes should be closely monitored in horses receiving parenteral nutrition as well as supplemental electrolyte solutions.

While dextrose and amino acids solutions may cause phlebitis, acidosis, and osmotic diuresis, amino acids solutions can result in uremia and hyperammonemia.[118] In addition, high concentrations of amino acids may reduce duodenal motility, migrating motor complexes, and small intestinal transit time.[16] Five percent dextrose solutions were noted to increase gastric reflux frequency and volume in horses treated with parenteral nutrition.[125]

3.4 Diets for Specific Diseases

3.4.1 Uncomplicated Colic

In the majority of cases of colic, a specific diagnosis is not determined. Vagotonia (gas colic) or mild impactions are the top suspects. Physical examination in these cases is typically unremarkable and advanced diagnostics are often unnecessary. Treatment, including oral fluids, mineral oil, and non-steroidal anti-inflammatory medications, is usually successful, with a full recovery in most cases in 12–24 h.

In cases of simple colic, feeding should be resumed as soon as normal borborygmi and fecal production are noted. Good quality forages should be provided for the first 12–24 h of refeeding in small amounts (0.5 kg or 1.1 lb) every 4–6 h. If there are no further signs of discomfort, feedings can gradually increase over 24–48 h to normal rations. Forages are the preferred diet in any horse, but alternatives to hay include complete pellets, alfalfa pellets, hay cubes, or hand grazing starting at a 15–20-minute duration. Mashes are often acceptable ways to increase water intake and palatability of feeds. Grains should be avoided for 10–14 days to avoid additional microbial disruption. The clinician should make an effort to reintroduce the type of feed that the horse will be fed after it recovers. If the feed that the horse is reintroduced to is different than their regular diet, changes should be made gradually over 7–10 days if the owner wishes to return to the original diet.

Most cases of uncomplicated colic do not recur. However, the diet, environment, and feeding schedule should be closely scrutinized to identify any predisposing factor that may have led to the colic. If a problem is identified, such as a change in feed supplier or recent travel, preventive measures can be recommended.

3.4.2 Equine Gastric Ulcer Syndrome

Equine gastric ulcer syndrome (EGUS) is a term that is used to encompass a variety of disease processes that result in ulceration of either or both the glandular and squamous portions of the stomach and signs of colic. Gastric ulceration results from an imbalance between ulcer promoting factors (hydrochloric acid, bile acids, pepsin) and protective factors (mucus, bicarbonate, mucosal blood flow, prostaglandin E2, epidermal growth factor, gastroduodenal motility).[166] Dietary factors that may contribute to EGUS include high concentrate diets, low roughage or poor quality fiber diets, meal feeding, and fasting.[161] Dietary recommendations for prevention of EGUS are centered on increasing the frequency of feedings, reducing the quantities of starches fed, and increasing the quality of forages provided.

Saliva and ingested feeds are the primary buffers for the acid produced in the stomach of the horse. Because of this, pasture turnout is often recommended as the best method to prevent and control gastric ulcers.[172–174] However, this may not eliminate ulcers, since horses naturally tend to eat less at certain times of the day. These foraging patterns have been suggested to be the cause of a circadian pattern to the pH of the proximal stomach in horses regardless of their housing.[175] This may be the reason that horses have been diagnosed

with gastric ulcers even when kept solely at pasture.[176] While the horse's voluntary intake is not under our control, free choice forages should still be provided, since intermittent feeding or feed withholding is an experimental model used to consistently produce gastric ulcers.[177,178]

Stall confinement and meal feeding are separate factors that have been associated with altered feed intake and gastric ulceration.[179] In one study, feeding meals greater than 6 h apart increased the likelihood of non-glandular ulceration, suggesting that continuous access to forages may be critical to reducing this risk.[169] This was supported by the results of a second study that found ulcers in 75% of horses fed twice daily and in 57.9% of horses fed three times daily.[181] Based on these findings, continuous feeding of alfalfa or good quality grass hay has been recommended for horses not on pasture to protect the non-glandular mucosa. The high protein and calcium content of alfalfa may provide better protection than grass hays alone. It is speculated that alfalfa has a direct buffering effect because of its high protein content or through a reduction in gastrin secretion.[181] This effect on pH was consistent, even when alfalfa was fed with concentrates such as oats, barley, or pelleted rations.[54,172] Based on these findings, alfalfa may be the forage of choice for horses at risk for, or diagnosed with, gastric ulcers.[174]

Grains should be kept at a minimum in horses with EGUS, due to their known association with the formation of gastric ulcers.[171] Soluble carbohydrates present in most cereals fed to horses are fermented in the stomach to volatile fatty acids. These fatty acids are able to penetrate the cells of the mucosa at a low pH, resulting in cell swelling and disruption.[182–184]

Concentrate diets are also known to increase the release of gastrin, the hormone responsible for acid secretion.[185] While gastric acid can be disruptive alone, the effects of volatile fatty acids are exacerbated by a pH less than 4.[182–184] In addition, grains have been shown to delay the secretion of gastrin, increasing the likelihood of inappropriate acid secretion after ingesta has passed. As an empty stomach is more likely to expose the non-glandular mucosa to acid and ulceration may be more likely when feeding grains.[186]

Grains should only be fed in amounts less than 0.5 kg/100 kg body weight and no less than every 6 h to reduce volatile fatty acids below the threshold for mucosal damage.[182] The grains selected should be low in starch, since a starch intake between 1–2 g/kg/meal was associated with a 2.6 times increase in the likelihood of ulcers (95% CI 1.3–5.2; P = 0.006) and an intake greater than 2 g/kg bodyweight per meal increased the likelihood by 3.2 times (95% CI 1.3–7.7; P = 0.009).[169] Hay, preferably alfalfa, should be available at all times. Fat supplements such as vegetable oils may be used as a substitute for concentrates to provide energy. While lipids were unable to prevent non-glandular ulceration, they may be useful in the therapy and prevention of glandular ulceration by reducing gastric acid and increasing prostaglandin production.[55,187]

Horses with colic are at no higher risk for gastric ulcers than the general population, but the likelihood that they will be withheld from feed due to their disease process may increase the chance of ulcer formation.[188] Horses with diseases that may require long periods without oral feeding (i.e., duodenitis/proximal jejunitis) are particularly at risk.[189] This strengthens the argument that horses with colic should be fed as soon as their medical conditions allow to reduce the risk of iatrogenic complications of feed withholding.

3.4.3 Duodenitis/Proximal Jejunitis

Duodenitis/proximal jejunitis (DPJ), also known as anterior enteritis, is an inflammatory disease resulting in hypersecretion in the proximal small intestine, gastrointestinal ileus, and copious nasogastric reflux. A full description of this disease process, diagnosis, and therapy can be found elsewhere.[190] While infectious organisms including *Salmonella* spp, *Clostridium perfringens*, and *Clostridium difficile* have been implicated, the exact cause is still unknown.[191–194] A suspected link with aflatoxicosis or fusariotoxicosis has also been made, based on necropsy findings of lesions consistent with DPJ. Therefore, it is important to be highly vigilant for mold in concentrates and other feeds containing corn.[195,196]

High concentrate diets were previously thought to increase the risk of DPJ, due to high concentrations of hydrolysable carbohydrates that fermented in the stomach and possibly the small intestine.[197] This link between grains and DPJ and has been statistically supported by a modest odds ratio of 1.3–1.62 (P < 0.001) in a case control study performed in Texas.[198] In this study, horses with DPJ were fed a median of 4.1 kg concentrate daily versus 2.7 kg in the control group.

Horses with DPJ were significantly more likely to have had access to pasture grazing in this same study,

with an odds ratio of 3.5–4.0 (P < 0.0005).[198] This connection to pasture grazing has caused comparisons to be made between DPJ and equine dysautonomia (Equine Grass Sickness), another cause of ileus in the horse associated with grazing pastures. Speculated causes of dysautomonia are similar to DPJ, including mycotoxins and *Clostridium* spp., supporting an infectious cause for both syndromes.[199–202]

Medical therapy for DPJ involves maintaining hydration with IV fluids, supporting oncotic pressure with plasma or colloids, providing anti-inflammatory medications, and prokinetics. Surgery should be considered if obstructive diseases of the small intestine cannot be ruled out or if medical management is unsuccessful.[203,204] If surgery is elected, decompression of the small intestine into the cecum or an incomplete bypass may be performed.[192,197,205,206] Both medical and surgical treatments have a good chance for full recovery if aggressive treatment is pursued, and the disease is allowed to run its course.[192,207]

Horses with DPJ are usually unable to take in enteral feed due to the severity of ileus resulting in significant volumes of gastric reflux. In addition, protein loss is often severe due to loss of the intestinal mucosal barrier and protein catabolism from prolonged cachexia. Based on the BCS at the time of diagnosis, parenteral nutrition should be considered for any horse identified as malnourished (low BCS), horses with increased demands (pregnancy, lactation) and any horse with DPJ that continues to reflux for more than 48 h (see Section 3.3.3 on parenteral nutrition). Parenteral nutrition should continue until the horse is voluntarily eating at least 60% of its resting energy requirements.

Enteral feeding can begin once progressive motility is confirmed by a lack of net gastric reflux and ultrasonographic confirmation of small intestinal contractions. Water is initially provided in small amounts (1–2 l every 2–4 h) to confirm progressive motility. If water is accepted without complication, then hay, softened complete feeds, or alfalfa pellets can be introduced slowly, starting at 25% of the daily ration divided into meals every 2–4 h. The horse should be reintroduced to full feed within 2–3 days. Vital parameters, appetite, attitude, and repeated ultrasonographic examination will assess the progression of feedings during reintroduction. Concentrates or fresh grasses with a high concentration of fermentable carbohydrates should be avoided. After recovery, grains should be avoided for the first two weeks and should be limited to meals less than 0.5 kg/100 kg body weight and in more than four feedings per day. Protein-rich forages, including alfalfa or vegetable oils, may be required to regain weight lost during the disease.

3.4.4 Small Intestinal Strangulation

Small intestinal strangulations result in obstruction of the blood supply as well as the intestinal lumen. Strangulating lesions can be caused by a number of conditions, including mesenteric lipomas, mesenteric rents, intussusceptions, and epiploic foramen entrapment, but all are directly unrelated to dietary factors. Clinical signs of strangulation include severe pain unresponsive to analgesics, small intestinal distention on rectal and ultrasound examination, peritoneal fluid changes, and variable amounts of nasogastric reflux depending on the duration and location of the obstruction. Definitive diagnosis of the strangulating lesion is confirmed during exploratory laparotomy and resection and anastomosis may be performed if the bowel is deemed non-viable.

The small intestine is extremely sensitive to the manipulation required in surgery as well as distention caused by obstruction and these factors may result in post-operative ileus. If ileus occurs after surgery, then enteral feeding is not possible. Therefore, parenteral feeding is often required to maintain body condition and provide supportive nutrition for recovery (see Section 3.3.3 on parenteral nutrition). The timing for initiating early parenteral nutrition is case dependent, due to preexisting conditions, concurrent diseases, BCS on presentation, and the financial considerations of the owner. Despite evidence of improved nutritional status of horses post-surgery that are provided parenteral nutrition, including lower total bilirubin and serum triglycerides, it is still unclear as to any benefits of providing parenteral nutrition to surgical colic cases, with the downside of increased cost to the client.[47,68] Based on the lack of clear evidence, most adult horses are simply held off feed until ileus subsides.

In an effort to prevent post-operative ileus, horses with small intestinal resections or enterotomies should be provided oral feed as soon as possible after surgery. Common practice has been to begin oral supplementation only when borborygmi are present and defecation has occurred, but human medicine is now recommending providing enteral feed even earlier.[65] Veterinary medicine is changing as well in that regard.

Freeman et al.[203,208] advocate reintroducing feed for any horse without signs of colic or nasogastric reflux on a set schedule post-surgery, rather than relying on defecation or intestinal sounds (see Table 3.9). On this plan, horses are first offered water in small amounts at 12–18 h after surgery, followed by alfalfa hay in handfuls, which slowly increases every 2–4 h over the next 24 h. The goal is to reintroduce the horse to at least 75% of full feed over 1–2 days. Softened complete feed, alfalfa pellets, or grass offered as small meals are viable alternatives to hay for horses when anastomosis function is questionable or severe mucosal edema is suspected. Vital signs, attitude, packed cell volume, and serum total solid concentration, as well as progressive gastrointestinal motility with a lack of nasogastric reflux are used to determine if feeding is progressing satisfactorily. Small feedings in a controlled manner increase gastrointestinal motility and reduce cost and complications including gastric ulceration.

Short bowel syndrome is defined as a malabsorptive disorder caused by strangulations with resections that result in a loss of >60% of the small intestine.[209] However, the length of small intestine that is necessary for adequate digestion and absorption may be variable, based on reports of individual cases where horses have survived with less (12.3–15.0 feet).[208,210] The small intestine is the primary site for absorption of carbohydrates, protein, and minerals, and the ileum is the specific site for fat-soluble vitamin absorption. However, the large intestine appears able to compensate post-operatively for the lack of absorption of proteins, carbohydrates, and B vitamins. In addition, the small intestine is capable of a compensatory adaptive hyperplasia that increases the efficiency of digestion by increasing the length, diameter, and surface area of the remaining intestine.[211–213]

Clinical findings of short bowel syndrome include weight loss, hepatic damage, capricious appetite, and diarrhea.[208,209] If recognized after surgery, the goal is to optimize large bowel fermentation with a highly digestible fiber source, such as alfalfa, beet pulp, or soybean hulls to support volatile fatty acid production.[214] If the ileum or greater than 75% of the small intestine has been resected, fat-soluble vitamins may need to be supplemented to the diet.[209] Supplementation with rice bran or corn oil may be required to provide additional energy to maintain body weight, but should be avoided in cases with ileal resection.[96,209] Complete pelleted feeds

Table 3.9 Refeeding schedule for post-operative small intestinal resections. The diet can be adjusted based on each individual horse's response to feedings, in that the interval between meals can be increased, the weight of feed decreased, or both for slower reintroductions. Any horse with positive net nasogastric reflux should be held off enteral feed and water until ileus resolves.

Amount to feed based on dietary needs of a 500-kg horse with a goal of achieving at least 75% of daily energy requirements (DER; 75% of DER = 12,300 kcal/day) 3–4 days post-celiotomy					
Day post-surgery	Hours post-surgery	Amount of feed required		Selected diets	
				Alfalfa hay (DE = 2,430 kcal/kg)	Complete pelleted feed* (DE = 2,695 kcal/kg)
		Weight of feed	Frequency	DE (kcal) fed during specified time period	
Day 1	0–12	none per os		0	0
	12–24	0.1 kg (0.2 lbs)	q 2–4h	729–1,458	809–1,617
Day 2	24–36	0.25 kg (0.55 lbs)	q 2–4h	1,823–3,645	2,021–4,043
	36–48	0.5 kg (1.1 lbs)	q 3–4h	3,645–4,860	4,043–5,390
Day 3	48–60	0.75 kg (1.65 lbs)	q 3–4h	5,468–7,290	6,064–8,085
	60–72	1.0 kg (2.2 lbs)	q 3–4h	7,290–9,720	8,085–10,780
Day 4	72–96	1.25 kg (2.75 lbs)	q 4–6h	12,150–18,225	13,475–20,212
Day 5 onward	Continue to modify diet so that the total ration meets DER for the specific patient. Feedings can be adjusted by changing the number of feedings and the amount of feed offered to obtain the total daily rations desired. All changes in type of diet, including the addition of supplements, should occur slowly over 1 week.				

* Purina Equine Senior®, Purina Mills, St. Louis, MO

provided in small frequent meals have also been successful in supporting horses with resections of up to 70% of the distal small intestine.[215] However, grains should be avoided if an extensive resection has been performed, due to the inability to adequately process starches.[26]

3.4.5 Ileal Impaction (Nonstrangulating Small Intestinal Obstruction)

Ileal impactions are most commonly observed in mature horses in the southeastern United States. This obstruction is linked to excessive non-fermentable fiber and fine stem character of poor quality coastal Bermudagrass hay, which may be related to factors such as maturity at harvesting, soil composition, curing, and storage.[15,216] Another risk factor commonly cited for ileal impactions is infection with *Anoplocephala perfoliata* tapeworms, which localize at the ileocecal junction and may result in obstruction of the ileocecal valve due to inflammation.[15,217]

Clinical signs of ileal impaction include moderate to severe signs of colic, depending on the duration and severity of the obstruction.[15,19,218] Early in the course of the disease, the impaction may be felt on transrectal palpation as a firm tubular structure entering the cecum on the right side of the abdomen.[219] As the obstruction progresses and becomes complete, the small intestine oral to the ileum fills with ingesta and multiple loops may be palpable per rectum and noted on ultrasound examination. Ileus results and gastric reflux may be obtained.[19,218]

Medical therapy is currently recommended, using intravenous fluids, gastric decompression, sedation, and analgesics.[219] Serial abdominocenteses can monitor the progress of medical therapy and if protein concentration and white blood cell count increase with no response to medical therapy, surgery is recommended. At surgery, the impaction is reduced into the cecum using external massage, often with direct intraluminal infusion with balanced electrolyte solutions or carboxymethylcellulose.[19,218] In some cases, an enterotomy may be useful to reduce the trauma caused by external manipulation. Post-operative ileus and adhesions are risks for any surgical procedure used to relieve an ileal impaction.

In most horses, ileal impactions will resolve with medical therapy within 12 h, therefore supportive care in the form of parenteral nutrition is rarely required.[219] In the acute phase of recovery, horses should be fed on a schedule as recommended for small intestinal strangulation, whether they have been managed medically or surgically, in that feeding can resume gradually as soon as the impaction appears to have resolved. Clinically, resolution would be noted as a lack of significant nasogastric reflux, good intestinal motility on ultrasound exam, absence of pain, and no palpable impaction or small intestinal distention. However, the ileum can become edematous or spasm due to inflammation from the impaction or surgical manipulation, making recurrence likely if feeding is too aggressive. Continued use of non-steroidal anti-inflammatory drugs during refeeding may reduce this risk and some clinicians have recommended withholding hay until 48 hours after resolution of clinical signs.[219] Personal observations have noted that large intestinal impactions may often be a coexisting problem and should be addressed prior to refeeding.

Due to the fact that ileal impactions have been definitely linked to coastal Bermudagrass hay, it is recommended after recovery to avoid feeding this forage.[15] If alternative hay sources are not available, then complete pelleted diets or pasture are viable alternatives to forage. If coastal Bermudagrass hay must be fed, it should be introduced gradually, and not fed as free choice round bales.[220] High quality, first cutting hays are recommended and water intake should be ensured.[20] In addition, feeding a pelleted ration or concentrates can increase gastrointestinal transit time and possibly reduce the risk of reimpaction.[217]

3.4.6 Ascending (Large) Colon Impactions

Ascending colon impactions are the most frequent cause of colic in the horse and have been proposed to be caused by a number of external factors, including decreased water intake, stress, feed quality, or dietary changes that result in dehydration of the colon ingesta.[222] Obstruction typically occurs at points in the large colon where narrowing occurs, including the pelvic flexure, left ventral colon, and the sternal and diaphragmatic flexures.[16,223] Clinical signs typically include mild to moderate colic with a reduction in fecal output. Transrectal palpation may note firm, mucus covered fecal balls and if an impaction is palpable in the large colon, then the diagnosis is confirmed. Therapy centers on the administration of fluids, laxatives, and judicious use of analgesics and antispasmotics.[223–225] The horse should be withheld from feed during treatment. Surgery is indicated if the impaction does not resolve in a timely manner, the abdomen becomes more distended, or if pain becomes intractable. At surgery, the impaction is usually relieved by lavage through a pelvic flexure enterotomy.

For horses treated with medical therapy alone, feeding should not be delayed once the impaction has cleared (see Table 3.10). Signs of resolution include absence of pain, a lack of abnormalities on transrectal palpation, adequate fecal production, and normal gastrointestinal transit time as noted by the passage of mineral oil. Good quality forages, ideally alfalfa hay, should initially be provided in small amounts (0.5 kg or 1.1 lb) 4–6 times daily, with a gradual increase over 24–48 h to normal rations.[45] Free choice hay may be preferable after successful reintroduction of feed to reduce the risk of gastric ulcers. Alternatives to hay during the acute phase, depending on the patient and clinician preference, include complete pellets, alfalfa pellets, or grazing, starting at 15 minute intervals. The goal is to have the horse back on a full ration within 1–3 days after reintroduction of feed (1.5–2.5% of body weight in forages). Grains should be avoided for 10–14 days after colic has resolved to avoid further disruptions in the microbial populations by undigested starches. Concentrates should be reintroduced slowly, starting with less than 1 kg (2.2 lb) per 500 kg horse twice a day and increasing gradually if needed by 0.5–0.75 kg increments per day.[45]

Table 3.10 Examples of refeeding schedules for mild ascending colon impactions, when colic resolves in 12–24 hours. The interval between meals can be increased, the weight of feed decreased, or both for slower reintroductions (over 3–4 days).

	Weight of feed	Frequency of feedings	Type of Feed		
			Hay only	Complete pelleted feed	Alfalfa pellet
			DE (kcal)/day	DE (kcal)/day	DE (kcal)/day
Day 1	0.5 kg (1.1 lb)	q 4–6 h	Alfalfa hay: 4,860–7,290 Grass hay: 4,360–6,540 Coastal Bermudagrass hay: 3,740–5,610	5,390–8,085	4,760–7,140
Day 2	1 kg (2.2 lb)	q 4–6 h	Alfalfa hay: 9,720–14,580 Grass hay: 8,720–13,080 Coastal Bermudagrass hay: 7,480–11,220	10,780–16,170	9,520–14,280
Day 3	Full ration	q 6–12 h	Full hay ration at normal intervals. Introduce additional feeds or supplements slowly over 1 week. No grain for 10–14 days.	Full pelleted ration at normal intervals, or introduce hay, supplements or grazing slowly over 1 week. No grain for 10–14 days.	Introduce hay, complete pellets, supplements, or grazing slowly over 1 week. No grain for 10–14 days.

If the horse has undergone a celiotomy to relieve impaction, then the feeding schedule should be identical for a resolved medically treated impaction. Most horses can return to feed as soon as complete recovery from anesthesia, usually 3–6 h after returning to the stall. Some clinicians prefer to withhold feed for 12–24 h after performing an enterotomy. However, a secure closure and good surgical technique will not delay reintroduction of feed and the colon lumen is large enough at the pelvic flexure so that any distention by feed should not stress the suture line. In addition, enterotomy and lavage has a disruptive effect on the large colon flora, which should be supported as soon as possible with a healthy substrate for fermentation.[226] Grass hay has been associated with a reduced risk of post-operative diarrhea in horses after enterotomy, therefore, grazing or grass hay are both recommended in the early postoperative period.[227] It is important to remember hospital biosecurity when grazing horses after colic, due to the unavoidable alterations in gastrointestinal flora and the risk of salmonellosis. This is especially important postoperatively for large intestinal problems, which doubles

the risk of diarrhea over other types of intestinal lesions ($P < 0.006$)[227] Enterotomy was also found to increase the risk an additional 1.5 times ($P = 0.042$).

For horses that are prone to impactions, prevention is centered on providing good quality forage and encouraging adequate water intake. Late season cuttings of hay that are high in fiber should be avoided, as well as forages known to be of poorer quality, including coastal Bermudagrass and straw. Green grass or alfalfa based diets may provide a laxative effect. Complete pelleted feeds will improve overall digestibility of the diet for horses with dental disease. Alfalfa pellets, alfalfa or hay cubes, or beet pulp may provide a highly digestible fiber source with shorter fiber length to improve digestibility. While the value of regular dental prophylaxis is still not completely known, proper occlusion will aid in reducing fiber length and possibly reduce the risk of impactions. Salt (NaCl or KCl) may be added to the feed to encourage water intake, up to 8 tablespoons a day. Alternatively, electrolyte water, molasses flavored water, or other flavorings may be added to provide interesting alternatives, alongside a plain water bucket.

3.4.7 Sand Impactions

Sand impactions are a specific type of intestinal obstruction resulting from the ingestion of sand, typically obtained from the environment. Feeding on the ground or in sandy arenas has been specifically implicated as risk factors. However, some horses with pica, especially foals, may intentionally ingest sand. In addition, naturally sandy soils in some regions (i.e., Florida, Georgia, and Arizona) provide ample opportunity during grazing for accidental ingestion, especially on short-cropped pastures.[228]

Clinical signs are often similar to feed impactions of the ascending colon,[229] but the irritating nature of sand may result in debridement of the mucosal lining, diarrhea, and signs of endotoxemia due to bacterial translocation.[230,231] Sand impactions can occur at multiple points throughout the digestive tract, including the stomach, cecum, small intestine, and ascending and small colon. However, sand impactions of the dorsal ascending colon are most often identified in horses at surgery.[229–231] Peritonitis or rupture of the large intestine or stomach may occur due to large volumes of sand or long standing impactions that damage the integrity of the intestinal wall.

Diagnosis of sand is often made based on a history of exposure and identification of sand in the ingesta. Sand may be palpated per rectum as a "gritty" feeling in the manure or as a palpable impaction. Fecal sedimentation may help to determine exposure to sand. It is performed by dissolving 3–4 fecal balls in water in a palpation sleeve and identifying sand sediment in the fingers of the glove. However, fecal floatation poorly correlates to the presence of sand in the intestines, due to a high proportion of false negatives, and does not allow for the determination of the amount of sand present in the colon.[232] In areas with sandy soil, it is common to see a small amount of sand when performing a fecal sedimentation test.

The volume of sand present is better demonstrated by abdominal radiographs as a mineralized opacity, but its sensitivity is low in larger horses, especially for sand impactions that are not in the ascending colon. The accumulation of sand can be graded 0–4 and a significant amount of sand is greater than 5 by 15 cm in length and pulls the large colon against the ventral body wall.[233] Ultrasound may be helpful in identifying the presence of sand, but it cannot replace radiography for assessment of volume.[234] While auscultation may identify characteristic "waves on a beach" sounds caudal to the xyphoid process in some horses, it is not sensitive for sand obstructions, especially if colic is reducing large intestinal motility.[235]

Treatment of colic due to sand impaction has centered on the use of fluid therapy, osmotic laxatives, and psyllium fiber (0.5–1.0 g/kg).[236] Psyllium husks contain mucilage, which absorbs water and is believed to act as a laxative. Psyllium gels when mixed with water, so it must be administered quickly through a nasogastric tube. Alternatively, psyllium can be mixed with 2 l of mineral oil, which suspends the psyllium and allows for easier administration by nasogastric tube. Between 2 and 4 l of water can be administered immediately after dosing with the psyllium-oil mixture.[237]

Treatment with psyllium has a variable response in the literature, even when combined with additional laxatives or mineral oil.[238] One study noted no difference between treatment with psyllium (0.5 g/kg), wheat bran (1 g/kg), or an 1:1 mineral oil/water mixture (8 g/kg) compared with no treatment at all when sand was administered via nasogastric tube at a dose of 0.5 g/horse.[239] Doses of psyllium up to 1.0 g/kg were also ineffective in horses with 10 g/kg of sand surgically placed into the cecum.[240] Another study noted a significant improvement, with twice the amount of sand cleared using 0.5 kg psyllium with 2 l of mineral oil, versus mineral oil alone.[241] However, the total amount of sand cleared after 5 days of treatment was only 51%. In horses unresponsive to psyllium, additional treatment with magnesium sulfate (1 g/kg for 3 days) was effective in resolving radiographic signs of impaction.[238]

Horses that do not respond to medical therapy and analgesia are surgical candidates and concurrent large colon displacements or volvulus are not uncommon findings at surgery.[229] Through a ventral midline celiotomy, the colon is carefully exteriorized, a pelvic flexure enterotomy is performed, and the sand siphoned from the site of impaction, commonly the right dorsal colon.[230,231] The gastrointestinal tract must be carefully examined for pressure necrosis, vascular compromise, and transmural damage. Short term survival is good for both medical and surgical treatment of sand impactions and long term survival is excellent.[230]

If the horse is treated for sand impaction with surgery and an enterotomy, the feeding schedule should be similar to that provided for surgical resolution of feed impactions. However, it is important to recognize that horses with conditions of the ascending colon treated by enterotomy and lavage are at a higher risk for developing diarrhea. Horses with sand colic are especially predisposed due to the mucosal irritating nature of the condition.[227] Based on positive results in clinical cases, administration of di-tri-octahedral smectite (0.5 kg/500 kg in 4 l water, q24h) for 3 days post-operatively may reduce diarrhea.[226] Di-tri-octahedral smectite may lessen damage to the colonic mucosa by neutralizing clostridial and *Bacteroides* spp. toxins.[242–244] It may also have a prolonged protective effect through regulation of gastrointestinal flora and intestinal secretions.[245,246] This is an important benefit for horses recovering from surgery, due to the disruption of intestinal flora and the mucus layer by an enterotomy.

It is unknown what volume of sand is significant in terms of causing clinical disease and the specific volume may be different for each individual horse. It is reasonable to assume that any volume of sand may alter the integrity and function of the gastrointestinal tract due to its abrasive nature and long term exposure may be even more damaging.[247]

While sand impactions can be treated, prevention of further ingestion of sand is a better option. Often, removing the horse from its environment is not possible, but reducing the exposure to sand can be attempted. Horses should not be fed on the ground and large tubs or rubber mats should be used to prevent feed from spilling onto sandy soils. Pastures should not be overgrazed and rested and reseeded to encourage better growth. Pastures should be reseeded with forage varieties that have a more extensive root system and are less likely to be pulled from the ground while the horse grazes. Psyllium, either as a generic powder or commercial pellets, may be used as a preventive (0.25 kg once daily for 1 week every month). Horses with continuous exposure could be treated daily with psyllium, but there is some concern that gastrointestinal flora may acclimate to this new fiber source and ferment the psyllium, reducing the effectiveness.[240] The most effective method of clearing sand from the gastrointestinal system is to provide up to 2.5% of body weight per day of hay. The bulk alone is capable of removing almost 95% of ingested sand and was more efficacious in a controlled trial than psyllium, mineral oil, or wheat bran.[239]

3.4.8 Enteroliths and Fecaliths

Enteroliths are intestinal concretions formed by the deposition of minerals, primarily magnesium, nitrogen, and ammonium phosphate salts, around a nidus of foreign material.[24 248,249] Concretions may also form around fibrous undigested feed material, which are classified as fecaliths. These mineralized masses are believed to develop in the ampulla of the right dorsal colon and may cause partial or complete obstruction as they are propelled aboral into the narrow transverse or descending colon. Signs of abdominal discomfort may abate if the enterolith is able to dislodge orally back into the right dorsal colon and these horses often have a history of recurrent and intermittent colic.

Any foreign material can serve as the center for calculus formation, including sand, pebbles, rope, cloth, hair, or other foreign material. Current research into enterolithiasis points to a multifactorial cause. However, the end result of all factors investigated is an intestinal environment that promotes the deposition of mineral due to a basic pH and the presence of minerals including magnesium, nitrogen, phosphorus, calcium, sulfur, sodium, and potassium.[21–23,250]

Genetics have been identified as a cause of enteroliths, in that certain breeds are predisposed, including Arabians, Morgans, American Saddlebreds, American Miniature Horses, and donkeys.[12,22,251,252] There is also an increased predilection among siblings.[251] This may be due to a genetic predisposition for a more alkaline large intestinal ingesta, which has been found in horses with enterolithiasis versus horses without enteroliths.[22,23]

Diet also plays a role, in that specific feeds have been found to produce an intestinal environment that favors enterolith formation. Alfalfa is rich in minerals, as well as protein, which can provide a source of ammonium nitrates.[253] Feeding greater than 50% alfalfa hay has been statistically linked to enterolith formation (OR = 4.74; 95% CI 1.44–15.63)[11] and results in higher colonic calcium, magnesium, phosphorus, and sulfur concentrations, and a more alkaline pH.[23] While it has never been definitively linked to enterolithiasis, wheat bran is also higher in protein, magnesium, and phosphate than most grains and is suspected to contribute to the problem.[11,12,22] Both soil and water are also a source of minerals. It is clear that horses in California are predisposed; however, enteroliths have been diagnosed in a number of other states and countries.[251]

Stall confinement for more than 50% of the day, low fiber diets, and feeding intermittent meals has been linked to enterolith formation.[11,12,22] It has been postulated that inactivity may affect the motility of the ampulla of the right dorsal colon, encouraging mineral deposition in horses that are stalled.[22,252] Grazing may provide both exercise and some dilution of the minerals ingested, along with production of short chain fatty acids for fiber fermentation, potentially reducing colon pH and the chance of crystallization.[22,254]

Diagnosis of enteroliths can be made at surgery, necropsy, or by abdominal radiography. Palpation may identify an enterolith in the small colon, but often it is too far cranial to allow detection per rectum. In some cases, the owners may report seeing small enteroliths passed in the feces, confirming the diagnosis. Horses typically present with a history of mild, recurrent colic with partial obstruction, but if complete, clinical signs will be similar to other forms of large intestinal obstruction. Advanced imaging may allow for diagnosis and early detection before complete obstruction occurs, but radiographs are less sensitive to identify enteroliths in the small colon and in horses with significant gas distention.[255] Definitive treatment is surgical to allow for removal through a large colon or descending colon enterotomy. However, prognosis may be improved if the surgery is elective, before obstruction and pressure necrosis occurs.

Since genetics cannot be controlled, the practitioner should focus on prevention through dietary changes in horses at high risk, including those with a previous history of enteroliths, horses boarding at facilities with a high incidence of the problem, and those related to horses diagnosed with enterolithiasis. Horses of specific breeds, including Arabians, American Miniature Horses, and ponies, should also be included in the high risk category if they have additional risk factors that would predispose them (environment, diet) or they have a history of chronic or recurrent colic.

Prevention should be centered on avoiding feeds that increase the risk of enterolith formation, including those that are high in magnesium and phosphorus. Alfalfa hay should be limited to less than 50% of the diet and hay grown in California should be avoided.[11] Grass or oat hays appear to be protective, possibly due to lower protein and magnesium levels and higher fiber content for the production of short chain fatty acids.[11] High protein diets also should be avoided unless required, due to the ammonium produced. Minerals may be removed from the water source using a water filter, but this is an expensive proposition, and in most cases the mineral content of the feed far outweighs any contribution from water sources.[243]

Protective treatments include those that acidify the colon contents. Calculi are formed in basic environments and if the colon is acidified by starch digesting bacteria, there is a chance that stone formation could slow or stop. Along that train of thought, there have been reports of in vivo dissolution of enteroliths using vinegar to reduce the colon pH.[21,24] While unproven as a preventive or therapy, there are additional reports that vinegar administration may reduce the risk of recurrence.[251] Approximately 1–2 cups (8–16 oz) per day of apple cider vinegar is recommended.[250,256]

Environmental factors are more difficult to control. While eliminating the source of a nidus for calculi formation is impossible, reducing the risk for ingestion of foreign bodies is recommended.[257] Regular treatment with psyllium (0.25–0.5 kg, once daily for 1 week per month) should be provided in endemic areas with sandy environments. Horses should be fed off the ground and feed placed in tubs or on rubber mats to reduce the ingestion of sand. Finally, based on evidence of a protective effect, pasture turnout should be provided.

3.4.9 Ascending Colon Displacement

The ascending colon is freely movable within the abdomen, since the right dorsal and transverse colons are the only point of attachment to the body wall. Displacements of the ascending colon may occur secondary to other disorders, such as fecal impactions, or as a primary problem due to management practices including feeding large amount of concentrates in infrequent meals.[41] Large concentrate boluses allow fermentable carbohydrates to reach the ascending colon, increasing the rate of fermentation and volatile fatty acid production.[258,259] In addition, normal motility patterns may be disrupted by large meals, increasing gas and fluid accumulation from altered fermentation.[39,260] However, an underlying motility disorder may be the ultimate cause in some types of displacements.[261]

Displacements are commonly grouped into right dorsal and left dorsal (nephrosplenic) displacements, as well as pelvic flexure retroversion, or non-strangulating volvulus at the cecocolic junction.[262–264] The exact position of the colon in the abdomen may vary; therefore, diagnosis may simply be large colon displacement. A left dorsal displacement is entrapment of the ascending colon over the nephrosplenic ligament. It is diagnosed on transrectal palpation by tracing a band of the left ventral colon into the dorsal left quadrant between the kidney and base of the spleen. Diagnosis is supported by the inability to locate the left kidney on ultrasound examination through the left flank.[104] Right dorsal displacement is dislocation of the colon into any number of configurations in the abdomen and is commonly diagnosed rectally by a tight band running between the cecum and right body wall. In some cases, the pelvic flexure is not palpable and the caudal abdomen feels empty due to retroflexion of the colon towards the diaphragm.

Clinical signs of displacement include intermittent mild to moderate abdominal pain with concurrent abdominal distention. Fecal production is also reduced. Obstruction of the lumen may result from the displacement of the colon itself or secondary to impaction that may be a concurrent problem. Distention can obstruct venous and lymphatic outflow, resulting in congestion and edema of the tissues, however, tissue damage is minor and resolves quickly once the displacement is corrected.

Medical management can be attempted using fluid therapy, analgesics, and handwalking to stimulate motility.[197] In cases with left dorsal displacement, phenylephrine and jogging may be attempted to contract the spleen and replace the colon, if the large colon is not severely distended with gas or impaction.[265] Trocarization may reduce the amount of gas distention in the abdomen. Alternatively, the horse can be rolled under anesthesia to attempt to replace the colon ventrally.[266,267]

Horses with significant distention per rectum, unrelenting pain, or an abnormal abdominocentesis should be taken to surgery immediately. A ventral midline celiotomy will allow for correction of most displacements. Alternatively, a standing flank approach may be performed to relieve left dorsal displacements, however, a full exploratory is not possible through a flank approach. A pelvic flexure enterotomy may be elected for relief of impactions.

Horses recovering from displacements are returned to feed in a similar manner to horses with ascending colon impactions once the displacement has resolved (see previous section on ascending colon impactions). If medical treatment was successful, confirmation that the colon has returned to its normal position can be made by transrectal palpation, adequate fecal production, and a lack of signs of colic for at least 12 h. Good quality forage is recommended when returning to feed and the long fiber provided by most hays is preferred to increase

the bulk of ingesta within the colon. It is believed that maintaining adequate fill of the ascending colon with ingesta will reduce the risk that gas distention will promote migration to an abnormal position in the abdomen.[264] If surgery and an enterotomy were performed, it is recommended to leave some ingesta in the lumen, to provide some weight to the colon. The remaining feed should also promote normal fermentation to reduce the risk of diarrhea.[227] Concentrates should be avoided for at least 10–14 days or eliminated from the diet to reduce the risk of soluble carbohydrates reaching the large intestine and resulting in abnormal gas production.

Prevention of large colon displacements is centered on providing adequate quantities of good quality fiber and ensuring adequate water intake. Concentrates should be eliminated from the diet or fed in only in small quantities (less than 0.5 kg/100 kg, no less than every 6 h). Because ascending colon impactions are often a concurrent problem, strategies recommended for prevention of impactions can be used for displacements as well. While the recurrence rate for nephrosplenic entrapment is low (between 7.5–8.1%) surgical ablation of the nephrosplenic space can reduce this risk.[268–270] A recent study noted an increased risk of recurrent colic after diagnosis and surgical treatment of right dorsal displacements, with a recurrence rate of 41.9% versus only 8.3% for left dorsal displacement.[260] Retroflexion of the pelvic flexure and non-strangulating volvulus also had higher rates of recurrent colic. However, the recurrence rate for a second right dorsal displacement was still similar to nephrosplenic displacement (about 7%). It is speculated that the cause of right dorsal displacement may be an underlying motility disorder, versus increased gas production proposed to cause left dorsal displacement.[263] This may be the cause of the increased risk of recurrence, which could undermine other preventive strategies. Based on these studies, colopexy may be recommended in cases with repeated displacements.[271]

3.4.10 Ascending Colon Volvulus (Large Colon Torsion)

Ascending colon volvulus is produced by the twisting of the colon on its mesenteric axis, typically in a counterclockwise direction at the level of the attachment of the right and left dorsal colons to the abdominal wall.[273] The cause of volvulus is still debated, but loss of abdominal fill after parturition or recent dietary changes have been blamed.[264] If the colon twists greater than 270° on its axis, both the vasculature and lumen can be occluded, resulting in strangulation of blood flow and significant abdominal hypertension due to fluid and gas distention within the lumen. After occlusion of the vasculature occurs, the colon suffers irreversible damage within 3–4h, therefore expedient therapy is essential to improve survival.[274] Examination of the horse is typically abbreviated, due to the severity of colic. Clinical findings include pain refractory to analgesics and a distended large intestine on rectal exam.

Treatment of volvulus involves detorsion of the large colon through a ventral midline celiotomy. After derotating the colon, viability is assessed by evaluating the colon for a return of a pink color to the serosal surface, active mucosal bleeding at a pelvic flexure enterotomy, mucosal edema and hemorrhage, arterial pulses in the colonic arteries noted by palpation or Doppler, muscular motility, or fluorescein uptake. The gold standard for assessment of viability is histopathology, but results are often only available after the horse has recovered from surgery or euthanized.[274] If the colon is deemed nonviable, it can be resected up to the level of the cecocolic fold, however, damage often extends farther than can be adequately removed.[276] In these cases, questionable bowel may remain in the abdomen, even with a resection, increasing the likelihood of dehiscence and fatal peritonitis.

Post-operative feeding of horses with volvulus is dependent on the degree of damage sustained by the colon. In horses treated quickly with minimal mucosal edema and mural hemorrhage, feeding can begin in the early post-operative period (between 6–12h after surgery). Usually a pelvic flexure enterotomy is performed and some surgeons prefer to wait at least 12–24h before testing the suture line with feed. If damage to the colon is minimal at surgery, the horse can be started on good quality forage, at a rate of 0.5kg every 4–6h. Alternatives to hay include complete rations or alfalfa pellets at the same rate, or grazing for 15–20min. The diet should be slowly increased over the next 1–3 days, until the full ration is reached (2.0–2.5% of body weight in hay). Grains should be avoided, due to the disruption of normal flora from both the ischemic event and lavage through the pelvic flexure enterotomy.[22]

In horses with large colon resection or if the colon remains in situ but has sustained extensive damage due to ischemia, it is recommended to postpone oral nutrition until 12–48h after surgery to reduce the risk of obstruction or failure of the anastomosis. This is especially true for horses with a questionable suture line due to inability to completely resect the involved colon. In horses with compromised intestine, endotoxemia, anorexia, and disruption of both fermentation and absorption may persist, and parenteral nutrition may be recommended. Once the horse is reintroduced to feed based on vital signs and appetite, a highly digestible diet is required due to the loss of surface area of the ascending colon.

The colon is the site for protein and cellulose digestion and phosphorus absorption, therefore adjustments should be made in the post-operative period to ensure the diet contains at least 12% protein, 0.4% phosphorus, and a quality fiber source (<28%).[277,278] Pelleted diets, including alfalfa pellets or complete rations, would seem ideal due to the reduction in transit time after resections, but were found to have reduced cellulose digestibility.[277,279] If pellets are included in the diet, these rations often must be fed at a rate above maintenance to prevent weight loss.[279] While grass hay is recommended to reduce the risk of post-operative diarrhea, it does not have the protein content to maintain body weight in horses with large colon resections or severe colon damage. Alfalfa hay is preferred and horses should receive at least 2% of body weight per day to maintain condition.[280] Despite reduced absorption, additional phosphorus supplements are not needed to maintain blood levels.[279] However, adequate water intake should be ensured after resection (up to 8l more than normal horses) due to increased loss of water in the feces.[279] Over time, the digestive tract appears to adapt through hypertrophy and special diets are not required.[279,281,282] In some horses, supplementing with oil or soybean meal may improve and maintain weight gain in the early post-operative period.[281]

Prevention of large colon volvulus is centered on surgical techniques. Recurrence rates in the literature vary between 5–50%, therefore, large colon resections or colopexy of the left ventral colon may be chosen to reduce this risk.[276,283,284] Dietary changes should be gradual and a forage based diet is recommended to reduce the amount of carbohydrates entering the colon. However, occupational risk for broodmares is a factor that often will not be eliminated.

3.4.11 Cecal Impactions

Impaction is the most common disorder resulting in colic related to the cecum.[285,286] If impaction is the primary problem, the cause is often multifactorial, associated with poor quality roughage, poor dentition, and reduced water intake.[287,288] Alternatively, cecal impactions can be secondary to treatment for a separate disorder, including orthopedic or ophthalmic disorders. Secondary impactions have been related to painful conditions, NSAIDs (or lack thereof), anesthetics, atropine administration, and stall rest.[286,288–293]

Cecal impactions are further classified by the physical character of the impaction.[289] Type 1 impactions consist of firm dry ingesta and are often comparable to ascending colon impactions in that they are often attributed to a mechanical obstruction. Type 2 impactions are characterized as an idiopathic stasis with ingesta having a normal to fluid-like consistency. These horses often have an edematous or thickened cecal wall with peritonitis and evidence of endotoxemia. However, there is often significant overlap between classifications.[264]

Clinical signs are subtle and often only noted as depression, anorexia, and reduced fecal output. Cecal impactions can rupture without any outward signs of discomfort, therefore fecal production of all hospitalized horses should be monitored carefully.[287,290,294] Diagnosis is by transrectal palpation, which will note either an ingesta or fluid filled cecum in the caudal right abdomen with taut cecal bands. Cecal impactions can be treated medically with intravenous and/or oral fluids and analgesics. Feed should be withheld.[15,287,288,290,295] However, surgical management may be indicated if the cecum is grossly distended, medical management is not progressing, or a type 2 stasis is suspected.[294]Some surgeons recommend early surgical intervention to improve survival.[287] At surgery, typhlotomy and lavage may be performed to relieve the impaction.[261,287,289,294,296] If impaction recurs, or if a type 2 impaction is diagnosed, a complete or incomplete ileocolostomy or jejunocolostomy may be advised, with or without occlusion of the distal small intestine.[261,273,294,297–299]

Feeding after cecal impaction is complicated by a high rate of recurrence.[290] Therefore, reintroduction to feed should be slow and gradual, especially in any horse when the inciting cause cannot be resolved (i.e., stall rest, pain) or cecal dysfunction is suspected. Only water should be offered in small amounts for the first 12–24 h after the impaction has resolved. Resolution is based on a normal rectal examination and adequate fecal output. Horses that tolerate oral fluids can be gradually reintroduced to feed. However, those that have had a bypass may require a slower reintroduction to feed, starting at 36–48 h post-surgery, due to the association between refeeding and colic.[298] Hand walking and limited hand grazing (5–15 m) may be allowed early on to stimulate motility, since complete fasting can reduce cecal motility further.[300] Once feed is introduced, low residue feeds including complete pelleted diets and alfalfa pellets are often preferred to reduce bulk within the large intestine and cecum. Reintroduction to hay should be gradual, starting with handfuls, and alfalfa is preferred due to its laxative effects. Coastal Bermudagrass hay should be avoided due to its association with intestinal impactions.[294]

Similar to ascending colon impactions, prevention is centered on providing good quality forage and encouraging adequate water intake. Quality fiber should be provided, as first cutting hays, fresh grass, or beet pulp. Laxative diets, including alfalfa-based diets or green grass, may be preferred, especially if the horse cannot be removed from the predisposing causes of cecal impactions. If possible, exercise should be encouraged and paddock or pasture turnout provided to increase cecal motility.[6,301] Affected horses should be dewormed against tapeworms due to the suspected association between tapeworms and cecal impaction.[287,296,302,303]

3.4.12 Cecocecal and Cecocolic Intussusception

Cecocecal intussusceptions result from invagination of the cecal apex into the cecal body. The cecal apex can continue into the right ventral colon to become a cecocolic intussusception. Cecal intussusceptions may result from changes in diet, bacterial infections, parasites, and medications that alter motility or result in inflammation.[290,291,304–306] Clinical signs are non-specific due to the variable degree of intussusception and obstruction of the flow of ingesta.[290,305,307] Horses may have a prolonged illness with mild to intermittent signs of colic, fever, or weight loss.[307] Physical exam findings are non-specific as well, but it is possible that the intussusception may be palpated on the right side of the abdomen or located with ultrasound examination.[305,307]

Treatment is surgical, involving manual reduction of the cecum from the intussusception followed by typhlotomy or amputation with the aid of a colotomy.[264,305,307,308]

Due to the often protracted nature of the disease, reduction may be impossible. A complete bypass is then performed using a ileocolostomy or jejunocolostomy with or without amputation of the cecum within the colon.[299,304,309,310]

Depending on the procedure performed, refeeding after intussusception can begin as soon as 24 h after surgery.[264] However, if a bypass procedure was elected, feeding should be delayed for 36–48 h due to the association of refeeding with signs of colic.[298] Water should be offered initially and if the horse tolerates liquids, then feed can be offered similar for horses after a large colon impaction. Small quantities of good quality hay are provided (0.5 kg or 1.1 lb, 4–6 times daily) and slowly increased over 2–3 days until the horse is on a full ration. Alternatives to hay include pelleted complete diets or alfalfa pellets. Grazing should be encouraged, starting at every 4 hours for 15 min, due to its effect on cecal motility.[300] Concentrates should be avoided for 10–14 days to prevent any negative effects on colonic microbial populations.

3.4.13 Descending (Small) Colon Obstructions

Fecal impactions are the most common cause of obstruction of the small colon, alongside enteroliths in regions that are endemic (see Section 3.4.8 for specific information on enteroliths).[285,311,312] Risk factors for fecal impaction are similar to those that result in impactions of other portions of the gastrointestinal tract. Poor quality roughage, poor dentition, parasitic damage, inactivity, dehydration, and motility disorders have all been implicated as contributing factors.[285,312–314] It is important to note that horses with small colon impactions have an increased risk of salmonellosis, but it remains unknown whether impaction is the cause or result of *Salmonella* spp. infection.[312,313,315]

Clinical signs of descending colon obstruction may include reduced fecal output, mild to moderate abdominal pain, abdominal distention, small volume diarrhea or scant feces, fever, and straining to defecate.[312,313] Diagnosis of obstruction is typically made on rectal palpation with a tubular impaction or foreign body noted in the lumen of the descending colon. If the obstruction is more oral or in the transverse colon, then only gas distension of the ascending colon and cecum will be noted on palpation. Radiographs may be helpful in visualizing enteroliths, however, they are not always visible.[255]

For feed impactions of the small colon, medical therapy includes IV and oral fluids, laxatives, and analgesics. Antibiotics or endotoxin antiserum may be indicated if the horse is leukopenic or endotoxemic.[312] Surgery is indicated if the horse is unresponsive to medical therapy or analgesics, abdominal fluid is abnormal, abdominal distention increases, or if the mass is believed to be a foreign body or enterolith. During a ventral midline celiotomy, a high enema can be administered to lavage the impaction with extraluminal massage. An enterotomy can also be performed to remove the impaction directly. If a foreign body or enterolith is present, it can be delivered per rectum with the aid of an enema. If the obstruction cannot be mobilized, an enterotomy can be performed in the taenia of the descending colon or in the pelvic flexure for removal or to retropulse it into the colon.[316] In addition, a large colon enterotomy should be performed to remove the majority of fecal matter oral to the obstruction to reduce the risk of reimpaction.[135]

If medical therapy resolves the small colon impaction, noted by adequate fecal output and absence of pain, feed can be reintroduced slowly in a manner similar for ascending colon impactions (see Section 3.4.6). Water is typically allowed for the first 12–24 h after resolution, followed by a slow reintroduction to feed. The main difference between refeeding an ascending and descending colon impaction is that pelleted diets are preferred initially to prevent reimpaction. Hay is generally reintroduced 3–4 days after resolution of the impaction.[315]

Horses treated surgically for descending colon obstruction are reintroduced to feed in a more conservative manner. This portion of the colon is more prone to stricture and dehiscence after enterotomy due to the size of the lumen, high concentration of collagenase enzymes, and the mechanical stress of fecal balls passing through the site.[318,319] It is also important to note that ileus may contribute to reimpaction, since time to first defecation is significantly delayed after surgery for descending colon impaction (30–40 h).[320] Due to this concern, horses should be held off feed for 36–48 h after surgery and then feed should be slowly reintroduced starting at 0.5 kg every 6 h and increasing gradually to a full ration over 2–4 days.[315,320] Low residue feeds, such as complete diets or alfalfa pellets, are preferred for the first 10–14 days after surgery to prevent reimpaction and wetting the feed into a slurry may be beneficial.[314] This diet can be continued indefinitely if luminal size is a concern.

Laxatives and oral fluids may also be helpful to maintain soft feces in the immediate post-operative period, along with a laxative diet (alfalfa or fresh grass). In addition, magnesium sulfate (0.2 g/kg/day) can be administered in the feed.

Small colon impactions can possibly be prevented by providing good quality roughage and adequate fresh water. Dental care should be provided and older horses with loss of adequate grinding surface should be provided a complete extruded feed rather than hay. In horses with suspected stricture, a pelleted diet should be fed as well. Prevention of enteroliths and fecoliths is described in the previous section. Horses that obstruct with a foreign body often outgrow the urge to eat inappropriate items, but the environment should be modified to reduce the risk. Often, good quality pasture will reduce the consumption of foreign material.[321]

3.4.14 Descending (Small) Colon Strangulations

Strangulation of the descending colon most commonly occurs due to a mesenteric lipoma, but volvulus, herniation, and intussusception have also been reported.[285,311,322–324] Clinical signs often include moderate to severe colic and abdominal distention, but signs of discomfort are often delayed. Rectal exam is similar to small colon obstruction in that large colon distention is noted, as well as a lack of fecal balls. Sometimes the clinician will be able to palpate the obstruction of the lumen, if it is far enough caudal. Abnormal rectal findings, progressive abdominal distention, and peritoneal fluid changes will indicate the need for surgery. Treatment involves resection of the affected colon, as well as a pelvic flexure enterotomy to lavage ingesta form the ascending colon.[325–327] Post-operative refeeding is similar to small colon obstructions treated surgically.

References

1. Bergman EN. Energy contributions of volatile fatty acids from the gastrointestinal tract in various species. Physiol Rev 1990;70:567–590.
2. Boyd LE, Carbonaro DA, Houpt KA. The 24-hour time budget of Prezwalski horses. Appl Anim Behav Sci 1988; 21:5–17.
3. Crowell-Davis SL, Houpt KA, Carnevale J. Feeding and drinking behaviour of mares and foals with free access to pasture and water. J Anim Sci 1985;60:883–889.
4. Durham AE. The role of nutrition in colic. Vet Clin North Am Equine Pract 2009;25:67–78.
5. Longland AC, Byrd BM. Pasture nonstructural carbohydrates and equine laminitis. J Nutr 2006;136:2099S–2102S.
6. Cohen ND, Gibbs PG, Woods AM. Dietary and other management factors associated with colic in horses. J Am Vet Med Assoc 1999;215:53–60.
7. Hoffman RM, Wilson JA, Kronfeld WL, et al. Hydrolyzable carbohydrates in pasture, hay, and horse feed: direct assay and seasonal variation. J Anim Sci 2001;79:500–506.
8. Longland AC, Cairns AJ, Humphreys MO. Seasonal and diurnal changes in fructan concentration in *Lolium perenne*: implications for the grazing management of equine predisposed to laminitis. Proc 16th Equine Nutr Physiol Soc Symp 1999;258–259.
9. Hudson JM, Cohen ND, Gibbs PG, et al. Feeding practices associated with colic in horses. J Am Vet Med Assoc 2001;219:1419–1425.
10. Hillyer MH, Taylor FGR, Proudman CJ, et al. Case control study to identify risk factors for simple colonic obstruction and distension colic in horses. Equine Vet J 2002;34:455–463.
11. Hassel DM, Aldridge BM, Drake CM, et al. Evolution of dietary and management risk factors for enterolithiasis among horses in California. Res Vet Sci 2008;85:476–480.
12. Cohen ND, Vontur CA, Rakestraw PC. Risk factors for enterolithiasis among horses in Texas. J Am Vet Med Assoc 2000;216:1787–1794.
13. Reeves MJ, Salman MD, Smith G. Risk factors for equine acute abdominal disease (colic): results from a multi-center case-control study. Prev Vet Med 1996;26:285–301.
14. Cohen ND, Peloso JG. Risk factor for history of previous colic and for chronic, intermittent colic in a population of horses. J Am Vet Med Assoc 1996;208:697–703.
15. Little D, Blikslager AT. Factors associated with development of ileal impaction in horses with surgical colic: 78 cases (1986–2000). Equine Vet J 2002;34:464–468.
16. White NA, Dabareiner RM. Treatment of impaction colics. Vet Clin North Am Equine Pract 1997;13:243–259.
17. Tinker MK, White NA, Thatcher CD, et al. Prospective study of equine colic risk factors. Equine Vet J 1997; 29:454–458.
18. Embertson RM, Colahan PT, Brown MP, et al. Ileal impaction in the horse. J Am Vet Med Assoc 1985;186:570–572.
19. Hanson RR, Wright JC, Schumacher J, et al. Surgical reduction of ileal impaction in the horse: 28 cases. Vet Surg 1998;27:555–560.
20. Pugh DG, Thompson JT. Impaction colics attributed to decreased water intake and feeding coastal Bermuda grass hay in a boarding stable. Equine Prac 1992;14:9–14.
21. Hintz HF, Lowe JE, Livesay-Wilkins P, et al. Studies on equine enterolithiasis. Proc Am Assoc Equine Pract 1988; 24:53–59.
22. Hassel DM, Rakestraw PC, Gardner IA, et al. Dietary risk factors and colonic pH and mineral concentrations in horses with enterolithiasis. J Vet Intern Med 2004;18:346–349.

23. Hassel DM, Spier SJ, Aldridge BM, et al. Influence of diet and water supply on mineral content and pH within the large intestine of horses with enterolithiasis. Vet J 2009;182:44–49.

24. Murray RC, Constantinescu GM, Green EM. Equine entero-liths. Compend Contin Educ Pract Vet 1992;14:1104–1113.

25. Shirazi-Beechey SP. Molecular insights into dietary induced colic in the horse. Equine Vet J 2008;40:414–421.

26. Dyer J, Fernandez-Castano Merediz E, Salmon SH, et al. Molecular characterization of carbohydrate digestion and absorption in equine small intestine. Equine Vet J 2002;34:349–358.

27. Roberts MC. Amylase activity in the small intestine of the horse. Res Vet Sci 1974;17:400–401.

28. Shirazi-Beechey SP. Molecular biology of intestinal glucose transport. Nutr Res Rev 1995;8:27–41.

29. Kienzle E, Radicke S, Landes E, et al. Activity of amylase in the gastrointestinal tract of the horse. J Anim Physiol Anim Nutr 1994;72:234–241.

30. Lorenzo-Figueras M, Morisset SM, Morisset J, et al. Digestive enzyme concentration and activities in healthy pancreatic tissue of horses. Am J Vet Res 2007;68:1070–1072.

31. Richards N, Choct M, Hinch GN, et al. Examination of the use of exogenous α-amylase and amyloglucoside to enhance starch digestion in the small intestine of horse. Anim Feed Sci Technol 2004;114:295–305.

32. Potter GD, Arnold FF, Householder DD, et al. Digestion of starch in the small or large intestine of the equine. Pferdeheilkunde 1992;1:107–11.

33. Goodson J, Tyznik WJ, Clin, JH, et al. Effects of an abrupt diet change from hay to concentrate on microbial numbers and physical environment in the cecum of the pony. Appl Environ Microbiol 1988;54:1946–1950.

34. Julliand V, de Fombelle A, Drogoul C, et al. Feeding and microbial disorders in horses: 3. Effects of three hay: grain rations on microbial profiles and activities. J Equine Vet Sci 2001;21:543–546.

35. Medina B, Girard ID, Jacotot E, et al. Effect of a preparation of Saccharomyces cerevisiae on microbial profiles and fermentation patterns in the large intestine of horses fed a high fiber or a high starch diet. J Anim Sci 2002; 80:2600–2609.

36. Drogoul C, de Fombelle A, Julliand V. Feeding and microbial disorders in horses 2: effect of three hay: grain ratios on digesta passage rate and digestibility in ponies. J Equine Vet Sci 2001;26:487–491.

37. de Fombelle A, Julliand V, Drogoul C, et al. Feeding and microbial disorders in horses: 1. Effects of an abrupt incorporation of two levels of barley in a hay diet on microbial profile and activities. J Equine Vet Sci 2001;21: 439–445.

38. Hintz HF, Argenzio RA, Schryver HF. Digestion coefficients, blood glucose levels and molar percentage of volatile acids in intestinal fluid of ponies fed varying forage-grain ratios. J Anim Sci 1971;33:992–995.

39. Clarke LL, Roberts MC, Argenzio RA. Feeding and digestive problems in horses: physiologic responses to a concentrated meal. Vet Clin North Am Equine Pract 1990;6:433–450.

40. Lopes MA, White NA, Crisman MV, et al. Effects of feeding large amounts of grain on colonic contents and feces in horses. Am J Vet Res 2004;65:687–694.

41. Morris D, Morris J, Ward S. Comparisons of age, breed, history and management in 229 horses with colic. Equine Vet J 1986;7(Suppl):129–133.

42. Hussein HS, Vogedes LA, Fernandez GC, et al. Effects of cereal grain supplementation on apparent digestibility of nutrients and concentrations of fermentation end-products in the feces and serum of horses consuming alfalfa cubes. J Anim Sci 2004;82:1986–1996.

43. Cohen ND, Matejka PL, Honnas CM, et al. Case-control study of the association between various management factors and development of colic in horses. J Am Vet Med Assoc 1995;206:667–673.

44. Mehdi S, Mohammad V. A farm-based prospective study of equine colic incidence and associated risk factors. J Equine Vet Sci 2006;26:171–174.

45. Geor RJ. Feeding Management of horses recovering from colic. Compend Contin Educ Pract 2007;2:344–355.

46. Vineyard KR, Gordon ME, Williamson KK, et al. Evaluation of the safety and performance of an enteral diet formulated specifically for horses. J Equine Vet Sci 2011;31:254–255.

47. Lopes MAF, White NA. Parenteral nutrition for horses with gastrointestinal disease: a retrospective study of 79 cases. Equine Vet J 2002;34:250–257.

48. Magdesian KG. Nutrition of critical gastrointestinal illness: feeding horses with diarrhea or colic. Vet Clin North Am Equine Pract 2003;19:617–644.

49. Naylor JM, Kronfeld DS, Acland H. Hyperlipemia in horses: effects of undernutrition and disease. Am J Vet Res 1980;41:899–905.

50. Anthony PS. Nutrition screening tools for hospitalized patients. Nutr Clin Pract 2008;23:373–382.

51. Atalay BG, Yagmur C, Nursa T, et al. Use of subjective global assessment and clinical outcomes in critically ill geriatric patients receiving nutrition support. JPEN J Parenter Enteral Nutr 2008;32:454–459.

52. Kuzu MA, Terzioğlu H, Genç V, et al. Preoperative nutritional risk assessment in predicting postoperative outcome in patients undergoing major surgery. World J Surg 2006;30:378–390.

53. Schiesser M, Müller S, Kirchhoff P, et al. Assessment of a novel screening score for nutritional risk in predicting complications in gastro-intestinal surgery. Clin Nutr 2008;27:565–570.

54. Sungurtekin H, Sungurtekin U, Okke D. Nutrition assessment in critically ill patients. Nutr Clin Pract 2008;23:635–641.

55. Cargile JL, Burrow JA, Kim I, et al. Effect of dietary corn oil supplementation on equine gastric fluid acid, sodium, and prostaglandin E2 content before and during pentagastrin infusion. J Vet Intern Med 2004;18:545–549.

56. Carroll CL, Huntington PJ. Body condition scoring and weight estimation of horses. Equine Vet J 1988;20:41–45.

57. Ellis JM, Hollands T. Accuracy of different methods of estimating the weight of horses. Vet Rec 1998;143:335–336.

58. Henneke D, Potter G, Kreider J, et al. Relationship between condition score, physical measurements and body fat percentage in mares. Equine Vet J 1983;15:371–372.

59. Carter RA, Goer RJ, Staniar WB, et al. Apparent adiposity assessed by standardized scoring systems and morphometric measurements in horses and ponies. Vet J 2009; 179:204–210.

60. Kienzle E, Schramme S. Body condition scoring and prediction of bodyweight in adult warm-blooded horses. Pferdeheilkunde 2004;20:517–524.

61. Burkholder WJ. Use of body condition scores in clinical assessment of the provision of optimal nutrition. J Am Vet Med Assoc 2000;217:650–654.

62. Gentry LR, Thompson DL, Gentry GT, et al. The relationship between body condition score and ultrasonic fat measurements in mares of high versus low body condition. J Equine Vet Sci 2004;24:198–203().

63. Atkinson M, Worthley LIG. Nutrition in the critically ill patient: Part I. Essential physiology and pathophysiology. Crit Care Resusc 2003;5:109–120.

64. Klein S. The myth of serum albumin as a measure of nutritional status. Gastroenterology 1990;99:1845–1846.

65. McClave SA, Martindale RG, Vanek VW, et al. Guidelines for the provision and assessment of nutrition support therapy in the adult critically ill patient: Society of Critical Care Medicine (SSCM) and American Society for Parenteral and Enteral Nutrition (A.S.P.E.N.). JPEN J Parenter Enteral Nutr 2009;33:277–316.

66. Soeters PB, von Meyenfeldt MF, Meijerink WJHJ, et al. Serum albumin and mortality. Lancet 1990;335:348–351.

67. Frape D. Pests and ailments related to grazing area, diet and housing. In: Frape D, ed. Equine nutrition and feeding. Singapore: Wiley Blackwell, 2010;334.

68. Durham AE, Phillips TJ, Walmsley JP, et al. Nutritional and clinicopathological effects of post operative parenteral nutrition following small intestinal resection and anastomosis in the mature horse. Equine Vet J 2004;36:390–396.

69. National Research Council, Committee on Nutrient Requirements of Horses: In: Nutrient requirements of horses. 6th ed., Washington, DC: National Academies Press, 2007.

70. Gupta AK, Mamta YP, Yadav MP. Effect of feed deprivation on biochemical indices in equids. J Equine Sci 1999; 10:33–38.

71. Benedict FG. A study of prolonged fasting. Carnegie Institute of Washington Publication 203, Washington, DC, 1915.

72. Rooney DK. Clinical nutrition. In: Reed S Bayly WM, eds. Equine internal medicine. WB Philadelphia: WB Saunders Co, 1998;216–250.

73. Frankenfield DC, Coleman A, Alam S, et al. Analysis of estimation methods for resting metabolic rate in critically ill adults. JPEN J Parenter Enteral Nutr 2008;33:27–36.

74. Haugen HA, Can LN, Li F. Indirect calorimetry: a practical guide for clinicians. Nutr Clin Pract 2007;22:377–388.

75. Reid CL. Nutritional requirements of surgical and critically ill patients: do we really know what they need? Proc Nutr Soc 2004;63:467–472.

76. Cruz AM, Cote N, McDonell WN, et al. Postoperative effects of anesthesia and surgery on resting energy expenditure in horses as measured by indirect calorimetry. Can J Vet Res 2006;70:257–262.

77. Damask MC, Askanazi J, Weissman C, et al. Artifacts in measurement of resting energy expenditure. Crit Care Med 1983;11:750–752.

78. Swinamer DL, Phang PT, Jones RL, et al. Twenty-four hour energy expenditure in critically ill patients. Crit Care Med 1987;15:637–643.

79. Brandi LS, Bertolini R, Santini L, et al. Effects of ventilator resetting on indirect calorimetry measurement in the critically ill surgical patient. Crit Care Med 1999;27:531–539.

80. Henneberg S, Soderberg D, Groth T, et al. Carbon dioxide production during mechanical ventilation. Crit Care Med 1987;15:8–13.

81. Mazan MR, Hoffman AM, Kuehn H, et al. Effect of aerosolized albuterol sulfate on resting energy expenditure determined by use of open-flow indirect calorimetry in horses with recurrent airway obstruction. Am J Vet Res 2003;64:235–242.

82. Mazan MR, Deveney EF, Dewitt S, et al. Energetic cost of breathing, body composition, and pulmonary function in horses with recurrent airway obstruction. J Appl Physiol 2004;97:91–97.

83. Green CJ, Frazer RS, Underhill S, et al. Metabolic effects of dobutamine in normal man. Clin Sci 1992;82:77–83.

84. Mansell PI, Fellows IW, Birmingham AT, et al. Metabolic and cardiovascular effects of infusions of low doses of isoprenaline in man. Clin Sci 1988;75:285–291.

85. Tattersfield AE, Wilding P: Agonists and ventilation. Thorax 1993;48:877–878.

86. Eccles RC, Swinamer DL, Jones RL, et al. Validation of a compact system for measuring gas exchange. Crit Care Med 1986;14:807–811.

87. Westenskow DR, Cutler CA, Wallace WD. Instrumentation for monitoring gas exchange and metabolic rate in critically ill patients. Crit Care Med 1984;12:183–187.

88. Pagan JD, Hintz HF. Equine energetics. I. Relationship between body weight and energy requirements in horses. J Anim Sci 1986;63:815–821.

89. Elia M. Changing concepts of nutrient requirements in disease implications for artificial nutritional support. Lancet 1995;345:1279–1284.

90. Barak N, Wall-Allonso E, Sitrin MD. Validation of the stress factors used for calculating energy expenditure in hospitalized patients. Clin Nutr 2001;20(Suppl):A120.

91. Kemper M, Beredijiklian P. A comparison of measured total energy expenditure to measured resting energy expenditure. Respir Care 1992;37:1291–1295.

92. Zimmel DN. Post-operative parenteral nutritional support for colics. Proc Am Coll Vet Surg Symp 2002;65–69.

93. Abutarbush S, Carmalt J, Shoemaker RW. Causes of gastrointestinal colic in horses in western Canada: 604 cases (1992 to 2002). Can Vet J 2005;46:800–805.

94. Donaghue S. Nutritional support of hospitalized animals. J Am Vet Med Assoc 1992;200:612–615.

95. Naylor JM. Feeding the sick horse. Proc Br Equine Vet Assoc Specialist Days Behav Nutr 1999;87–90.

96. Geor RJ. Nutritional support of the sick adult horse. In: Pagan JD, Geor RJ, eds. Advances in equine nutrition II. Nottingham University Press, Nottingham, 2001;403–418.

97. Brown R, Houpt K, Schryver H. Stimulation of food intake in horses by diazepam and promazine. Pharmacol Biochem Behav 1976;5:495–497.

98. Asai Y, Matsui A, Osawa T, et al. Digestible energy expenditure in grazing activity of growing horses. Equine Vet J 30(Suppl): 1999;490–492.

99. Pagan JD: Recent research developments from Kentucky Equine Research. In: Pagan JD, ed. Advances in equine nutrition III. Nottingham: Nottingham University Press, 2003;1–10.

100. Harris P. Feeding management of elite endurance horses. Vet Clin North Am Equine Pract 2009;25:137–153.

101. Rodiek AV, Stull CL. Glycemic index of ten common horse feeds. J Equine Vet Sci 2007;27:205–211.

102. Hernandez G, Velasco N, Wainstein C, et al. Gut mucosal atrophy after a short enteral fasting period in critically ill patients. J Crit Care 1999;14:73–77.

103. Rokyta R, Matejovic M, Krouzecky A, et al. Enteral nutrition and hepatosplanchnic region in critically ill patients – friends or foes? Physiol Res 2003;52:31–37.

104. Saito H, Trocki O, Alexander JW, et al. The effect of route of nutrient administration on the nutritional state, catabolic hormone secretion, and gut mucosal integrity after burn injury. JPEN J Parenter Enteral Nutr 1987;11:1–7.

105. Mechanik JI, Brett EM. Nutrition support of the chronically critically ill patient. Crit Care Med 2002;18:597–618.

106. Mosenthal AC, Xu D, Deitch EA. Elemental and intravenous total parenteral nutrition diet-induced gut barrier failure is intestinal site specific and can be prevented by feeding nonfermentable fiber. Crit Care Med 2002; 30:396–402.

107. Hallebeek JM, Beynen AC. A preliminary report on a fat-free diet formula for nasogastric enteral administration as treatment for hyperlipaemia in ponies. Vet Q 2001; 23:201–205.

108. Gottschlich MM, Jenkins ME, Mayes T, et al. An evaluation of the safety of early vs delayed enteral support and effects on clinical, nutritional and endocrine outcome after severe burns. J Burn Care Rehab 2002;23:401–415.

109. Schroeder D, Gillanders L, Mahr K, et al. Effects of immediate postoperative enteral nutrition on body composition, muscle function and wound healing. JPEN J Parenter Enteral Nutr 1991;15:376–383.

110. Fascetti AJ, Stratton-Phelps M. Clinical assessment of nutritional status and enteral feeding in the acutely ill horse. In: Robinson NE, ed., Current therapy in equine medicine 5. Philadelphia: WB Saunders Co, 2003;705–710.

111. Buechner-Maxwell VA, Elvinger F, Thatcher CD, et al. Physiologic response of normal adult horses to a low residue liquid diet. J Equine Vet Sci 2003;23:310–317.

112. Golenz MR, Knight DA, Yvorchuk-St. Jean KE. Use of a human enteral feeding preparation for treatment of hyperlipemia and nutritional support during healing of an esophageal laceration in a miniature horse. J Am Vet Med Assoc 1992;200:951–953.

113. Sweeney RW, Hansen TO. Use of a liquid diet as the sole source of nutrition in six dysphagic horses and as a dietary supplement in seven hypophagic horses. J Am Vet Med Assoc 1990;197:1030–1032.

114. Hardy J, Stewart RH, Beard WL, et al. Complications of nasogastric intubation in horses: nine cases (1987–1989). J Am Vet Med Assoc 1992;201:483–489.

115. Lopes MAF. How to provide nutritional support via esophagostomy. Proc Am Assoc Equine Pract 2001;47:252–256.

116. Stick JA, Derksen FJ, Scott EA. Equine cervical esophagostomy: Complications associated with duration and location of feeding tubes. Am J Vet Res 1981;42:727–732.

117. Geor RJ. Nutritional considerations for the colic patient. Proc Am Assoc Equine Pract-AAEP Equine Colic Focus Meet 2005;55–64.

118. Spurlock SL, Ward MV. Parenteral nutrition in equine patients: principles and theory. Compend Contin Educ Pract Vet 1991;13:461–468.

119. Braunschweig CL, Levy P, Sheean PM, et al. Enteral compared with parenteral nutrition: a meta-analysis. Am J Clin Nutr 2001;74:534–542.

120. Westman EC: Is dietary carbohydrate essential for human nutrition? Am J Clin Nutr 2002;75:951–953.

121. Heyland DK, MacDonald S, Keefe L, et al. Total parenteral nutrition in the critically ill patient: a meta-analysis. J Am Med Assoc 1998;280:2013–2019.

122. Joseph SE, Heaton N, Potter D, et al. Renal glucose production compensates for the liver during the anhepatic phase of liver transplantation. Diabetes 2000;49: 450–456.

123. Kreymann KG, Berger MM, Deutz NE, et al. ESPEN guidelines on enteral nutrition: intensive care. Clin Nutr 2006;25:210–223.

124. Mithieux G. New data and concepts on glutamine and glucose metabolism in the gut. Curr Opin Clin Nutr Metab Care 2001;4:267–271.

125. Bier DM, Brosnan JT, Flatt JP, et al. Report of the IDECG Working Group on lower and upper limits of carbohydrate and fat intake. Eur J Clin Nutr 1999;53(Suppl): S177–S178.

126. Durham AE, Phillips TJ, Walmsley JP, et al. Study of the clinical effects of postoperative parenteral nutrition in 15 horses. Vet Rec 2003;153:493–498.

127. Singer P, Berger MM, Van den Berghe G, et al. ESPEN guidelines on parenteral nutrition: intensive care. Clin Nutr 2009;29:387–400.

128. Finfer S, Chittock DR, Su SY, et al. NICE-SUGAR study investigators, intensive versus conventional glucose control in critically ill patients. N Engl J Med 2009;360: 1283–1297.

129. Van den Berghe G, Wilmer A, Milants I, et al. Intensive insulin therapy in mixed medical/surgical ICU – benefit versus harm. Diabetes 2006;55:3151–3159.

130. Dunkel BM, Wilkins PA. Nutrition and the critically ill horse. Vet Clin North Am Equine Pract 2004;20:107–126.

131. Covelli HD, Black JW, Olsen MS, et al. Respiratory failure precipitated by high carbohydrate loads. Ann Intern Med 1987;95:579–581.

132. Silberman H, Silberman AW. Parenteral nutrition, biochemistry and respiratory gas exchange. JPEN J Parenter Enteral Nutr 1986;10:151–154.

133. Dabrowski GP, Rombeau JL. Practical nutritional management in the trauma intensive care unit. Surg Clin North Am 2000;80:921–932.

134. Hawker FH. How to feed patients with sepsis. Curr Opin Crit Care 2000;6:247–252.

135. Carr EA, Holcombe SJ. Nutrition of critically ill horses. Vet Clin North Am Equine Pract 2009;25:93–108.

136. Adam S, Forrest S. ABC of intensive care. Br Med J 1999;319:175–178.

137. Ishibashi N, Plank LD, Sando K, et al. Optimal protein requirements during the first 2 weeks after the onset of critical illness. Crit Care Med 1998;26:1529–1535.

138. Waitzberg DL, Plopper C, Terra RM, et al. Postoperative total parenteral nutrition. World J Surg 1999;23:560–564.

139. Hansen TO, White NA, Kemp DT. Total parenteral nutrition in four healthy adult horses. Am J Vet Res 1988;49:122–124.

140. Biolo G, Tipton KD, Klein S, et al. An abundant supply of amino acids enhances the metabolic effect of exercise on muscle protein. Am J Physiol 1997;273:E122–E129.

141. Biolo G, Ciocchi B, Lebenstedt M, et al. Short-term bed rest impairs amino acid induced protein anabolism in humans. J Physiol 2004;558:381–388.

142. Streat SJ, Beddoe AH, Hill GL. Aggressive nutritional support does not prevent protein loss despite fat gain in septic intensive care patients. J Trauma 1987;27:262–266.

143. Kaminski DL, Adams A, Jellinek M. The effect of hyperalimentation on hepatic lipid content and lipogenic enzyme activity in rats and man. Surgery 1980;88:93–100.

144. Roggero P, Gianni ML, Morlacchi L, et al. Blood urea nitrogen concentration in low-birth-weight preterm infants during parenteral and enteral nutrition. J Pediatr Gastroenterol Nutr 2007;51:213–215.

145. Rosmarin DK, Wardlaw GW, Mirtallo J. Hyperglycemia associated with high, continuous infusion rates of total parenteral nutrition dextrose. Nutr Clin Pract 1996;11: 151–156.

146. Talpers SS, Romberger DJ, Bunce SB, et al. Nutritionally associated increased carbon dioxide production. Excess total calories vs high proportion of carbohydrate calories. Chest 1992;102:551–555.

147. Krishnan JA, Parce PB, Martinez A, et al. Caloric intake in medical ICU patients: consistency of care with guidelines and relationship to clinical outcomes. Chest 2003; 124:297–305.

148. Villet S, Chiolero RL, Bollmann MD, et al. Negative impact of hypocaloric feeding and energy balance on clinical outcome in ICU patients. Clin Nutr 2005;24:502–509.

149. McCowen KC, Friel C, Sternberg J, et al. Hypocaloric total parenteral nutrition: effectiveness in prevention of hyperglycemia and infectious complications – a randomized clinical trial. Crit Care Med 2000;28:3606–3611.

150. Magdesian KG. Parenteral nutrition in the mature horse. Equine Vet Educ 2010;22:364–371.

151. Hollis AR, Boston RC, Corley KT. Blood glucose in horses with acute abdominal disease. J Vet Intern Med 2007;21:1099–1103.

152. Krinsley SJ. Association between hyperglycemia and increased hospital mortality in a heterogeneous population of critically ill patients. Mayo Clin Proc 2003;78:1471–1478.

153. White NA. Parenteral nutrition. Proc Am Coll Vet Surg 1999;9:114–115.

154. Coppack SW. Pro-inflammatory cytokines and adipose tissue. Proc Nutr Soc 2001;60:349–356.

155. Frayn KN; Neuroendocrine control of metabolism activity after injury: implications for nutritional care. Nutrition 1987;3:201–202.

156. Sapolsky RM, Romero LM, Munck AU; How do glucocorticoids influence stress responses? Integrating permissive, suppressive, stimulatory, and preparative actions. Endocr Rev 2000;21:55–89.

157. Taylor FGR, Hillyer MH. The differential diagnosis of hyperglycaemia in horses. Equine Vet Educ 1992;4:135–138.

158. Dempsey DT. Complications of parenteral and enteral nutritional support. In: Torosian MH, ed. Nutrition for hospitalized patients. New York: CRC Press, 1995;353–379.

159. Butters M, Miller W, Bittner R. Effect of enteral and parenteral nutrition on glucose tolerance in the early post operative phase. Infusionstherapie 1990;17:257–260.

160. Ralston SL. Insulin and glucose regulation. Vet Clin North Am Equine Pract 2002;18:295–304.

161. Divers TJ. Perioperative partial and total parenteral nutrition. In: White NA, Moore JN, eds, Current techniques in equine surgery and lameness. London: WB Saunders Company, 1998;19–21.

162. McKenzie HC. Equine hyperlipidemias. Vet Clin North Am Equine Pract 2010;27:59–72.

163. Cheluvappa R, Denning GM, Lau GW, et al. Pathogenesis of the hyperlipidemia of gram-negative bacterial sepsis may involve pathomorphological changes in liver sinusoidal endothelial cells. Int J Infect Dis 2010;14: e857–e867.

164. Ali A, Walentik C, Mantych GJ, et al. Iatrogenic acute hypermagnesemia after total parenteral nutrition infusion mimicking septic shock syndrome: two case reports. Pediatrics 2003;112:e70–e72.

165. Gielkins HA, Van den Biggelaar A, Vecht J, et al. Effect of intravenous amino acids on interdigestive antroduodenal motility and small bowel transit time. Gut 1999;44: 240–245.

166. Sanchez LC. Diseases of the stomach. In: Reed SM, Bayly WM, Sellon DC, eds, Equine internal medicine. 2nd ed. St. Louis, MI: Saunders Elsevier, 2004;863–873.

167. Jonsson H, Egenvall A. Prevalence of gastric ulceration in Swedish Standardbreds in race-training. Equine Vet J 2006;38:209–213.

168. Lester GD. Gastrointestinal diseases of performance horses. In: Hinchcliff KW, Kaneps AJ, Geor RJ, eds, Equine Sports Medicine and Surgery. Philadelphia: Saunders Elsevier, 2004;1037–1043.

169. Luthersson N, Hou Nielsen K, Harris P, et al. Risk factors associated with equine gastric ulceration syndrome (EGUS) in 201 horses in Denmark. Equine Vet J 2009; 41:625–630.

170. Merritt AM. The equine stomach: A personal perspective. Proc Am Assoc Equine Pract 2003;49:75–102.

171. Vatistas NJ, Sifferman RL, Holste J, et al. Induction and maintenance of gastric ulceration in horses in simulated race training. Equine Vet J 1999;29(Suppl):40–44.

172. Buchanan BR, Andrews FM; Treatment and prevention of equine gastric ulcer syndrome. Vet Clin Equine Pract 2003;19:575–597.

173. Reese RE, Andrews FM. Nutrition and dietary management of equine gastric ulcer syndrome. Vet Clin North Am Equine Pract 2009;25:79–92.

174. Videla R, Andrews FM. New perspectives in equine gastric ulcer syndrome. Vet Clin North Am Equine Pract 2009; 25:283–301.

175. Husted L, Sanchez LC, Olsen SN, et al. Effect of paddock versus stall housing on 24 hour gastric pH within the proximal and ventral equine stomach. Equine Vet J 2008;40:337–341.

176. le Jeune SS, Nieto JE, Dechant JE, et al. Prevalence of gastric ulcers in Thoroughbred broodmares in pasture: A preliminary report. Vet J 2009;181:251–255.

177. Murray MJ, Schusser GF. Measurement of 24-h gastric pH using an indwelling pH electrode in horses unfed, fed, and treated with ranitidine. Equine Vet J 1993;25: 417–421.

178. Murray MJ. Equine model of inducing ulceration in alimentary squamous epithelial mucosa. Dig Dis Sci 1994;12:2530–2535.

179. Murray MJ, Eichorn ES. Effects of intermittent feed deprivation, intermittent feed deprivation with ranitidine administration, and stall confinement with ad libitum access to hay on gastric ulceration in horses. Am J Vet Res 1996;57:1599–1603.

180. Feige K, Furst A, Eser MW. Effects of housing, feeding, and use on equine health with emphasis on respiratory and gastrointestinal disease. Schweiz Arch Tierheilkd 2002;144:348–355.

181. Nadeau JA, Andrews FM, Mathew AG, et al. Evaluation of diet as a cause of gastric ulcers in horse. Am J Vet Res 2000;61:784–790.

182. Andrews FM, Buchanan BR, Smith SH, et al. In vitro effects of hydrochloric acid and various concentrations of acetic, propionic, butyric, or valeric acids on bioelectric properties of equine gastric squamous mucosa. Am J Vet Res 2006;67:1873–1882.

183. Nadeau JA, Andrews FM, Patton CS, et al. Effects of hydrochloric, acetic, butyric and propionic acids on pathogenesis of ulcers in the non-glandular portion of the stomach of horses. Am J Vet Res 2003;64:404–412.

184. Nadeau JA, Andrews FM, Patton SC, et al. Effects of hydrochloric, valeric and other volatile fatty acids on pathogenesis of ulcers in the non-glandular portion of the stomach of horses. Am J Vet Res 2003;64:413–417.

185. Smyth GB, Young DW, Hammon LS. Effects of diet and feeding on past-prandial serum gastrin and insulin concentrations in adult horses. Equine Vet J 1988; 7(Suppl):56–59.

186. Sandin A, Girma K, Sjoholm B, et al. Effects of differently composed feeds and physical stress on plasma gastrin concentration in horses. Acta Vet Scand 1998;39:265–272.

187. Frank N, Andrews FM, Elliott SB, et al. Effects of dietary oils on the development of gastric ulcers in mares. Am J Vet Res 2006;66:2006–2011.

188. Rabuffo TS, Hackett ES, Grenager N, et al. Prevalence of gastric ulcerations in horses with colic. J Equine Vet Sci 2009;29:540–545.

189. Dukti SA, Perkins S, Murphy J, et al. Prevalence of gastric squamous ulceration in horses with abdominal pain. Equine Vet J 2006;38:347–349.

190. McConnico RS. Duodenitis-proximal jejunitis (anterior enteritis, proximal enteritis). In: Reed SM, Bayly WM, Sellon DC, eds, Equine internal medicine. 2nd ed. St. Louis, MI: Saunders Elsevier, 2004;873–878.

191. Arroyo LG, Stampfli HR, Weese JS. Potential role of *Clostridium difficile* as a cause of duodenitis-proximal jejunitis in horses. J Med Microbiol 2006;55:605–608.

192. Edwards GB. Duodenitis-proximal jejunitis (anterior enteritis) as a surgical problem. Equine Vet Educ 2000;12:411–414.

193. Griffiths NJ, Walton JR, Edwards GB. An investigation of the toxigenic types of *Clostridium perfringens* in horses with anterior enteritis: preliminary results. Anaerobe 1997;3:121–125.

194. Merritt AM, Robbins J, Brewer B. Is *Salmonella* infection a cause of the acute gastric dilitation/ileus syndrome in horses? Proc 1st Equine Colic Res Symp 1982;119–124.

195. Schumacher J, Seahorn TL, Cohen ND. Duodenitis/ proximal jejunitis in horses. Compend Contin Educa Pract Vet 1994;16:1197–1206.

196. Schumacher J, Mullen J, Shelby R, et al. An investigation of the role of *Fusarium moniliforme* in duodenitis/proximal jejunitis of horses. Vet Hum Toxicol 1995;37:39–45.

197. Huskamp B. Diagnosis of gastroduodenitis and its surgical treatment by a temporary duodenocaecostomy. Equine Vet J 1985;17:314–316.

198. Cohen ND, Toby E, Roussel A, et al. Are feeding practices associated with duodenitis-proximal jejunitis? Equine Vet J 2006;38:526–531.

199. Hunter LC, Miller JK, Poxton IR. The association of *Clostridium botulinum* type C with equine grass sickness: a toxicoinfection? Equine Vet J 1999;31:492–499.

200. McCarthy HE, French NP, Edwards GB, et al. Equine grass sickness is associated with low antibody levels to *Clostridium botulinum*: A matched case-control study. Equine Vet J 2004;36:123–129.

201. Poxton IR, Hunter LC, Brown R, et al. Clostridia and equine grass sickness. Rev Med Microbiol 1997;8:S49–S51.

202. Robb J, Doxey DL, Milne EM, et al. The isolation of potentially toxigenic fungi from the environment of horses with grass sickness and mal seco. In: Hahn C, Gerber V, Herholz C, et al., eds. Grass sickness, equine motor neuron disease and related disorders: Proc 1st Int Workshop. 1995;52–541.

203. Freeman DE, Hammock P, Goetz BT, et al. Short- and long-term survival and prevalence of postoperative ileus after small intestinal surgery in the horse. Equine Vet J 2000;32(Suppl):42–51.

204. Johnston JK, Morris DD. Comparison of duodenitis/proximal jejunitis and small intestinal obstruction in horses: 68 cases (1977–1985). J Am Vet Med Assoc 1987;191:849–854.

205. Gillis JP, Taylor TS, Puckett MJ. Gastrojejunostomy for management of acute proximal enteritis in a horse. J Am Vet Med Assoc 1994;204:633–635.

206. White NA, Tyler DE, Blackwell RB. Haemorrhagic fibrinonecrotic duodenitis-proximal-jejunitis: 20 cases (1977–1984). J Am Vet Med Assoc 1987;190:311–315.

207. Underwood C, Southwood LL, Knight D. Complications and survival associated with surgical compared with medical management of horses with duodenitis-proximal jejunitis. Equine Vet J 2008;40:373–378.

208. Freeman DE, Schaeffer DJ. Comparison of complications and long-term survival rates following hand-sewn versus stapled side-to-side jejunocecostomy in horses with colic. J Am Vet Med Assoc 2010;237:1060–1067.

209. Tate LP, Ralston SL, Koch CM, et al. Effects of extensive resection of the small intestine in the pony. Am J Vet Res 1983;44:1187–1191.

210. Vachon AM, Fischer AT. Small-intestinal herniation through the epiploic foramen-53 cases (1987–1993). Equine Vet J 1995;27:373–380.

211. Chaves M, Smith MW, Williamson RCN; Increased activity of digestive enzymes in ileal enterocytes adapting to proximal small bowel resection. Gut 1987;28:981–987.

212. O'Connor TP, Lam MM, Diamond J. Magnitude of functional adaptation after intestinal resection. Am J Physiol 1999;276:R1265–R1275.

213. Quigley EM, Thompson JS. The motor response to intestinal resection: Motor activity in the canine small intestine following distal resection. Gastroenterology 1993;105:791–798.

214. Frederico LM, Jones SL, Blikslager AT. Predisposing factors for small colon impaction in horses and outcome of medial and surgical treatment: 44 cases (1999–2004). J Am Vet Med Assoc 2006;229(10):1612–1616.

215. Lewis LD. Sick horse feeding and nutritional support. In: Lewis LD, ed., Equine clinical nutrition. Baltimore: Lea and Febiger, 1995;396–419.

216. Lee RD, Harris G, Murphy TR. Bermudagrasses. In Georgia. Univ of Georgia Coop Ext Service Bull, 2010; B911:1–11.

217. Proudman CJ, French NP, Trees AJ. Tapeworm infection is a significant risk factor for spasmodic colic and ileal impaction colic in the horse. Equine Vet J 1998;30:194–199.

218. Parks AH, Doran RE, White NA, et al. Ileal impaction in the horse: 75 cases. Cornell Vet 1989;79:83–91.

219. Hanson RR, Schumacher J, Humberg J, et al. Medical treatment of horses with ileal impaction: 10 cases (1990–1994). J Am Vet Med Assoc 1996;208:898–900.

220. Blikslager AT: Treatment of gastrointestinal obstruction–stomach impaction, ileal impaction, and cecal impaction. Proc Am Assoc Equine Pract-AAEP Equine Colic Focus Meet. Ithaca, NY: International Veterinary Information Service (www.ivis.org), 2005.

221. Hintz HF, Loy RG. The effects on pelleting on the nutritive value of horse rations. J Anim Sci 1966;25:1059–1062.

222. White NA. Epidemiology and etiology of colic. In: White NA, ed. The equine acute abdomen. Philadelphia: Lea and Febiger, 1990;50–64.

223. Dabareiner RM, White NA. Large colon impactions in horses: 147 cases (1985–1991). J Am Vet Med Assoc 1995;206:679–685.

224. Hallowell G. Retrospective study assessing efficacy of treatment of large colonic impactions. Equine Vet J 2008;40:411–413.

225. Lopes MA, Moura GS, Filho JD. Treatment of large colonic impaction with enteral fluid therapy. Proc Am Assoc Equine Pract 1999;45:99–102.

226. Hassel DM, Smith PA, Nieto JE, et al. Di-tri-octahedral smectite for the prevention of post-operative diarrhea in equids with surgical disease of the large intestine: Results of a randomized clinical trial. Vet J 2009;182:210–214.

227. Cohen ND, Honnas CM. Risk factors associated with development of diarrhea in horses after celiotomy for colic: 190 cases (1990–1994). J Am Vet Med Assoc 1996;209:810–813.

228. Colahan P. Sand colic. In: Robinson NE, ed. Current therapy in equine medicine 2. Philadelphia: WB Saunders, 1987;55–58.

229. Specht TE, Colahan PT. Surgical treatment of sand colic in equids: 48 cases (1978–1985). J Am Vet Med Assoc 1988;193:1560–1564.

230. Granot N, Milgram J, Bdolah-Abram T, et al. Surgical management of sand impactions in horses: a retrospective study of 41 cases. Aust Vet J 2008;86:404–407.

231. Ragle CA, Meagher DM, Lacrox CA, et al. Surgical treatment of sand colic: results in 40 horses. Vet Surg 1989;18:48–51.

232. Edens LM, Cargile JL. Medical management of colic. In: Robinson NE, ed. Current therapy in equine medicine 4. Philadelphia: WB Saunders, 1997;182–191.

233. Kendall A, Ley C, Egenvall A, et al. Radiographic parameters for diagnosing sand colic in horses. Acta Vet Scand 2008;20:17–23.

234. Korolainen R, Ruohoniemi M. Reliability of ultrasonography compared to radiography in revealing intestinal sand accumulations in horses. Equine Vet J 2002;34:499–504.

235. Ragle CA, Meagher DM, Schrader JL, et al. Abdominal auscultation in the detection of experimentally induced gastrointestinal sand accumulation. J Vet Int Med 1989;3:12–14.

236. Ethell MT, Dart AJ, Hodgson DR, et al. Alimentary system. In: Rose RJ, Hodgson DR, eds. Manual of equine practice. Philadelphia: Saunders, 1993;319.

237. Blikslager AT, Jones SL. Obstructive diseases of the gastrointestinal tract. In: Reed SM, Bayly WM, Sellon DC, eds, Equine internal medicine. 2nd ed. St. Louis, MI: Saunders Elsevier, 2004;992–936.

238. Ruohoniemi M, Kaikkonen R, Raekallio M, et al. Abdominal radiography in monitoring the resolution of sand accumulations from the large colon of horses treated medically. Equine Vet J 2001;33:50–64.

239. Lieb S: Sand removal from the GI tract of equine. Proc 15th Equine Nutr Physiol Symp, 1997;335.

240. Hammock PD, Freeman DE, Baker GJ. Failure of psyllium mucilloid to hasten evacuation of sand from the equine large intestine. Vet Surg 1998;27:547–554.

241. Hotwagner K, Iben C. Evacuation of sand from the equine intestine with mineral oil, with and without psyllium. J Anim Physiol Anim Nutr 2008;92:86–91.

242. Lawler JB, Hassel DM, Magnuson RJ, et al. Adsorptive effects of di-tri-octahedral smectite on Clostridium perfringens alpha, beta, and beta-2 exotoxins and equine colostral antibodies. Am J Vet Res 2008;69:233–239.

243. Traub-Dargatz JL. Adsorptive effects of di-tri-octahedral smectite on *Clostridium perfringens* alpha, beta, and beta-2 exotoxins and equine colostral antibodies. Am J Vet Res 2008;69:233–239.

244. Weese JS, Cote NM, de Gannes RV. Evaluation of in vitro properties of di-tri-octahedral smectite on Clostridial toxins and growth. Equine Vet J 2003;35:638–641.

245. Albengres E, Urien S, Tillement JP, et al. Interactions between smectite, a mucus stabilizer, and acid and basic drugs. Eur Clin Pharmacol 1985;28:601–605.

246. Yao-Zong Y, Shi-Rong L, Delvaux M. Comparative efficacy of dioctahedral smectite (Smecta) and a probiotic preparation in chronic functional diarrhea. Dig Liver Dis 2004;36:824–828.

247. Bertone JJ, Traub-Dargatz JL, Wrigley RW, et al. Diarrhea associated with sand in the gastrointestinal tract of horses. J Am Vet Med Assoc 1988;193:1409–1412.

248. Blue MG, Wittko RW. Clinical and structural features of equine enteroliths. J Am Vet Med Assoc 1981;179:79–82.

249. Hassel DM, Schiffman PS, Snyder JR. Petrographic and geochemic evaluation of equine enteroliths. Am J Vet Res 2001;62:350–358.

250. Hintz HF, Hernandez TM, Soderholm V, et al. Effect of vinegar supplementation on pH of colonic fluid. Proc Equine Nutr Physiol Sym 1989;11:116–118.

251. Hassel DM, Langer D, Snyder JR, et al. Evaluation of enterolithiasis in horses: 900 cases (1973–1996). J Am Vet Med Assoc 1999;214:226–230.

252. Hassel DM. Enterolithiasis. Clin Techniques Equine Pract 2002;1:143–147.

253. Lloyd K, Hintz HF, Wheat JD, et al. Enteroliths in horses. Cornell Vet 1987;77:172–186.

254. Stevens CE. Physiological implications of microbial digestion in the large intestine of mammals: relation to dietary factors. Am J Clin Nutr 1978;31:S161–S168.

255. Yarbrough TB, Langer DL, Snyder JR, et al. Abdominal radiography for diagnosis of enterolithiasis in horses: 141 cases (1990–1992). J Am Vet Med Assoc 1994;205:592–595.

256. Hintz HF. Equine Nutrition Update. Proc Am Assoc Equine Pract 2000;46:62–79.

257. Rose JA, Rose EM. Colonic obstructions in the horse: radiographic and surgical considerations. Proc Am Assoc Equine Pract 1987;23:95–101.

258. Argenzio RA. Functions of the equine large intestine and their interrelationship in disease. Cornell Vet 1975;65:303–330.

259. Clarke LL, Argenzio RA, Roberts MC. Effects of meal feeding on plasma volume and urinary electrolyte clearance in ponies. Am J Vet Res 1990;51:571–576.

260. Ruckebusch Y. Motor functions of the large intestine. Adv Vet Sci Comp Med 1981;25:345–369.

261. Smith LJ, Mair TS. Are horses that undergo an exploratory laparotomy for correction of a right dorsal displacement of the large colon predisposed to post operative colic, compared to other forms of large colon displacement? Equine Vet J 2010;42:44–46.

262. Hackett RP. Displacement of the large colon. In: Mair TS, Divers TJ, Ducharme NG, eds. Manual of equine gastroenterology. St. Louis: WB Saunders, 2002;284–288.

263. Hardy J. Specific diseases of the large colon. In: White NA, Moore JN, Mair TS, eds. The equine acute abdomen. Jackson, WY: Teton New Media, 2008;628–644.

264. Rakestraw PC, Hardy J. Large intestine. In: Auer JA, Stick JA, eds. Equine surgery, 3rd ed. St. Louis: Saunders, 2006;436–478.

265. Van Harreveld PD, Cox J, Biller DS. Phenylephrine HCl as a treatment of nephrosplenic entrapment in a horse. Equine Vet Educ 1999;11:282–284.

266. Boening K, von Saldern F. Nonsurgical treatment of left dorsal displacement of the large colon of horses under general anesthesia. Proc Equine Colic Res Symp, 1986;325.

267. Kalsbeek HC. Further experiences with non-surgical correction of nephrosplenic entrapment of the colon in the horse. Equine Vet J 1989;6:442–443.

268. Baird AN, Cohen ND, Taylor TS, et al. Renosplenic entrapment of the large colon in horses: 57 cases (1983–1988). J Am Vet Med Assoc 1991;198:1423–1426.

269. Farstvedt E, Hendrickson D. Laparoscopic closure of the nephrosplenic space for prevention of recurrent nephrosplenic entrapment of the ascending colon. Vet Surg 2005;34:642–645.

270. Hardy J, Minton M, Robertson JT, et al. Nephrosplenic entrapment in the horse: a retrospective study of 174 cases. Equine Vet J 2000;32(Suppl):95–97.

271. Hance SR, Embertson RM. Colopexy in broodmares: 44 cases (1986–1990). J Am Vet Med Assoc 1992;201: 782–787.

272. Quinteros DD, Garcia-Lopez JM, Provost PJ. Complete caecal bypass without ileal transection for caecal impaction in horses: seven clinical cases (1997–2007). Aust Vet J 2010;88:434–438.

273. Snyder JR, Pascoe JR, Olander HJ, et al. Strangulating volvulus of the ascending colon in horse. J Am Vet Med Assoc 1989;195:757–764.

274. Snyder JR, Olander HJ, Pascoe JR, et al. Morphologic alterations observed during experimental ischemia of the equine large colon. Am J Vet Res 1988;49:801–809.

275. Van Hoogmoed L, Snyder JR, Pascoe JR, et al. Use of pelvic flexure biopsies to predict survival after large colon torsion in horses. Vet Surg 2000;29:572–577.

276. Hughes FE, Slone DE. Large colon resection. Vet Clin North Am Equine Pract 1997;13:341–350.

277. Bertone AL, Ralston SL, Stashak TS. Fiber digestion and voluntary intake in horses after adaptation to extensive large colon resection. Am J Vet Res 1989;50:1628–1632.

278. Ralston SL, Sullins KE, Stashak TS. Digestion in horses after resection of ischemic insult to the large colon. Am J Vet Res 1986;47:2290–2293.

279. Bertone AL, Van Soest PJ, Stashak TS. Digestion, fecal and blood variables associated with extensive large colon resection in the horse. Am J Vet Res 1989;50:253–258.

280. Bertone AL. Large colon resection. Vet Clin North Am Equine Pract 1989;5:377–393.

281. Driscoll N, Baia P, Fischer AT, et al. Large colon resection and anastomosis in horses: 52 cases. Equine Vet J 2008;40:342–347.

282. Ellis CM, Lynch TM, Slone DE, et al. Survival and complication safer large colon resection and end-to end anastomosis for strangulating large colon volvulus in seventy three horses. Vet Surg 2008;37:786–790.

283. Harrison IW. Equine large intestinal volvulus: a review of 124 cases. Vet Surg 1988;17:77–81.

284. Markel MD. Prevention of large colon displacements and volvulus. Vet Clin North Am Equine Pract 1989;5:395–405.

285. Dart AJ, Snyder JR, Pascoe JR, et al. Abnormal; conditions of the equine descending (small) colon: 102 cases (1979–1989). J Am Vet Med Assoc 1992;200:971–978.

286. Edwards GB. Caecal diseases that result in colic. In: Mair T, Divers T, Ducharme N, eds. Manual of equine gastroenterology. London: WB Saunders, 2002;267–278.

287. Campbell ML, Colahan PC, Brown MM, et al. Cecal impaction in the horse. J Am Vet Med Assoc 1984;184:950–952.

288. Collatos C, Romano S. Cecal impaction in horses: causes, diagnosis and medical treatment. Compend Contin Educ Pract Vet 1993;15:976–981.

289. Daberiener R, White NA. Diseases and surgery of the cecum. Vet Clin North Am Equine Pract 1997;13:303–315.

290. Dart AJ, Hodgson DR, Snyder JR. Caecal disease in equids. Aust Vet J 1997;75:552–557.

291. Edwards G. The clinical presentation and diagnosis of caecal obstruction in the horse. Equine Vet Educ 1992;4:237–240.

292. Lester GD, Bolton JR, Cullen LK, et al. Effects of general anesthesia on myoelectric activity of the intestine in horses. Am J Vet Res 1992;52:1553–1557.

293. Little D, Redding WR, Blikslager AT. Risk factors for reduced postoperative fecal output in horses: 37 cases (1997–1998). J Am Vet Med Assoc 2001;218:414–420.

294. Plummer A, Rakestraw PC, Hardy J, et al. Outcome of medical and surgical treatment of cecal impaction in horses: 114 cases (1994–2004). J Am Vet Med Assoc 2007;231:1378–1385.

295. Huskamp B, Scheidemann W. Diagnosis and treatment of chronic recurrent caecal impaction. Equine Vet J 2000;32(Suppl):65–68.

296. Roberts CT, Slone DE. Caecal impactions managed surgically by typhlotomy in 10 cases (1988–1998). Equine Vet J 2000;32(Suppl):74–76.

297. Craig DR, Pankowski RL, Car BD, et al. Ileocolostomy: a technique for surgical management of equine cecal impactions. Vet Surg 1987;16:451–455.

298. Gerard MP, Bowman KF, Blikslager AT, et al. Jejunocolostomy or ileocolostomy for treatment of cecal impactions in horses: nine cases (1985–1995). J Am Vet Med Assoc 1996;209:1287–1290.

299. Lores M, Ortenburger A. Use of cecal bypass via side-to-side ileocolic anastomosis without ileal transaction for treatment of cecocolic intussusception in three horses. J Am Vet Med Assoc 2008;232:574–577.

300. Ross MWW, Cullin KK, Rutkowski JA. Myoelectric activity of the ileum, cecum and right ventral colon in ponies during interdigestive, nonfeeding, and digestive periods. Am J Vet Res 1990;51:561–566.

301. Sullins KE. Disease of the large colon. In: White NA, ed. The equine acute abdomen. Philadelphia: Lea & Febiger, 1990;375–391.

302. Beroza GA, Barclay WP, Phillips TN, et al. Cecal perforation and peritonitis associated with Anaplocephala perfoliata infection in three horses. J Am Vet Med Assoc 1983; 183:804–806.

303. Proudman CJ, Edwards GB. Are tapeworms associated with equine colic? A case control study. Equine Vet J 1993; 25:224–226.

304. Boussauw BH, Domingo R, Wilderjans H, et al. Treatment of irreducible caecocolic intussusceptions in horses by jeujuno(ileo)-colostomy. Vet Rec 2001;149:16–18.

305. Gaughan EM, Hackett RP. Cecocolic intussusceptions in horses: 11 cases (1979–1989). J Am Vet Med Assoc 1990; 197:1373–1375.

306. Gaughan EM, van Harreveld P. Cecocecal and cecocolic intussusceptions in horses. Compend Contin Educ Pract Vet 2000;22:616–621.

307. Martin BBJ, Freeman DE, Ross MW, et al. Cecocecal and cecocolic intussusceptions in horse: 30 cases (1976–1996). J Am Vet Med Assoc 1999;214:80–84.

308. Hubert JD, Hardy J, Holcombe SJ, et al. Cecal amputation via a right ventral colon enterotomy for correction of nonreducible cecocolic intussusception in 8 horses. Vet Surg 2000;29:317–325.

309. Tyler R. Cecocolic intussusception in a yearling Thoroughbred filly and its surgical management by ileocolostomy. Equine Vet Educ 1992;4:229–232.

310. Ward JL, Fubini SL. Partial typhlectomy and ileocolostomy for treatment of non-reducible cecocolic intussusceptions in a horse. J Am Vet Med Assoc 1994;205:325–328.

311. Edwards GB. Diseases and surgery of the small colon. Vet Clin North Am Equine Pract 1997;13:359–375.

312. Rhoads W, Barton M, Parks AH. Comparison of medical and surgical treatment for impaction of the small colon in horses: 84 cases (1986–1996). J Am Vet Med Assoc 1999;214:1042–1047.

313. Ruggles A, Ross MW. Medical and surgical management of small colon impaction in horses: 28 cases (1984–1989). J Am Vet Med Assoc 1991;199:1762–1766.

314. Schumacher J, Mair T. Small colon obstruction in the mature horse. Equine Vet Educ 2002;14:19–28.

315. Freeman DE. Duodenitis-proximal jejunitis. Equine Vet Educ 2000;12:415–426.

316. Taylor T, Valdez H, Norwood G. Retrograde flushing for relief of obstruction of the transverse colon in the horse. Equine Pract 1979;2:22–28.

317. Plummer A. Impactions of the small and large intestines. Vet Clin North Am Equine Pract 2009;25:317–327.

318. Hawley PR, Faulk WP, Hunt TK, et al. Collagenase activity in the gastrointestinal tract. Br J Surg 1970;57:896–900.

319. Stashak T. Techniques of enterotomy, decompression, and intestinal resection and anastomosis. Vet Clin North Am Large Anim Pract 1982;4:147–165.

320. Prange T, Holcombe SJ, Brown, JA, et al. Resection and anastomosis of the descending colon in 43 horses. Vet Surg 2010;39:748–753.

321. Gay CC, Spiers VC, Christie BA, et al. Foreign body obstruction of the small colon in six horses. Equine Vet J 1979;11:60–63.

322. Kirker-Head C, Stekel R. Volvulus of the small colon in a horse. Mod Vet Pract 1988;69:14–16.

323. Rhoads WS, Parks AH. Incarceration of the small colon through a rent in the gastrosplenic ligament in a pony. J Am Vet Med Assoc 1999;214:226–228.

324. Ross MW, Stephens PR, Reinmer JM. Small colon intussusception in a broodmare. J Am Vet Med Assoc 1988;192:372–374.

325. Bristol DG, Cullen J. A comparison of three methods of end to end anastomosis in the equine small colon. Cornell Vet 1988;78:325–337.

326. Hanson RR, Nixon AJ, Calderwood-Mays M, et al. Evaluation of three techniques for end-to-end anastomosis of the small colon in horses. Am J Vet Res 1988;49:1613–20.

327. Hanson RR, Nixon AJ, Calderwood-Mays M, et al. Comparison of staple and suture techniques for end-to-end anastomosis in horses. Am J Vet Res 1988;49:1621–1628.

328. Reid CL, Campbell IT, Little RA. Muscle wasting and energy balance in critical illness. Clin Nutr 2004;23:273–280.

329. Naylor JM, Freeman DE, Kronfeld DS, et al. Alimentation of hypophagic horses. Compend Contin Educ Pract Vet 1992;6:S93–S99.

330. Bedenice D. Evidence-based medicine in equine critical care. Vet Clin North Am Equine Pract 2007;23:293–316.

4 Muscular system

Stephanie J. Valberg, DVM, PhD, Diplomate ACVIM, ACVSMR

The most basic aim of veterinary clinical nutrition is to design diets that prevent diseases by meeting the minimum daily requirements for essential nutrients. Two neuromuscular disorders that are impacted by nutritional deficiencies include myodegeneration due to selenium deficiency[1] and equine motor neuron disease due to vitamin E deficiency.[2] More recently, equine research has embraced nutrigenomics, in which a horse's nutritional requirements are tailored to its individual genetic make-up. Equine nutrigenomics has been applied to the dietary management of genetic disorders such as polysaccharide storage myopathy (PSSM), recurrent exertional rhabdomyolysis (RER), and hyperkalemic periodic paralysis (HYPP). This chapter will focus on dietary management of these disorders as well as general dietary recommendations for horses with sporadic forms of tying up or exertional rhabdomyolysis (ER).

4.1 Myopathies Associated with Nutritional Deficiencies

4.1.1 Nutritional Myodegeneration due to Selenium Deficiency

Nutritional myodegeneration (NMD; white muscle disease, nutritional muscular dystrophy) occurs in foals due to a dietary deficiency of selenium.[1,3–5] The nutritional deficiency usually arises *in utero* when selenium deficient diets are consumed by dams during gestation. In some, but not all cases, there may also be a deficiency of vitamin E.

4.1.1.1 Prevalence

The prevalence of NMD depends on whether forage fed to pregnant mares was grown on selenium-deficient soil and if mares received supplemental dietary selenium. Selenium deficient areas occur throughout a large portion of the United States and other countries.[4,6]

Forages and grains produced in the northeastern and eastern seaboards and northwestern regions of the United States are particularly deficient. Forage types within an area will also vary in their selenium content. Legumes and rapidly growing forage have lower selenium content than grasses. Regardless, as selenium is now usually added to equine concentrates, the incidence of NMD has declined markedly since the 1980s. Vitamin E deficiency occurs most commonly when horses do not have regular access to green pastures and when they are fed hay deficient in vitamin E due to prolonged or poor storage.

4.1.1.2 Pathophysiology

During normal cellular metabolism, highly reactive forms of oxygen (free radicals) are produced. Vitamin E is active within the cell membrane as a lipid-soluble antioxidant that scavenges free radicals that otherwise might react with unsaturated fatty acids to form lipid hydroperoxides. In contrast, the selenium containing enzyme glutathione peroxidase (GSH-Px) destroys hydrogen peroxide and lipoperoxides that have already been formed and converts them to water or relatively harmless alcohols. A deficiency in selenium and vitamin E in highly metabolically active skeletal and cardiac muscle results in oxidant damage to muscle cell membranes and mitochondria leading to a loss of cellular integrity.[4,7] The most rapidly growing or active foals in the herd are often affected.

4.1.1.3 Clinical Signs

Foals may present with signs of heart failure including sudden death or depression, rapid heart rate, difficulty breathing, and foamy nasal discharge. Foals may have skeletal muscle degeneration primarily and these foals have firm painful muscles on palpation, muscle weakness, trembling of the limbs, and stiffness. Affected foals will lie down frequently and have difficulty rising. If the tongue and pharyngeal muscles are affected,

Nutritional Management of Equine Diseases and Special Cases, First Edition. Edited by Bryan M. Waldridge.
© 2017 John Wiley & Sons, Inc. Published 2017 by John Wiley & Sons, Inc.

then milk may be seen from the nostrils and foals may develop aspiration pneumonia.

4.1.1.4 Diagnosis

Suspicion of NMD arises when foals have associated clinical signs and elevated serum muscle enzyme activities such as creatine kinase (CK) and aspartate transaminase (AST). With severe muscle degeneration, hyperkalemia, hyperphosphatemia, hyponatremia, hypochloremia, and myoglobinuria may be present.[5] Confirmation of NMD requires analysis of whole blood selenium and serum vitamin E concentrations. Normal equine whole blood selenium concentrations range from 0.07 to greater than 0.1 ppm (µg/g) and normal equine serum vitamin E concentrations range from 2–5 ppm.[8] Recent supplementation or selenium/vitamin E injections can confuse interpretation of circulating concentrations of selenium or vitamin E. Measuring GSH-Px activity formed in the red blood cells during erythropoiesis may be of value in such cases. Adequate GSH-Px activity is greater than 20–50 U/mg of hemoglobin per minute in horses, however, this range varies between laboratories.[9] Tissue biopsies and tissue specimens obtained at necropsy provide an accurate indication of selenium and vitamin E storage. Normal liver concentrations of selenium are 1.05–3.50 µg/g DM for horses.[10] Muscle biopsies show evidence of acute myodegeneration and scattered calcification within myofibers.

Vitamin E deteriorates rapidly in plasma samples and, therefore, plasma samples for α-tocopherol analysis need to be put on ice immediately, protected from light by wrapping in tin foil, and frozen (−21 °F, −70 °C) if analysis is to be delayed. The critical plasma concentration of vitamin E (α-tocopherol) for NMD is 1.1–2.0 ppm (µg/g).[2]

The precise interrelationships between selenium, vitamin E, other metabolic factors, and triggering mechanisms in NMD are not fully understood because many animals deficient in selenium or vitamin E have no evidence of muscle disease. In certain situations, deficiencies of both selenium and vitamin E are necessary for disease to occur. In other animals, NMD can occur when a deficiency of only one of the nutrients is present and the other is normal in blood and tissues.

4.1.1.5 Treatment

Foals with NMD affecting skeletal but not cardiac muscle often respond favorably to treatment and rest. Improvement is evident after a few days, and within 3–5 days,

affected animals can often stand and walk. The cardiac form of NMD is usually not compatible with life. Therapy includes supplementation with selenium and vitamin E as well as general supportive care. Injectable selenium products are available with concentrations varying from 1–5 mg of selenium/ml, with all products containing 50 mg/ml (68 IU) of vitamin E as d,l-α-tocopheryl acetate.[9] The label dose for selenium is 0.055–0.067 mg/kg, IM (2.5–3.0 mg/45 kg body weight). Dosage of injectable products administered should not be greatly increased above the label dose to prevent inadvertent selenium toxicosis.

The vitamin E in selenium/vitamin E combination products is added as a preservative and is, therefore, insufficient for vitamin E supplementation.[9] Oral supplementation with water-soluble natural (d-α-tocopherol) products rapidly achieve normal blood levels.[8] Recommended daily vitamin E supplementation for sick foals is 10 IU/kg body weight.[8]

4.1.1.6 Dietary Prevention

Prevention and control of NMD is achieved by supplementation of selenium and vitamin E to pregnant dams. Oral supplementation of adult horses with 1 mg of selenium per day increases blood selenium concentrations above levels known to be associated with NMD.[11] Supplementation of pregnant mares is advised in areas known to be selenium deficient; however, only limited selenium may cross the placenta.[3] Supplementation during lactation increases the levels of selenium in milk and thus provides a potential means of selenium supplementation in foals; however, evidence in cattle indicates that this increased level of selenium in milk may not meet nutrient requirements.[6,12,13]

4.1.2 Equine Motor Neuron Disease and Vitamin E Deficiency

Equine Motor Neuron Disease (EMND) is a chronic degenerative disorder of motor neurons arising from the spinal cord and brain stem nuclei that innervate skeletal muscle fibers.[14,15] Long-standing dietary vitamin E deficiency is one of several intrinsic and environmental factors that contribute to EMND.[16,17]

4.1.2.1 Prevalence

EMND occurs worldwide and particularly affects horses with limited access to green pasture.[16–18] However, low serum vitamin E concentrations and clinical signs of

EMND have been documented in horses grazing lush grass-based pastures in Europe.[19,]

4.1.2.2 Pathophysiology

EMND affects neurons supplying highly oxidative type 1 muscle fibers.[15,20] A chronic deficiency of vitamin E predisposes motor neurons with high oxidative activity to lipid peroxidation over time leading to permanent neuronal damage. In naturally-occurring EMND, there appears to be an individual susceptibility to oxidative stress in at risk horses, with clinical signs developing in only a subset of horses maintained in high risk environments. Horses with naturally occurring EMND require at least 18 months of a vitamin E deficiency before developing clinical signs.[21] In addition, excessive dietary copper, a potential pro-oxidant, is a risk factor for EMND development.[22] Other proposed pathologic causes of EMND include low bioavailability of dietary vitamin E, excess utilization of vitamin E caused by exposure to environmental oxidants, such as iron, cadmium, and lead, failure of absorption or retention of vitamin E, a familial predisposition, or decreased absorption due to intestinal epithelial absorptive dysfunction.[8]

4.1.2.3 Clinical Signs

Classic clinical signs of EMND include weight loss, muscle atrophy, muscle weakness, muscle fasciculation, frequent weight shifting of hind limbs, excessive recumbency, elevated tail head, and abnormally low head and neck carriage.[15] Horses often stand with their limbs underneath their abdomen, like an elephant standing on a ball.

4.1.2.4 Diagnosis

A definitive diagnosis is based upon postmortem demonstration of degeneration and loss of motor neurons from the ventral horns of the spinal cord.[20] Antemortem diagnosis of EMND is based upon histopathology and low serum vitamin E concentration. Histologic evidence of EMND includes degeneration of myelinated axons from a biopsy of the ventral branch of the spinal accessory nerve or neurogenic atrophy of predominantly type 1 muscle fibers in a biopsy of the sacrocaudalis dorsalis medialis muscle.[2,15,21]

4.1.2.5 Treatment

For EMND affected cases, 5000–7000 IU/day of d-α-tocopherol is recommended.[8] It is important to note that there are synthetic and natural forms of vitamin E supplements and they differ in their bioavailability. For treatment of EMND, the micellized form of natural RRR-α-tocopherol (d-α-tocopherol) is recommended due to the rapid restoration of adequate tissue levels of vitamin E using this formulation.[23,24] For absorption of the esterified form (acetate), the ester group has to be removed and the α-tocopherol portion made water-soluble by the action of bile salts (micellization).[8] These additional digestive steps may limit α-tocopherol absorption in the horse.

With vitamin E treatment, approximately 40% of cases demonstrate clinical improvement within 6 weeks and some may appear normal within 3 months.[14] It should be noted, however, that return to performance may result in deterioration. Divers[14] reports that approximately 40% of cases will stabilize but remain permanently impaired while 20% will have continual progression of clinical signs. Early recognition of signs of muscle atrophy and low dietary vitamin E are essential if signs of EMND can be reversed.

The diet should consist of good quality grass or alfalfa hay and pasture. Vitamin E content varies markedly among equine dietary constituents with the highest levels in fresh grass and declining concentrations with processing and storage. Most pasture grasses, especially orchard grass supply approximately 50–80 IU of vitamin E/kg dry matter, however, this can be highly variable.

4.1.2.6 Prevention

Horses without access to green forage should be supplemented with 1 IU/kg body weight/day of vitamin E to prevent EMND and higher levels are recommended for horses in heavy exercise. It is important to account for the 2:1 ratio of activity of RRR-α-tocopherol compared to all-rac-α-tocopherol acetate when considering vitamin E supplementation.[8] For example, if pure RRR-α-tocopherol is the supplement provided to a 500-kg adult sedentary horse (recommended dose of 1 IU/kg), only 250 IU can be administered whereas if a synthetic all-rac-α-tocopherol supplement is provided, 500 IU should be administered because it is less biologically active. These respective dosages will provide the same active amount of α-tocopherol.

4.1.3 Vitamin E Deficient Myopathy

Some horses with clinical signs of EMND and vitamin E deficiency are not diagnosed with EMND because they lack evidence of neurogenic atrophy in the sacrocaudalis dorsalis muscle. A recent study suggests that these horses have a vitamin E deficient myopathy characterized by abnormal staining of mitochondria in sacrocaudalis dorsalis muscle biopsy specimens.[25] Thus there may be a specific myogenic presentation of vitamin E deficiency. Horses with this vitamin E deficient myopathy show a remarkable response to treatment with vitamin E, unlike horses with EMND.

4.1.3.1 Pathophysiology

Affected horses have low muscle vitamin E concentrations which may produce weakness due to a reversible manifestation of mitochondrial oxidative stress. Loss of muscle mass and weakness is a feature of mitochondrial myopathies in horses[26] and humans. A recent study in mice suggests that a mitochondrial stress response may induce gene expression that mimics starvation in a normal nutritional state.[27] Thus, vitamin E deficient myopathy may be an entity unto itself or possibly a predecessor to development of EMND.

4.1.3.2 Clinical Signs

Affected horses share the same clinical features of muscle weakness and atrophy with EMND. Horses show a decrease in performance due to exercise intolerance, generalized locomotor muscle wasting, muscle fasciculations, weight shifting, and increased recumbency.

4.1.3.3 Diagnosis

Acquired vitamin E deficient myopathy is diagnosed by confirming low serum or muscle vitamin E concentrations and identifying an abnormal moth-eaten staining pattern in nicotinaminde adenine dinucleotide tetrazolium reductase stain of frozen biopsies of the sacrocaudalis dorsalis muscle.[25] In many, but not all, cases serum vitamin E concentrations are low ($<2\,\mu g/ml$). The distinction between this disorder and EMND is the presence of myopathic changes and mitochondrial abnormalities rather than neurogenic atrophy in sacrocaudalis dorsalis muscle. Gluteus medius muscle biopsy samples are normal.

4.1.3.4 Treatment

Acquired vitamin E deficient myopathy is highly responsive to treatment with natural (d-α-tocopherol) vitamin E ($5000\,IU/500\,kg$, PO, q24h) and a very gradual reintroduction to exercise once strength returns.[25]

4.1.4 Sporadic Exertional Rhabdomyolysis

Sporadic exertional rhabdomyolysis (ER) is a term used to describe horses that sporadically have a disruption of innately normal muscle during exercise due to management practices such as dietary imbalances, change in exercise, viral infections, or trauma. Horses usually have a history of adequate performance prior to onset of muscle pain and successfully return to performance following a reasonable period of rest, provision of a balanced diet, and a gradual training program. Horses with these sporadic occurrences may be of any age, breed, or sex, and involved in a wide variety of athletic disciplines. Episodes of muscle pain may recur over a short period of time prior to resolving the external perturbations that affect muscle function. In many cases, horses are initially presumed to have sporadic ER. However, if over time episodes of muscle pain recur despite the best management, further investigation may lead to a diagnosis of a form of chronic ER.

4.1.4.1 Causes and Dietary Management of Sporadic ER

1 *Overexertion*

A history of an increase in work intensity without a foundation of consistent training for a higher level of intensity is usually the basis for suspecting a training imbalance as a cause of ER.

2 *Heat and electrolyte exhaustion*

Prolonged exercise in hot, humid weather can lead to heat exhaustion ($105–108\,°F$ [$41–42\,°C$]) and myoglobinuria, especially during endurance competitions. Acute hyponatremia, hypokalemia, hypochloremia, and hypocalemia are apparent in blood samples and immediate intravenous fluid therapy treatment is required.[28] Commercial electrolyte mixtures containing a 2:1:4 ratio of Na:K:Cl are recommended prior to and during prolonged endurance rides to prevent depletion.[29]

3 *Chronic electrolyte imbalances*

Chronic imbalances are much more difficult to accurately assess than acute depletion. Work by Harris[29] established renal fractional excretions as a technique to evaluate electrolyte concentrations in horses. Blood and urine samples are obtained concurrently and creatinine and electrolyte concentrations are measured in both. [Serum creatinine]/[urine creatinine] multiplied by [urine electrolyte]/[serum electrolyte] $\times 100$ provides the renal fractional excretion of a given electrolyte. This technique is complicated by marked electrolyte variations that occur because of diet, time of day, sampling technique, and among individuals.[30] Furthermore, the high calcium crystal content in equine urine makes acidification of samples necessary to accurately assess urinary calcium and magnesium concentrations. In the United Kingdom, a number of horses with ER had low fractional excretions of sodium and daily dietary supplementation of 60 g (2 oz) NaCl resulted in abatement of clinical signs. Other horses had high phosphorus excretion suggesting a dietary calcium: phosphorus imbalance. Decreasing bran while providing a daily calcium supplement (60 g CaCO$_3$) was helpful in reducing clinical signs of ER.[31] Hypokalemia has also been suggested to play a role in chronic ER, although it is not a common finding in horses consuming adequate quantities of forage. Supplementation with good quality forage or 30 g of KCl/day (lite salt) is recommended for horses with low renal fractional excretion of potassium.

4 *Selenium and vitamin E deficiency*

In some areas, soil selenium can be particularly low and soil factors may impair adequate selenium uptake from the diet. In addition, inadequate vitamin E intake can arise when horses have restricted green pasture or turn out. While it is not readily documented that deficiencies of antioxidants such as vitamin E and selenium cause sporadic ER, it seems reasonable that inadequate antioxidant levels may predispose horses to muscle soreness. Adequate blood selenium concentration is usually considered to be >0.07 µg/ml. Veterinarians in selenium deficient areas often anecdotally report a higher degree of success in treating a variety of myopathies by providing selenium supplementation above that normally recommended for horses (0.2–0.3 mg/kg/dry matter) and that higher doses of oral selenium are required to maintain adequate blood levels. Adequate serum vitamin E concentration is 2.0–5.0 µg/ml.[9] Adequate daily intake of vitamin E ranges from 500–1000 IU per day, depending on exercise intensity. In addition to the vitamin E provided by green grasses and well-cured hay, supplemental vitamin E from commercially prepared diets and supplements may be necessary to achieve adequate antioxidant status. With extreme exertion such as endurance riding, antioxidants such as vitamin E may have a key protective role in preventing muscle damage. A beneficial effect of supplementing beyond daily requirements, particularly for horses performing less intense exercise remains equivocal.

4.2 Nutrigenomics

4.2.1 Chronic Forms of Exertional Rhabdomyolysis

Horses that have repeated episodes of ER from a young age, or from the time of purchase, or when they are put back into training after a long period of rest, may have an underlying intrinsic abnormality of muscle function. Many horses with intrinsic muscle defects will have repeated episodes of ER with minimal exercise even when the dietary and training recommendations for sporadic ER are followed. Five specific intrinsic causes of ER have been identified to date:

1 Recurrent exertional rhabdomyolysis (RER)
2 Malignant Hyperthermia (MH)
3 Type 1 polysaccharide storage myopathy (PSSM1)
4 Type 2 polysaccharide storage myopathy (PSSM2)
5 Idiopathic chronic exertional rhabdomyolysis.

The idiopathic group represents other causes of ER that have yet to be identified. In all these intrinsic forms of chronic ER, it appears that there are specific environmental stimuli that are necessary to trigger muscle necrosis in genetically susceptible animals. Horses cannot be cured of their susceptibility to this condition but if the specific form of ER is identified, changes in management can be implemented in order to minimize episodes of rhabdomyolysis.

4.2.1.1 Recurrent Exertional Rhabdomyolysis

RER describes a subset of ER that is believed to be due to an abnormality in the regulation of muscle contraction and relaxation.[32–34] Research into RER has primarily been performed in Thoroughbreds and to a lesser extent, Standardbred horses.[33,35–37] Scientific studies of RER have used a small number of horses that share common clinical signs of ER and have abnormal muscle contracture tests.[33,38,39] Broader epidemiologic and genetic studies have assumed that the same pathophysiologic basis for ER exists in the majority of Thoroughbred and Standardbred horses with similar clinical signs. Whether this is true are not will require more research. There are reports of some Arabian horses and Warmblood horses[40] with ER that may also suffer from RER based on their overlapping histories, clinical signs, muscle biopsy findings, and response to management.

4.2.1.2 Pathogenesis

Rhabdomyolysis in type 2 muscle fibers is triggered suddenly during exercise in RER horses which results in a sharp rise in serum myoglobin and CK activity.[41] Clinically, the triggering event is often associated with excitement in a horse that already has an underlying nervous temperament.[35–37] In Standardbreds, ER commonly begins after 15–30 min of jogging at 5 m/s, although clinical signs may not be apparent until after exercise.[35,41] In Thoroughbreds exercising on the treadmill, ER most commonly develops with intervals of walk, trot, and canter and is less common if horses are allowed to gallop.[42,43] At the racetrack, ER occurs commonly when RER horses are held back to a paced gallop.[36] During eventing, RER commonly occurs after the excitement of the steeplechase or early in the cross country phase when horses are held to a predetermined speed. RER rarely occurs when horses are allowed to achieve maximal exercise speeds such as racing. A day or more of rest before this type of exercise results in higher serum CK activity post exercise.[35,43]

Lactic Acid

There is no basis for an association between RER and a lactic acidosis. Thoroughbreds and Standardbreds rarely develop ER during near maximal exercise[35,36,44] when muscle lactate concentrations reach 240 mmol/kg dry weight[45] and plasma lactate concentrations are as high as 25 mM/l. Standardbred horses experience ER during jogging when muscle lactate concentrations are less than 24 mmol/kg dry weight.[46] Similarly, plasma lactate concentrations in RER Thoroughbred horses are less than 1.5 mM/l when performing walk, trot, and canter treadmill exercise that induces high serum CK activity.[42]

Intracellular Calcium Regulation

More recent research suggests that horses with RER may have an inherent abnormality in intramuscular calcium regulation that is intermittently manifested during exercise.[39,47] Myoplasmic calcium concentrations are tightly controlled by channels and pumps in the sarcoplasmic reticulum and usually unaffected by normal serum calcium concentrations or minor fluctuations in dietary calcium. Basal muscle intracellular

calcium concentrations in RER horses are similar to healthy horses based on assays in muscle cell cultures.[47] Higher intracellular calcium concentrations have been measured in horses of unspecified breeds during an episode of ER, however, this also could be secondary to any insult that impairs energy generation or cell membrane integrity.[48] To specifically study shuttling of calcium between the sarcoplasmic reticulum and myoplasm within the muscle cell, technically complex procedures such muscle contracture testing, calcium imaging in muscle cell cultures, and calcium release by isolated muscle membrane preparations have been evaluated. In spite of many detailed investigations of a small number of horses, the exact defect in regulating muscle contraction in RER horses has yet to be identified. RER appears to be a novel defect in muscle excitation-contraction coupling, calcium regulation, or contractility whose basis is yet to be defined. Alternatively, the increased sensitivity of RER horses in contracture testing may be a nonspecific indicator of an abnormality in other pathways governing muscle contraction.

4.2.1.3 Prevalence and Risk Factors

In Thoroughbred racehorses, the prevalence of RER is remarkably similar around the world with estimates ranging from 4.9% in the US,[36] 5.4% in Australia,[49] and 6.7% in the UK.[37,50] The annual incidence of ER in Standardbred racehorses in Sweden is 6.4%.[35] Exercise obviously increases the prevalence of RER in horses and episodes are observed more frequently once horses achieve a level of fitness.[35,36] In Standardbreds and Thoroughbreds, mares more commonly have RER than males particularly in Thoroughbreds less than 3 years of age.[35–37] Temperament has a strong effect on the expression of RER in both Standardbreds and Thoroughbreds, with nervous horses, particularly fillies, having a higher incidence of rhabdomyolysis than calm horses.[35–37] A genetic susceptibility to RER appears to exist in Thoroughbred horses and RER-affected Thoroughbreds may pass the trait along to 50% or more of their offspring.[51,52] No specific genetic defect has of yet been identified in horses with RER.

4.2.1.4 Diagnosis

A presumptive diagnosis of RER is based on clinical signs of muscle pain and the presence of risk factors commonly associated with RER. Muscle histopathology is nonspecific in RER horses; either there are no abnormalities or evidence of centrally located nuclei in mature muscle fibers and potentially waves of myofiber degeneration or regeneration.[34] There is a notable absence of abnormal amylase-resistant polysaccharide, although increased subsarcolemmal amylase-sensitive glycogen may be present.[53] Serum CK and AST activities serve as the basis for detecting muscle degeneration and they often show intermittent abnormal elevations that return to normal relatively quickly during the course of training.

4.2.1.5 Management

Prevention of rhabdomyolysis in horses susceptible to RER is complex and multiple factors need to be changed to decrease episodes. These factors include environment, exercise regime, and diet. In addition, medication may be needed at times to prevent further episodes of muscle damage. Since excitement and nervousness often trigger rhabdomyolysis,[35–37] stressful situations in the environment that can be modified need to be identified. This may involve a change to a smaller barn with fewer horses and fewer handlers, compatible companions, and a more consistent daily routine. Providing daily turn out with other horses seems to be very beneficial for RER horses and may decrease anxiety and thereby the likelihood of rhabdomyolysis. Although a period of rest is recommended for sporadic forms of ER until serum CK normalizes, it is not recommended for horses with RER. Daily exercise is important to prevent episodes of rhabdomyolysis and therefore when serum CK is about <3,000 U/L, horses are returned to regular daily exercise.

Supplements

Horses require daily dietary supplementation with sodium and chloride either in the form of loose salt (30–50 g/day) or a salt block. Additional electrolyte supplementation is indicated in hot humid conditions. A myriad of supplements is sold that are purported to decrease lactic acid build up in skeletal muscle of RER horses. These include sodium bicarbonate, B vitamins, branched chain amino acids, and dimethylglycine. Since lactic acidosis is no longer implicated as a cause for rhabdomyolysis, it is difficult to find a rationale for their use.

Medications

Low doses of tranquillizers, such as acepromazine, prior to exercise have been used in RER horses prone to excitement.[54] Dantrolene sodium acts to decrease release of calcium from the ryanodine receptor in skeletal muscle and is used to treat MH.[55] Controlled and field studies have also shown that oral dantrolene can significantly decrease signs of rhabdomyolysis in RER horses. Phenytoin also has been reported to be effective in preventing rhabdomyolysis in horses with RER.[56] Various hormones, ranging from thyroxine to progesterone and testosterone, have been given to horses with RER, however, there are no scientific studies to validate their use. Some mares appear to exhibit signs of rhabdomyolysis during estrus and it may well be of benefit in these horses to suppress estrus behavior using progesterone injections. Testosterone and anabolic steroids have been used to prevent signs of RER in racehorses, but their use is regulated.

Adjunct Therapies

Massage, myofascial release, mesotherapy, stretching, aqua-treadmills, and hot/cold therapy performed by experienced therapists may be of benefit in individual cases.[57–59] Their use may promote relaxation, normal muscle tension, and build muscle strength.

4.2.1.6 Dietary Management of RER

It is clear that diet impacts the expression of RER such that Thoroughbred horses fed more than 2.5 kg of grain are more likely to show signs of ER (Figure 4.1).[42] A nutritionally balanced diet, appropriate caloric intake, and adequate vitamins and minerals are the core elements of managing RER. For RER affected Thoroughbreds and Standardbreds in training, usually the challenge is supplying enough calories in a highly palatable form to meet their daily energy demands. This is in part because racehorses often require >30 MCal of digestible energy (DE) a day (5 kg sweet feed, 1.5% of body weight in hay) and because of their nervous temperament they may be more discriminating in their eating habits. Out of the total daily calories required by RER horses, research suggests that less than 20% DE be supplied by nonstructural carbohydrates (NSC = starch and sugar) and at least 20% of DE be supplied by fat (Table 4.1).[43,60]

Selection of Forage

Thoroughbred horses do not appear to show the same significant increase in serum insulin concentrations in response to consuming 17% NSC hay as seen in Quarter Horses.[61] This fact combined with the high caloric requirements of racehorses may mean that it is not as important to select hay with very low NSC content in RER Thoroughbreds as it is in PSSM horses. Anecdotally some trainers find horses with RER have more frequent episodes of ER on alfalfa hay. The nervous disposition of some RER horses may predispose them to gastric ulcers and thus frequent provision of hay with a moderate NSC and mixed alfalfa content may be indicated.

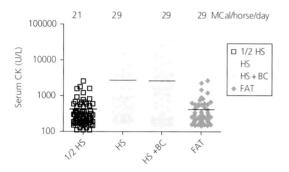

Figure 4.1 Serum CK activity 4h after 30min of exercise for 5 days a week in 5 RER susceptible Thoroughbreds when fed four different diets. ½ HS represents 2.5kg of high starch sweet feed (40% DE from NSC, 3% DE from fat) fed with grass hay for a total daily DE of 21 MCal/day. HS represents 5kg of high starch sweet feed fed with grass hay for a total daily DE of 29 MCal/day. HS+BC represents 5kg of high starch sweet feed with 4% sodium bicarbonate added. FAT represents a low starch, high fat feed (Re•Leve®, Kentucky Equine Research, Versailles, KY, 10% DE from NSC and 20% DE from fat) fed with grass hay for a total of 29 MCal/day. Note that horses fed a low caloric diet (1/2 HS) or a high caloric fat diet (FAT) have lower post exercise serum CK activity than horses fed a high calorie, high starch diet with or without sodium bicarbonate added.

Low Starch High Fat Concentrates

When RER Thoroughbreds are fed a moderate caloric intake (24 MCal/day) in the form of high starch concentrates (2.5kg of corn/oats/wheat middlings/molasses) they show very little elevation in serum CK activity with exercise (Figure 4.1).[42] Most Thoroughbred racehorses, however, are fed at least 5kg/day of high starch concentrate at 30 MCal or more/horse/day and at this level of feeding, post-exercise serum CK activity rises significantly.[36] The discovery that substitution of fat for starch in a high calorie ration significantly reduces muscle damage in exercising RER horses was a major advance in nutritional management of RER.[43] Practically, however, it was difficult to achieve the desired caloric intake of racehorses because the maximum amount of fat that finicky Thoroughbreds will happily consume is often limited to 600ml of vegetable oil or 5lb (2.3kg)/day of balanced rice bran. Management of RER horses was significantly improved when a palatable means to provide the amount of fat required by fit finicky RER Thoroughbreds was developed. A controlled trial using a specialized feed developed for RER (Re•Leve®, Kentucky Equine Research, Versailles, KY [13% fat by weight and 9% NSC]) determined that NSC should be no greater than 20% of daily DE and 20–25% of daily DE should be provided by fat for optimal management of RER horses fed 30 MCal or more/day.[43] No beneficial effect on serum CK activity occurred when 4.2% sodium bicarbonate was added to a high starch pellet feed (Figure 4.1).[43] The amount of fat in the diet of an RER horse depends upon its caloric requirements. Over and above hay at 1.5–2.0% of body

Table 4.1 Feeding recommendations for a 500-kg horse with exertional rhabdomyolysis due to RER or PSSM.

Exercise	RER			PSSM		
	light	moderate	intense	light	moderate	intense
Caloric intake (MCal)	20	25	33	18	23	30
Daily digestible energy from NSC (%)	15–20	15–20	15–20	<10	<10	<10
Daily digestible energy from fat (%)	15	15–20	20–25	15	15–20	15–20
Selenium (mg/day)	2.2	2.8	3.1	2.2	2.8	3.1
Vitamin E (mg/day)	1,400	1,800	2,000	1,400	1,800	2,000
Daily amount fed of a 12% NSC, 10% fat concentrate feed (kg)*	2.5	3.5	5	2	3	4
Grass hay <12% NSC by weight (kg)	7.5–10	7.5–10	7.5–10	7.5–10	7.5–10	7.5–10
Sodium chloride (g)	34	34	41	34	34	41

NSC is nonstructural carbohydrate

*Re•Leve®, Kentucky Equine Research, Versailles, KY, formulated for horses with exertional myopathies

weight and 2.5 kg of grain, any additional calories required should be supplied by fat.

The benefit of a higher fat diet does not appear to be a change in muscle metabolism. Pre- and post-exercise muscle glycogen and lactate concentrations are the same in RER horses fed a low starch, high fat diet compared to a high starch diet.[62] Rather, low starch, high fat diets in RER horses may decrease muscle damage by assuaging anxiety and excitability, which are tightly linked to developing rhabdomyolysis is susceptible horses. High fat low starch diets fed to fit RER horses produce lower glucose, insulin, and cortisol responses and led to a calmer demeanor and lower pre-exercise heart rates (Figure 4.2).[63] Neurohormonal changes may develop in response to high serum glucose, insulin, and cortisol concentrations resulting in an anxious demeanor. While a calm demeanor is desired during training, some racehorse trainers feeding low starch high fat feeds prefer to supplement with a titrated amount of grain 3 days prior to a race to potentially increase liver glycogen and increase a horse's energy during the race.

4.2.1.7 Expectations
Studies in RER horses show that significant reductions or normalization of post-exercise serum CK activity occurs within a week of commencing a low starch high fat diet.[43] Days off training in a stall are discouraged because post-exercise CK activity is higher following two days of rest compared to when working on consecutive days with the same amount of sub-maximal exercise.

4.2.2 Polysaccharide Storage Myopathy
PSSM was first recognized as a specific muscle disease in Quarter Horse-related breeds in 1992.[64] However, there are individual cases of abnormal polysaccharide inclusions reported in equine muscle dating back to 1979.[65–67] The remarkable feature of the first horses reported to have PSSM was two-fold higher muscle glycogen concentrations than normal horses and abnormal granular amylase-resistant inclusions in histologic sections of muscle.[64] Similar biopsy findings were reported in Belgian and Percheron draft horses in 1997.[68] Since that time, many hundreds of horses from a variety of breeds have been diagnosed with PSSM.[40,53,69,71–81]

Several acronyms and synonyms are used for polysaccharide storage myopathy besides PSSM[82] including

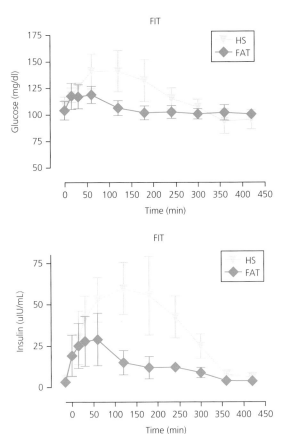

Figure 4.2 Postprandial glucose and insulin response (mean ± SE) for four fit RER horses after consuming a high NSC meal of 4 kg of sweet feed (HS: 40% DE from NSC, 3% DE from fat) or 4.0 kg of a low starch, high fat commercial concentrate (FAT: Re•Leve®, Kentucky Equine Research, Versailles, KY; 10% DE from NSC and 20% DE from fat). Note the lower glycemic and insulinemic response of RER horses fed the low starch, high fat feed.

Equine Polysaccharide Storage Myopathy (EPSM[83] and EPSSM[81]). Considerable controversy existed as to whether these others encompassed one muscle condition or several muscle conditions.[83,84,97] In 2008, a mutation in the glycogen synthase 1 gene was found to be highly associated with the presence of amylase-resistant polysaccharide in skeletal muscle from Quarter Horses with PSSM.[85] Genetic testing of hundreds of horses previously diagnosed with PSSM by muscle biopsy revealed that the majority of cases of PSSM were characterized by amylase-resistant polysaccharide in skeletal muscle with this genetic mutation.[86] However, some cases previously diagnosed with PSSM by muscle biopsy, particularly those with excessive amylase-sensitive glycogen, did not possess the genetic mutation. This suggested that there are at least two forms of PSSM.[86,87] For clarity, the form of PSSM caused by a glycogen synthase 1 (*GYS1*) gene mutation is now termed type 1 (PSSM1) whereas the form of PSSM that is not caused by the *GYS1* mutation and whose origin is yet unknown is now termed type 2 (PSSM2).[87] PSSM1 is likely the same disorder described as "Azoturia" or "Monday Morning Disease" in working horses in the nineteenth and twentieth centuries.[88–90]

4.2.2.1 Type 1 PSSM
Prevalence
The *GYS1* mutation responsible for type 1 PSSM is present in over 20 different horse breeds. It is estimated to have emerged as far back as 1600 years ago when the great horse was being developed from European draft and light horse breeds to carry knights with heavy armor into battle.[85] The highest prevalence of PSSM appears to occur in draft horses derived from Continental European breeds.[91] In contrast, the prevalence of PSSM is very low in United Kingdom-derived breeds such as Shires and Clydesdales.[92] Type 1 PSSM occurs in about 6–10% of Quarter Horses, American Paint, and Appaloosa horses.[93,94] The highest frequency of type 1 PSSM occurs in halter Quarter Horses (28% affected) and the lowest frequency in racing Quarter Horses.[94] The prevalence of type 1 PSSM is very low in light horse breeds such as Arabians and Thoroughbreds.

Pathophysiology
Glycogen is formed by the enzymes glycogen synthase that provides straight α 1 → 4 glycosidic linkages and a glycogen branching enzyme that adds branched α 1 → 6 glycosidic linkages to the glycogen molecule. The autosomal dominant *GYS1* mutation produces a gene product, glycogen synthase, which has an arginine substitution for histidine at codon 309.[85] The effect of this amino acid substitution is a higher than normal activity of glycogen synthase, both at rest and when activated by glucose 6-phosphate. As a result, skeletal muscle of PSSM horses has 1.5–4.0 fold higher concentration of glycogen than normal horse muscle.[95] A less branched abnormal polysaccharide eventually accumulates in PSSM muscle by 18 months of age.[69] The abnormal polysaccharide appears to be the result of a

much higher ratio of glycogen synthase to glycogen branching enzyme activity in PSSM muscle resulting in accumulation of a less branched abnormal glycogen molecule. The accumulation of abnormal polysaccharide is, in itself, not the cause of muscle dysfunction in PSSM since foals as young as 1 month of age may show evidence of muscle damage prior to the formation of abnormal polysaccharide in skeletal muscle fibers. Rather, the persistent glycogen synthase activity in type 1 PSSM horse muscle appears to disturb the normal flux of muscle energy metabolism during exercise. The overactive glycogen synthase enzyme in type 1 PSSM horse muscle results in a shift in energy metabolism towards storage of glycogen and fatty acids and away from utilization of these substrates.[80] A deficit in cellular energy within individual muscle fibers of type 1 PSSM horses has been found after only 6–15 min of exercise.[96] A diet high in NSC further exacerbates clinical signs of PSSM.[97] This may potentially be the result of elevation of serum insulin by a high NSC meal which activates abnormally regulated glycogen synthase enzyme activity, further exacerbating regulation of energy flux in skeletal muscle with the *GYS1* defect.

The precise link between diet, enhanced glycogen synthase activity, and muscle cell damage has not been fully elucidated. Glycogen synthase activation is reciprocally linked to inactivation of myophosphorylase, the enzyme necessary for release of glucose-1-phosphate from glycogen. Constitutively, active glycogen synthase further stimulated by insulin could impair release of glucose for energy metabolism by inactivating myophosphorylase. In addition, high grain diets favor fatty acid synthesis within the muscle cell as a result of increased muscle citrate concentrations.[98] If fatty acids within myofibers are directed toward synthesis rather than metabolism, this could further decrease substrates for energy metabolism in the muscle cell. During the first 20 min of exercise, muscles are dependent on glycogen for energy. If the mutation disrupts glycogen availability and impairs the availability of fatty acids, then exercise intolerance may arise.

Acute Clinical Signs
Horses usually show signs of PSSM at 6 years of age on average, however, this can range from 1–14 years of age. Some horses with type 1 PSSM are asymptomatic. In general, owners describe horses with type 1 PSSM as

having a calm and sedate demeanor. Acute clinical signs include tucking up of the abdomen, fasciculations in the flank, muscle stiffness, sweating, reluctance to move forward, and overt muscle contractures. The hindquarters are frequently most affected, but back muscles, abdominal, and forelimb muscles may also be involved. Signs of pain can last for more than 2 h and about 10% of cases become recumbent. Muscle pain often occurs with less than 20 min of exercise at a walk and trot, especially when horses are unfit at the commencement of training or after horses have had a substantial period of rest. A diet high in NSC exacerbates theses signs. During an acute episode of ER, horses with type 1 PSSM often have markedly elevated serum CK activity (>35,000 U/L) and myoglobinuria may be present. Severe colic-like pain after exercise and myoglobinuric renal failure are less common presenting complaints. Some owners report a seasonal incidence of acute clinical signs, which some have attributed to the quality of grass available at the time.

Chronic Clinical Signs
Light Breeds
Chronic signs of type 1 PSSM in riding horses include a lack of energy when under saddle, reluctance to move forward, stopping, stretching out as if to urinate, and a sour attitude towards exercise. Horses may have a combination of low grade reluctance to exercise, poor performance, and repeated episodes of ER. The range of severity of clinical signs of PSSM can be wide with some horses being asymptomatic and others completely incapacitated. Serum CK activities are often elevated in untreated Quarter Horses, even when horses are rested. While horses are symptomatic, CK will usually increase by 1,000 U/L or more 4 h after 15 min of exercise at a trot. The median CK and AST activity for all PSSM Quarter Horses with muscle biopsies submitted to the University of Minnesota was 2,809 and 1,792 U/L, respectively. Affected Quarter and Paint Horse foals and weanlings may develop rhabdomyolysis without exercise.

A small number of Quarter Horses and Paint horses have both the *GYS1* mutation and a genetic mutation for MH (*RYR1*), which results in particularly severe signs of ER and a limited response to diet and exercise changes.[99] During an episode of ER, excessively high body temperatures may develop and sudden death can occur in horses with the *RYR1* mutation.

Draft Horse and Draft Crosses
The average age of draft horses diagnosed with PSSM is about 8 years of age.[70] Many draft horses with PSSM are asymptomatic. Signs of severe rhabdomyolysis and myoglobinuria may occur in horses fed high grain diets and exercised irregularly with little turn out or in horses that undergo general anesthesia.[100] Other signs of PSSM in draft horses include progressive weakness and muscle loss resulting in difficulty rising in horses with normal serum CK activity. Pronounced weakness is more prevalent in homozygotes for the *GYS1* mutation. Gait abnormalities, such as excessive limb flexion, fasciculations, and trembling are also reported in draft horses. Although the condition Shivers was previously attributed to PSSM, a recent study found no causal association between these two conditions.[70] The median serum CK and AST activities in draft horses from which muscle biopsies were sent to the University of Minnesota was 459 and 537 U/L, respectively.

Diagnosis
A genetic test for the *GYS1* mutation can be performed on whole blood or hair root samples in North America at the University of Minnesota Veterinary Diagnostic Laboratory (www.vdl.umn.edu/vdl/ourservices/neuromuscular. html) and in Europe by Laboklin (www.laboklin.co.uk/laboklin/GeneticDiseases.jsp). MH testing is performed at the University of Minnesota and the University of California, Davis.

Muscle biopsy can also provide a means to diagnose type 1 PSSM. Muscle biopsy procedures, submission guidelines, and interpretation are provided by the Michigan State University Equine Neuromuscular Diagnostic Laboratory (http://cvm.msu.edu/research/faculty-research/valberg-laboratory). The distinctive features of type 1 PSSM in muscle biopsy samples are numerous subsarcolemmal vacuoles and dense, crystalline periodic acid Schiff's (PAS) positive, amylase resistant inclusions in fast twitch fibers.[87] Genetic testing provides the gold standard for diagnosis because a false negative diagnosis of type 1 PSSM by muscle biopsy may occur if biopsy samples are small or if horses are less than 1 year of age.

4.2.2.2 Type 2 PSSM
There is much less known about type 2 PSSM because, as it turns out, previous research on PSSM has largely involved horses with type 1 PSSM. Current knowledge of type 2 PSSM is based on retrospective evaluation of

cases diagnosed with PSSM by muscle biopsy[40] that are now known be free of the *GYS1* mutation and a few years of prospective clinical study.

Prevalence

Approximately 28% of PSSM cases that are diagnosed by muscle biopsy in Quarter Horses do not have the *GYS1* mutation.[75] Type 2 PSSM seems to be more common in higher performance horses such as barrel racing, reining, and cutting horses compared to the high prevalence of type 1 PSSM in halter horses. About 80% of cases of PSSM diagnosed by muscle biopsy in Warmbloods have type 2 PSSM. Breeds affected include Dutch Warmbloods, Swedish Warmbloods, Hanoverians, Friesians, Selle Francais, Westfalian, Canadian Warmblood, Irish Sport Horse, Gerdlander, Hussien, and Icelandic horses. Many other light breeds have also been diagnosed with type 2 PSSM including Morgans, Standardbreds, and Thoroughbreds. Type 2 PSSM also occurs in Arabians, however, in the author's experience, this breed is distinct in that Arabians often have amylase-resistant rather than amylase sensitive polysaccharide but are negative for the *GYS1* mutation.

Pathophysiology

The cause of type 2 PSSM is currently unknown. It may well be that there are a group of conditions that have separate etiologies but share common findings of glycogen accumulation and poor performance. A heritable predisposition is suspected in Quarter Horses but is yet to be proven.

Acute Clinical Signs

Horses with type 2 PSSM do not necessarily have the same calm temperament as horses with type 1 PSSM. In adults, acute clinical signs of rhabdomyolysis are similar between type 1 and type 2 PSSM. Muscle atrophy after rhabdomyolysis is a common complaint in Quarter Horses with type 2 PSSM and may not be preceded by exercise. There are more Quarter Horses less than 1 year of age reported with type 2 PSSM than type 1 PSSM and affected foals may present with an inability to rise or a stiff hind limb gait.

Chronic Clinical Signs

Chronic signs of type 2 PSSM are often most closely related to poor performance rather than recurrent ER and elevations in serum CK activity. An undiagnosed

gait abnormality, sore muscles, drop in energy level, and willingness to perform after 5–10 min of exercise are common complaints in Quarter Horses with type 2 PSSM. Warmbloods with type 2 PSSM have painful firm back and hindquarter muscles, reluctance to collect and engage the hindquarters, poor rounding over fences, gait abnormalities, and slow onset of atrophy. The mean onset of clinical signs in Warmbloods is between 8–11 years of age with median CK and AST activity being 323 and 331 U/L, respectively.

Diagnosis

Type 2 PSSM must be diagnosed by muscle biopsy where increased or abnormal PAS-positive, usually amylase-sensitive material is apparent, particularly in subsarcolemmal locations. Determination of what constitutes an abnormal amount of amylase-sensitive glycogen can be subjective. False positive diagnosis is possible for type 2 PSSM in highly trained horses that normally have higher muscle glycogen concentrations or in formalin fixed sections that show a greater deposition of subsarcolemmal glycogen even in healthy horses. Other histopathological features that may be present with both type 1 and type 2 PSSM include muscle necrosis, macrophage infiltration of myofibers, regenerative fibers, and fiber atrophy. Some laboratories grade polysaccharide accumulation as mild, moderate, or severe where mild accumulation represents a category which has a higher chance of being a false positive diagnosis. Mild PSSM cases in particular should receive a full physical examination to ensure that there are no other underlying causes for performance problems, such as orthopedic disease.

Management of Type 1 and Type 2 PSSM

Owners need to be aware that any horse diagnosed with PSSM will always have an underlying predilection for muscle soreness. The best that can be done is to manage horses in the most appropriate fashion to minimize clinical signs. With adherence to both the diet and exercise recommendations provided below, at least 70% of horses show notable improvement in clinical signs and many return to acceptable levels of performance.[40,71,83] There is, however, a wide range in the severity of clinical signs shown by horses with PSSM; those horses with severe or recurrent clinical signs will require more stringent adherence to diet and exercise recommendations in order to regain muscle function.

Rest

PSSM horses that are confined for days to weeks following an episode of rhabdomyolysis often have persistently elevated serum CK activity.[69] In contrast, PSSM horses kept on pasture with little grain supplementation often show few clinical signs of rhabdomyolysis and have normal serum CK activity.[69] As a result, a common recommendation for horses with PSSM is to limit stall confinement to less than 48 h after an episode of rhabdomyolysis and then provide turnout in paddocks of gradually increasing size. Providing horses with as much free exercise as possible on pasture appears to be beneficial in the long term. If pasture is lush, then a grazing muzzle may be needed.[76] Following an acute episode, excitable horses may require tranquilization prior to turn-out to avoid excessive galloping. Hand-walking horses recovering from an episode of PSSM for more than 5–10 min at a time may trigger another episode of rhabdomyolysis.

Exercise

The beneficial response to low starch fat supplemented diets only occurs if dietary change is instituted in conjunction with a regular incremental exercise program.[97] Regular daily exercise in PSSM horses over a 3-week period has been shown to produce a dramatic decrease in serum CK responses to exercise whereas stall confinement often causes elevations in serum CK activity post-exercise.[69,97] One common adaptation to daily training is an increase in oxidative capacity in skeletal muscle. The oxidative capacity of skeletal muscle in PSSM Quarter Horses was found to be very low based on markers such as citrate synthase activity and a β-fatty acid oxidative marker, β-hydroxyacl CoA dehydrogenase.[97] The activity of these enzymes, however, was equally low in control Quarter Horses. Whether the beneficial effect of daily exercise on PSSM horses is a result of improved oxidative enzyme capacities, enhanced substrate flux, or both has not been elucidated.

Important principles to follow when starting exercise programs in PSSM horses include; (1) provide adequate time for adaptation to a new diet prior to commencing exercise, (2) recognize that the duration of exercise, not the intensity, is of primary importance, (3) ensure the program is gradually introduced and consistently performed, and (4) minimize days without some form of exercise. If horses have experienced a moderate to marked episode of rhabdomyolysis recently, then 2 weeks of turn-out and diet change are often beneficial prior to recommencing exercise. Exercise should be very relaxed and the horse should have a long, low frame without collection. For many horses this is most readily done in a round pen or on a lunge line, but can be done under saddle if needed. Successive daily addition of increasing 2-min intervals of walk and trot beginning with only 4 min of exercise and working up to 30 min after 3 weeks is often recommended.[101,102] Horses that have minor elevations in CK activity 4 h after a 15-min exercise test may begin with 15 min of exercise. Owners often do not recognize that walking the horse for 10 min or more initially can trigger muscle soreness in PSSM horses. Advancing the horse too quickly often results in an episode of rhabdomyolysis and repeated frustration for the owner. Work can usually begin under saddle after 3 weeks of ground work and can gradually be increased by adding 2-min intervals of collection or canter to the initial relaxed warm-up period at a walk and trot. Unless a horse shows an episode of overt rhabdomyolysis during the initial first 4 weeks of exercise, re-evaluating serum CK activity is not helpful for the first month. This is because it is very common to have subclinical elevations in CK activity when exercise is re-introduced and a return to normal levels often requires 4–6 weeks of gradual exercise.[102] Keeping horses with PSSM fit seems the best prevention against further episodes of rhabdomyolysis.

Supplements

There are no specific supplements that have been shown to benefit horses with PSSM. Chromium which is reported to increase glucose absorption may be contraindicated in PSSM horses. Carnitine may replenish muscle carnitine stores if depleted and assist in transport of fat into the mitochondria. A deficiency of plasma carnitine has not been identified in type 1 PSSM horses. Plasma free carnitine concentration ranges from 10.24–27.11 µM/l (normal 13.20–25.63 µM/l) in horses with type 1 PSSM.

Dietary Management of PSSM

The basis for designing PSSM diets is the belief that lowering the daily starch and sugar intake and increasing dietary fat content will decrease the glucose load, increase the availability of non-esterified fatty acids for muscle metabolism, and lower serum insulin concentration.[97,98,103]

The end results of these dietary changes decrease uptake of glucose into muscles cells, decrease substrate available for and the stimulation of glycogen synthesis, and normalize substrate flux. Owners report that this type of diet improves clinical signs of muscle pain, stiffness and exercise tolerance in draft horses, warmbloods, Quarter Horses, and other breeds.[40,71,74,83] Quarter Horses naturally have very little lipid stored within muscle fibers. Dietary change appears to have lesser impact on alleviating gait changes such as Shivers.[40]

The horse's caloric requirement at an ideal body weight is the most important consideration in designing the diet for PSSM. This is because many horses with PSSM are easy keepers and may be overweight at the time of diagnosis. Adding excessive calories in the form of fat to an obese horse may produce metabolic syndrome and is contraindicated. If necessary, caloric intake should be reduced by using a grazing muzzle during turn out, feeding low NSC hay at 1.0–1.5% of body weight, and a low calorie ration balancer to meet vitamin and mineral requirements, and gradually introducing daily exercise. Rather than providing dietary fat to an overweight horse, fasting for 6 h prior to exercise can elevate plasma free fatty acids and alleviate any restrictions in energy metabolism in muscle.

Selection of forage Quarter Horses have been shown to significantly increase serum insulin concentrations in response to consuming 17% NSC hay, whereas insulin concentrations are fairly stable when fed 4% or 12% NSC hay (Figure 4.3).[98] Because insulin stimulates the already overactive glycogen synthase enzyme in the muscle of type 1 PSSM horses, selecting hay with 12% or less NSC is advisable. The degree to which the NSC content of hay should be restricted below 12% depends upon the caloric requirements of the horse. Feeding a 4% NSC hay allows room to add an adequate amount of fat without exceeding the daily caloric requirement and promoting excessive weight gain. For example, a 500-kg horse on a routine of light exercise generally requires 18 MCal/day of DE. If fed at 2% of body weight, a 12% NSC mixed grass hay almost meets the daily caloric requirement by providing 17.4 MCal/day. Thus with a 12% NSC hay, there is only room for 0.6 MCal of fat per day (72 ml of vegetable oil) to provide 18 MCal of energy. In contrast, a 4% NSC Blue Grama hay would provide 13.5 MCal/day that allows a reasonable addition of 4.5 MCal of fat per day (538 ml of vegetable oil).

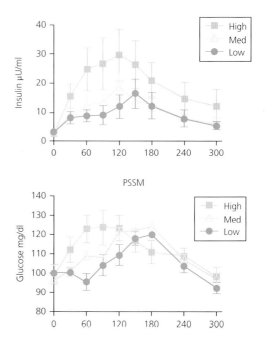

Figure 4.3 Postprandial glucose and insulin concentrations (mean ± SE) for seven type 1 PSSM-affected horses fed hay with either a high (17% NSC), medium (11% NSC), or low (4.4% NSC) NSC content. Glycemic and insulinemic responses for PSSM horses were significantly higher when fed high NSC hay than medium or low NSC hay.

Selection of fat sources High fat diets increase plasma free fatty acid concentrations and thus the availability of fats for oxidation in skeletal muscle.[97] Long chain fat diets also appear to increase glycogenolytic/glycolytic and oxidative flux in PSSM type 1 muscle as shown by higher glucose-6-phosphate, lower lactate, and higher pyruvate concentrations in muscle of PSSM type 1 horses fed and trained on a commercial high fat diet (Re-Leve®, Kentucky Equine Research, Versailles KY) compared to sweet feed.[98] Thus, one means to overcome limitations in delivery of oxidative substrates in PSSM type 1 horses is to provide ample long chain fat in the diet. The major sources of dietary fat for horses are vegetable based, including vegetable oils and rice bran. Animal based fat includes tallow, lard, and fish oil. Vegetable oils are highly unsaturated, very digestible (90–100%), and very energy dense. Suitable oils include soybean, corn, safflower, canola, flaxseed, linseed, peanut, and coconut. Controlled research studies in exercising PSSM horses have shown a decrease in muscle pain and serum CK activity in response to the

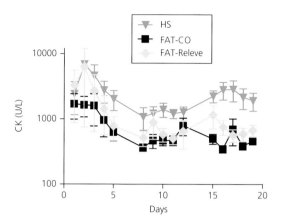

Figure 4.4 Three isocaloric diets were formulated to provide a total digestible energy of 24 MCal/day, either in the form of hay supplemented with grain (HS), corn oil with hay cubes (FAT-CO: 1.5 ml/kg/day), or 2.5 kg of a low starch, high fat concentrate (FAT-RE: Re•Leve®, Kentucky Equine Research, Versailles, KY). The oil provided 30% of digestible energy (DE) from fat whereas Re•Leve® provided 15% of DE from fat. Type 1 PSSM horses (n=8) were fed each diet for 3 weeks and exercised for up to 20 min at a walk and trot for 5 days per week. Note that 15% DE from fat significantly reduced serum CK activity in PSSM horses that were exercised and that it was not necessary to provide over 25% of DE from fat to have a significantly lower serum CK activity compared to the grain diet.

addition of corn oil,[71,83,98] soybean oil, and rice bran (Re•Leve®, Kentucky Equine Research, Versailles, KY) (Figure 4.4).[97,98] The amount of oil added in these trials constituted at least 13% of daily DE. Some veterinarians have advocated feeding as much as 25% of DE as fat to PSSM horses.[84] As discussed before, the principle consideration should be whether this provides excessive calories and additional weight gain because feeding 13% DE as fat may well be effective in reducing muscle pain (Table 4.1).

Limited research has been performed on the specific form of oil to feed PSSM horses. An odd carbon-7 chain fat (triheptanoin) fed to PSSM horses had a detrimental effect on muscle pain, exercise tolerance, and serum CK activity. Whereas in the same study, long chain fats fed as corn oil or a rice bran and soy oil supplemented feed had a beneficial effect on lowering serum CK activity.[98] Whether there is any direct beneficial effect on skeletal muscle of providing energy in the form of omega-3 versus omega-6 fatty acids has yet to be determined. Corn oil, sunflower oil, and safflower oil are high in omega-6 fatty acids and lower in omega-3 fatty acids.

Soybean and canola oils are moderately high in omega-6 and omega-3 fatty acids. Flax seed, linseed, and fish oils contain more omega-3 than omega-6 fatty acids. It is usually cost-prohibitive to provide sufficient dietary energy using omega-3 fatty acids. Soybean and canola oils provide a relatively affordable caloric alternative with moderately high omega-6 fatty acid content or a mixture of oils with flax or fish oil can be provided. Due to the potential additional oxidant stress of fats, vitamin E (1000–5000 U/day) should be fed to horses receiving high oil diets.

Low starch high fat concentrates While oils are energy dense and inexpensive, they have the disadvantages of being messy, unpalatable to some horses, prone to rancidity in warm temperatures, and difficult to feed in large amounts. As such, a number of concentrates have been developed that contain fats. An important principle is that starch and sugar components are low enough and fat supplementation is high enough to ensure that the calories supplied by NSC comprise no more than 10–15% of the daily total dietary DE and the calories supplied by fat comprise about 12–15% of daily DE (Table 4.1).[60,97] Common fat sources used in such concentrates include, in addition to the oils mentioned before, stabilized rice bran or animal fats. Rice bran and its products are palatable to most horses, have a moderate NSC content ~25% by weight, contain ~20% fat by weight as well as vitamin E, and are naturally high in phosphorus.[60] The NSC component of rice bran can vary if the manufacturing process is not careful to exclude the white rice grain. Commercial rice bran products occur as a powder or an extruded pellet and are considerably more stable in warm temperatures compared to animal fat and vegetable oils. A number of well-balanced low starch high fat commercial diets are suitable for horses with PSSM.[60,97] Some commercial feeds meet the recommended nutritional needs of PSSM horses all in one pelleted ration. These feeds typically contain at least 10–15% fat by weight and are less than 20% NSC by weight. Some feed companies offer similar nutritional content by blending two or more manufactured feeds or by supplementing with oils or rice bran. At present, the NSC content of equine feed products is not consistently listed on the feed tag and consultation with the feed manufacturer is necessary to obtain this information. Nutritional support is available through most feed manufacturers in designing an appropriate diet. There is a great deal of variation in individual tolerance to dietary starch. However, horses with more severe clinical signs of PSSM appear to require the greatest restriction in starch intake.

Expectations

The beneficial effect of low starch high fat diets also requires that horses are trained daily to enhance the enzymes involved in fat and glucose metabolism. It is important to note that a horse diagnosed with PSSM will always have an underlying predilection for muscle soreness and the best that can be done is to manage affected horses to minimize clinical signs. With adherence to both dietary and exercise recommendations, 70–75% of Quarter Horses and Warmbloods show notable improvement in clinical signs and many return to acceptable levels of performance.[40,71,76,84] However, there is a wide range in the severity of clinical signs with PSSM. Horses with severe or recurrent clinical signs will require more stringent adherence to diet and exercise recommendations in order to regain muscle function. PSSM horses that also have the mutation for MH do not respond as well to diet and exercise recommendations and may continue to develop ER with the possibility of a fatal episode.[99]

4.2.3 Hyperkalemic Periodic Paralysis

HYPP (or HPP) is not an exertional muscle disorder and it is not associated with significantly abnormal elevations in serum CK activity. Rather, HYPP occurs in resting horses and is characterized by muscle trembling in association with a rise in serum potassium concentrations. HYPP is an autosomal dominant trait in Quarter Horses or related breeds that are descended from the stallion Impressive and is associated with heavy muscling. Almost 60% of halter Quarter Horses have the genetic mutation, whereas few if any racing Quarter Horses are affected. HYPP also occurs in Paint Horses, Appaloosas, and Quarter Horse crossbreds.

4.2.3.1 Pathophysiology

Depolarization of the muscle cell membrane occurs with rapid opening of the sodium channel, an influx of sodium, and an efflux of potassium. Repolarization of the muscle cell membrane requires that the sodium channel closes and potassium re-enters the muscle cell. Horses with HYPP have a mutation in the α-subunit of the skeletal muscle sodium channel which can result in the channel being stuck in the open position that produces uncontrolled muscle twitching and trembling and depolarization block and paralysis in severe cases.[104] Horses with HYPP have similar potassium and sodium absorption, excretion, and balance compared to horses without HYPP, making it unlikely that those factors are responsible for the classic HYPP symptoms.[105,106] Rather, it appears that in both HYPP or unaffected horses, diets that contain more than 1.1% potassium (as fed) produce an increase in serum potassium concentration over 4 mmol/l within 4–6 h after the meal, likely causing entry of sodium into the mutant sodium channels and persistent depolarization of the muscle.[105,106] As muscle depolarizes, potassium is released into the circulation, resulting in even higher serum potassium concentration and further malfunction of the mutant sodium channel. Potassium excretion by the kidneys and re-uptake of potassium into cells (via the Na/K ATPase pump) usually resolves the situation. If plasma potassium concentrations continue to rise, then cardiac arrhythmias and sudden death may occur.

When most horses are fed diets containing 1.1% potassium, few postprandial changes in plasma potassium occur and signs of HYPP are minimized.[105] There is an individual variation in potassium response to a meal which may explain why some HYPP horses seem to be more prone to HYPP episodes than others. Other stressful factors such as fasting, transport, showing, clipping, anesthesia, or veterinary procedures may induce an HYPP episode in susceptible horses. For many HYPP-positive horses, however, the attacks come about without provocation.

4.2.3.2 Clinical Signs

It should be noted that many HYPP-positive horses show few or no signs of the disease in their lifetime. In other horses, intermittent episodes occur that are characterized by prolapse of the third eyelid, abnormal whinny, sweating, muscle twitches, and whole body tremors.[107] Profound weakness, difficulty breathing, collapse, and temporary paralysis may develop. Sudden death may occur. Clinical signs are twice as common in the daytime than at night.[106] Horses that are homozygous for HYPP have more severe clinical signs. Homozygous foals often have difficulty nursing, swallowing, and breathing due to pharyngeal collapse and facial and tongue muscle hypertonicity.[108]

4.2.3.3 Dietary Management

Limiting dietary potassium intake is key to management and prevention of episodes.[105,106] The objective is to feed less than 33 g of potassium per meal and feed multiple small meals or allow horses to eat continuously. This limits the amount of potassium available for absorption into the bloodstream at any given time.[106] Feeds can be submitted for nutritional analysis and feed labels checked for potassium content.

Forages

Potassium is abundant in the normal equine diet, particularly in forages (Table 4.2). Since fiber is an important dietary constituent for horses, continuous rather than meal feeding of fiber sources is a beneficial strategy to help limit major fluctuations in serum potassium concentration. For HYPP horses, total potassium in the diet should not exceed 1.1% or 33 g/day for an average sized horse. To achieve this low level of dietary potassium, forage choices narrow considerably. Hay should be tested to ensure that concentrations are <2%. Legumes, particularly alfalfa and first cutting of hay, tend to be higher in potassium and should be used sparingly or not at all in the diets of HYPP-positive horses. Grass forages generally contain 1–2% potassium and can be paired with a low-potassium cereal grain and an all-purpose vitamin and mineral supplement. HYPP horses should be turned out on grass pastures with low legume content. Beet pulp is a highly fermentable fiber source that is low in

Table 4.2 Potassium Content of Common Horse Feeds. Potassium content varies in all feedstuffs and these values are guidelines only. Data from ADM Alliance Nutrition, Inc. (www.admani.com/horse/Equine%20Library/Horse%20Potassium%20In%20Feed.htm).

	Potassium (%)	Potassium (g/lb of feed)
High potassium feeds		
Electrolyte supplements	~30	136
Sugar beet and cane molasses	6	27
Some kelp supplements	>4	>18
Alfalfa hay	1.4–2.4	6.4–10.9
Soybean meal	2	9.1
Reed canary grass	2.6	11.8
Orchard grass	2.4–2.6	10.9–11.8
Medium Potassium Feeds		
Clover hay	1.6–1.9	7.3–8.2
Fescue hay	1.7–2.1	7.7–9.5
Rice bran	1.8	8.1
Timothy	1.4–2.1	6.4–9.5
Brome	1.7	7.7
Coastal bermudagrass	1.2–1.9	5.5–8.2
Kentucky bluegrass	1.4	6.4
Oat hay	1.4	6.4
Low Potassium Feeds		
Pure fats and oils	0	0
Beet pulp (without molasses)	0.2–0.3	0.9–1.4
Corn	0.3	1.4
Oats	0.4	1.8
Barley	0.5	2.3
Pasture grass (23% DM)	0.3–0.8	1.4–3.6
Wheat	0.4	1.8
Wheat middlings	1.0	4.5
Wheat bran	1.2	5.5
Soybean hulls	1.2	5.5

potassium and commonly included as a low potassium forage alternative in rations for HYPP-affected horses.

Concentrates

Oats are ideal whereas commercially prepared sweet and pelleted feeds that contain molasses or soybean meal should be avoided as they are higher in potassium (Table 4.2).

Supplements

Even though mineral supplements likely contain potassium, when fed in recommended amounts the total diet will not contain excessive potassium. In contrast, most commercial electrolytes are unsuitable for HYPP horses as they usually contain high levels of potassium.

References

1. Dill SG, Rebhun WC. White muscle disease in foals. Comp Cont Educ Pract Vet 1985;7:S627–S636.
2. Divers TJ, Mohammed HO, Cummings JF, et al. Equine motor neuron disease: findings in 28 horses and proposal of a pathophysiological mechanism for the disease. Equine Vet J 1994;26:409–415.
3. Maylin GA, Rubin DS, Lein DH. Selenium and vitamin E in horses. Cornell Vet 1980;70:272–289.
4. McMurray CH, Rice DA. Vitamin E and selenium deficiency diseases. Irish Vet J 1982;36:57–67.
5. Perkins G, Valberg SJ, Madigan JM, et al. Electrolyte disturbances in foals with severe rhabdomyolysis. J Vet Intern Med 1998;12:173–177.
6. National Research Council. Nutrient requirements of beef cattle. National Academy Press: Washington, DC, 1976.
7. Moncada S, Vane JR. Arachidonic acid metabolites and the interactions between platelets and blood-vessel walls. N Engl J Med 1979;300:1142–1147.
8. Finno CJ, Valberg SJ. A comparative review of vitamin E and associated equine disorders. J Vet Intern Med 2012;26;1251–1266.
9. Valberg SJ. Diseases of muscle. In: Smith BP, ed. Large animal internal medicine, 3rd ed. St Louis: Mosby, 2002;1272–1273.
10. Taylor RF, Puls R, MacDonald KR. Bovine abortions associated with selenium deficiency in western Canada. Proc Am Assoc Vet Lab Diagnost 1979;22:77–84.
11. Roneus B. Glutathione peroxidase and selenium in the blood of healthy horses and foals affected by muscular dystrophy. Nord Vet Med 1982;34:350–353.
12. Campbell DT, Maas J, Weber DW, et al. Safety and efficacy of two sustained-release intrareticular selenium supplements and the associated placental and colostral transfer of selenium in beef cattle. Am J Vet Res 1990;51:813–817.
13. Koller LD, Whitbeck GA, South PJ. Transplacental transfer and colostral concentrations of selenium in beef cattle. Am J Vet Res 1984;45:2507–2510.
14. Divers T, Mohammed H. Equine motor neuron disease. In: Robinson NE, Sprayberry KA, eds. Current therapy in equine medicine 6. St Louis: Saunders, 2009;615–617.
15. Divers TJ, Mohammed HO, Cummings JF. Equine motor neuron disease. Vet Clin North Am Equine Pract 1997;13:97–105.
16. De la Rúa-Doménech R, Mohammed HO, Cummings JF, et al. Association between plasma vitamin E concentration and the risk of equine motor neuron disease. Vet J 1997;154:203–213.
17. De la Rúa-Doménech R, Mohammed HO, Cummings JF, et al. Intrinsic, management, and nutritional factors associated with equine motor neuron disease. J Am Vet Med Assoc 1997;211:1261–1267.
18. De la Rúa-Doménech R, Mohammed HO, Cummings JF, et al. Incidence and risk factors of equine motor neuron disease: an ambidirectional study. Neuroepidemiology 1995;14:54–64.
19. McGorum BC, Mayhew IG, Amory H, et al. Horses on pasture may be affected by equine motor neuron disease. Equine Vet J 2006;38:47–51.
20. Valentine BA, de Lahunta A, George C, et al. Acquired equine motor neuron disease. Vet Pathol 1994;31:130–138.
21. Mohammed HO, Divers TJ, Summers BA, et al. Vitamin E deficiency and risk of equine motor neuron disease. Acta Vet Scand 2007;49:17.
22. Divers TJ, Cummings JE, de Lahunta A, et al. Evaluation of the risk of motor neuron disease in horses fed a diet low in vitamin E and high in copper and iron. Am J Vet Res 2006;67:120–126.
23. Higgins JK, Puschner B, Kass PH, et al. Assessment of vitamin E concentrations in serum and cerebrospinal fluid of horses following oral administration of vitamin E. Am J Vet Res 2008;69:785–790.
24. Pusterla N, Puschner B, Steidl S, et al. Alpha-tocopherol concentrations in equine serum and cerebrospinal fluid after vitamin E supplementation. Vet Rec 2010;166:366–368.
25. Bedford HE, Valberg SJ, Firshman AM, et al. Histopathologic findings in the sacrocaudalis dorsalis medialis muscle of horses with vitamin E-responsive muscle atrophy and weakness. J Am Vet Med Assoc 2013;242:1127–1137.
26. Valberg SJ, Carlson GP, Cardinet GH, et al. Skeletal muscle mitochondrial myopathy as a cause of exercise intolerance in a horse. Muscle Nerve 1994;17:305–312.
27. Tyynismaa H, Carroll CJ, Raimundo N, et al. Mitochondrial myopathy induces a starvation-like response. Hum Mol Genet 2010;19:3948–3958.
28. Carlson GP. Medical problems associated with protracted heat and work stress in horses, in Proceedings. Assoc Equine Sports Med 1985;84–99.

29. Harris P, Colles C. The use of creatinine clearance ratios in the prevention of equine rhabdomyolysis: a report of four cases. Equine Vet J 1988;20:459–63.

30. Schott HC, McGlade KS, Molander HA, et al. Body weight, fluid, electrolyte, and hormonal changes in horses competing in 50- and 100-mile endurance rides. Am J Vet Res 1997;58:303–309.

31. McKenzie EC, Valberg SJ, Godden SM, et al. Comparison of volumetric urine collection versus single-sample urine collection in horses consuming diets varying in cation-anion balance. Am J Vet Res 64: 2003;284–291.

32. Harris PA, Snow DH. Role of electrolyte imbalances in the pathophysiology of the equine rhabdomyolysis syndrome. In: Persson S, Lindholm A, Jeffcott LB, eds. Equine exercise physiology 3. Davis CA: ICEEP, 1991;435–442.

33. Beech J. Chronic exertional rhabdomyolysis. Vet Clin North Am Equine Pract 1997;13:145–168.

34. Beech J, Lindborg S, Fletcher JE, et al. Caffeine contractures, twitch characteristics and the threshold for Ca$^{(2+)}$-induced Ca2+ release in skeletal muscle from horses with chronic intermittent rhabdomyolysis. Res Vet Sci 1993;54:110–117.

35. Valberg SJ, Mickelson JR, Gallant EM, et al. Exertional rhabdomyolysis in quarter horses and thoroughbreds: one syndrome, multiple aetiologies. Equine Vet J Suppl 1999;30:533–538.

36. Isgren CM, Upjohn MM, Fernandez-Fuente M, et al. Epidemiology of exertional rhabdomyolysis susceptibility in standardbred horses reveals associated risk factors and underlying enhanced performance. PLoS One 2010;5(7):e11594.

37. MacLeay JM, Sorum SA, Valberg SJ, et al. Epidemiologic analysis of factors influencing exertional rhabdomyolysis in Thoroughbreds. Am J Vet Res 1999;60:1562–1566.

38. McGowan CM, Fordham T, Christley RM. Incidence and risk factors for exertional rhabdomyolysis in thoroughbred racehorses in the United Kingdom. Vet Rec 2002;151:623–626.

39. Hildebrand SV, Arpin D, Cardinet G. Contracture test and histologic and histochemical analyses of muscle biopsy specimens from horses with exertional rhabdomyolysis. J Am Vet Med Assoc 1990;196:1077–1083.

40. Lentz LR, Valberg SJ, Balog EM, et al. Abnormal regulation of muscle contraction in horses with recurrent exertional rhabdomyolysis. Am J Vet Res 1999;60:992–999.

41. Hunt LM, Valberg SJ, Steffenhagen K, et al. An epidemiological study of myopathies in Warmblood horses. Equine Vet J 2008;40:171–177.

42. Valberg S, Jonsson L, Lindholm A, et al. Muscle histopathology and plasma aspartate aminotransferase, creatine kinase and myoglobin changes with exercise in horses with recurrent exertional rhabdomyolysis. Equine Vet J 1993;25:11–16.

43. MacLeay JM, Valberg SJ, Pagan JD, et al. Effect of ration and exercise on plasma creatine kinase activity and lactate concentration in Thoroughbred horses with recurrent exertional rhabdomyolysis. Am J Vet Res 2000;61:1390–1395.

44. McKenzie EC, Valberg SJ, Godden SM, et al. Effect of dietary starch, fat, and bicarbonate content on exercise responses and serum creatine kinase activity in equine recurrent exertional rhabdomyolysis. J Vet Intern Med 2003;17:693–701.

45. Valberg S, Haggendal J, Lindholm A. Blood chemistry and skeletal muscle metabolic responses to exercise in horses with recurrent exertional rhabdomyolysis. Equine Vet J 1993;25:17–22.

46. Valberg SJ. Metabolic response to racing and fiber properties of skeletal muscle in standardbred and thoroughbred horses. J Equine Vet Sci 1987 January 1;7:6.

47. Valberg S, Gustavsson BE, Lindholm A, et al. Blood chemistry and skeletal muscle metabolic responses during and after different speeds and durations of trotting. Equine Vet J 1989;21 91–95.

48. Lentz LR, Valberg SJ, Herold LV, et al. Myoplasmic calcium regulation in myotubes from horses with recurrent exertional rhabdomyolysis. Am J Vet Res 2002;63:1724–1731.

49. Lopez JR, Linares N, Cordovez G, et al. Elevated myoplasmic calcium in exercise-induced equine rhabdomyolysis. Pflugers Arch 1995;430:293–295.

50. Cole FL, Mellor DJ, Hodgson DR, et al. Prevalence and demographic characteristics of exertional rhabdomyolysis in horses in Australia. Vet Rec 2004;155:625–630.

51. Upjohn MM, Archer RM, Christley RM, et al. Incidence and risk factors associated with exertional rhabdomyolysis syndrome in National Hunt racehorses in Great Britain. Vet Rec 2005;156:763–766.

52. Dranchak PK, Valberg SJ, Onan GW, et al. Inheritance of recurrent exertional rhabdomyolysis in thoroughbreds. J Am Vet Med Assoc 2005;227:762–767.

53. MacLeay JM, Valberg SJ, Sorum SA, et al. Heritability of recurrent exertional rhabdomyolysis in Thoroughbred racehorses. Am J Vet Res 1999;60:250–256.

54. Quiroz-Rothe E, Novales M, Guilera-Tejero E, et al. Polysaccharide storage myopathy in the M. longissimus lumborum of showjumpers and dressage horses with back pain. Equine Vet J 2002;34:171–176.

55. Freestone JF, Wolfsheimer KJ, Kamerling SG, et al. Exercise induced hormonal and metabolic changes in Thoroughbred horses: effects of conditioning and acepromazine. Equine Vet J 1991;23:219–223.

56. Wang R, Zhong X, Meng X, et al. Localization of the dantrolene-binding sequence near the FK506-binding protein-binding site in the three-dimensional structure of the ryanodine receptor. J Biol Chem 2011;286:12202–12212.

57. Beech J, Fletcher JE, Lizzo F, et al. Effect of phenytoin on the clinical signs and in vitro muscle twitch characteristics in horses with chronic intermittent rhabdomyolysis and myotonia. Am J Vet Res 1988;49:2130–2133.

58. Tiidus PM. Manual massage and recovery of muscle function following exercise: a literature review. J Orthop Sports Phys Ther 1997;25:107–112.

59. Weerapong P, Hume PA, Kolt GS. The mechanisms of massage and effects on performance, muscle recovery and injury prevention. Sports Med 2005;35:235–56.

60. Zainuddin Z, Newton M, Sacco P, et al. Effects of massage on delayed-onset muscle soreness, swelling, and recovery of muscle function. J Athl Train 2005;40:174–180.

61. McKenzie EC, Firshman AM. Optimal diet of horses with chronic exertional myopathies. Vet Clin North Am Equine Pract 2009;25:121–135.

62. Borgia LA. Resistance training and the effect of feeding carbohydrates and oils on healthy horses and horses with polysaccharide storage myopathy. PhD dissertation, University of Minnesota (2010).

63. MacLeay JM, Valberg SJ, Pagan JD, et al. Effect of diet on thoroughbred horses with recurrent exertional rhabdomyolysis performing a standardised exercise test. Equine Vet J Suppl 1999;30:458–462.

64. Finno CJ, McKenzie E, Valberg SJ, et al. Effect of fitness on glucose, insulin and cortisol responses to diets varying in starch and fat content in Thoroughbred horses with recurrent exertional rhabdomyolysis. Equine Vet J Suppl 2010;38:323–328.

65. Valberg SJ, Cardinet GH, III, Carlson GP, et al. Polysaccharide storage myopathy associated with recurrent exertional rhabdomyolysis in horses. Neuromuscul Disord 1992; 2:351–359.

66. Andrews FM, Spurgeon TL, Reed SM. Histochemical changes in skeletal muscles of four male horses with neuromuscular disease. Am J Vet Res 1986;47:2078–2083.

67. Arighi M, Hulland TJ. Equine exertional rhabdomyolysis. Compend Cont Educ Pract Vet 1984;6:S726–S732.

68. Cardinet GH, Holliday TA. Neuromuscular diseases of domestic animals: a summary of muscle biopsies from 159 cases. Ann N Y Acad Sci 1979;317:290–313.

69. Valentine BA, Credille KM, Lavoie JP, et al. Severe polysaccharide storage myopathy in Belgian and Percheron draught horses. Equine Vet J 1997;29:220–225.

70. De La Corte FD, Valberg SJ, MacLeay JM, et al. Developmental onset of polysaccharide storage myopathy in 4 Quarter Horse foals. J Vet Intern Med 2002;16: 581–587.

71. Firshman AM, Baird JD, Valberg SJ. Prevalences and clinical signs of polysaccharide storage myopathy and shivers in Belgian draft horses. J Am Vet Med Assoc 2005;227:1958–1964.

72. Firshman AM, Valberg SJ, Bender JB, et al. Epidemiologic characteristics and management of polysaccharide storage myopathy in Quarter Horses. Am J Vet Res 2003;64: 1319–1327.

73. Herszberg B, McCue ME, Larcher T, et al. A GYS1 gene mutation is highly associated with polysaccharide storage myopathy in Cob Normand draught horses. Anim Genet 2009;40:94–96.

74. Johlig L, Valberg SJ, Mickelson JR, et al. Epidemiological and genetic study of exertional rhabdomyolysis in a warmblood horse family in Switzerland. Equine Vet J 2011;43:240–245.

75. McCue ME, Ribeiro WP, Valberg SJ. Prevalence of polysaccharide storage myopathy in horses with neuromuscular disorders. Equine Vet J Suppl 2006;36:340–344.

76. McGowan CM, Menzies-Gow NJ, McDiarmid AM, et al. Four cases of equine polysaccharide storage myopathy in the United Kingdom. Vet Rec 2003;152:109–112.

77. Stanley RL, McCue ME, Valberg SJ, et al. A glycogen synthase 1 mutation associated with equine polysaccharide storage myopathy and exertional rhabdomyolysis occurs in a variety of UK breeds. Equine Vet J 2009;41:597–601.

78. Valentine BA. Polysaccharide storage myopathy: a common metabolic disorder of horses. Vet Pathol 2002;39:630.

79. Valentine BA, Cooper BJ. Incidence of polysaccharide storage myopathy: necropsy study of 225 horses. Vet Pathol 2005;42:823–827.

80. Valentine BA, Habecker PL, Patterson JS, et al. Incidence of polysaccharide storage myopathy in draft horse-related breeds: a necropsy study of 37 horses and a mule. J Vet Diagn Invest 2001;13:63–68.

81. Valentine BA, McDonough SP, Chang YF, et al. Polysaccharide storage myopathy in Morgan, Arabian, and Standardbred related horses and Welsh-cross ponies. Vet Pathol 2000;37:193–196.

82. Valberg SJ, MacLeay JM, Billstrom JA, et al. Skeletal muscle metabolic response to exercise in horses with "tying-up" due to polysaccharide storage myopathy. Equine Vet J 1999;31:43–47.

83. Valentine BA, Van Saun RJ, Thompson KN, et al. Role of dietary carbohydrate and fat in horses with equine polysaccharide storage myopathy. J Am Vet Med Assoc 2001;219: 1537–1544.

84. Valentine BA, Hintz HF, Freels KM, et al. Dietary control of exertional rhabdomyolysis in horses. J Am Vet Med Assoc 1998;212:1588–1593.

85. McCue ME, Valberg SJ, Miller MB, et al. Glycogen synthase (GYS1) mutation causes a novel skeletal muscle glycogenosis. Genomics 2008;91:458–466.

86. McCue ME, Valberg SJ, Lucio M, et al. Glycogen synthase 1 (GYS1) mutation in diverse breeds with polysaccharide storage myopathy. J Vet Intern Med 2008;22: 1228–1233.

87. McCue ME, Armien AG, Lucio M, et al. Comparative skeletal muscle histopathologic and ultrastructural features in two forms of polysaccharide storage myopathy in horses. Vet Pathol 2009;46:1281–1291.

88. Carlström B. Uber die atiologie und pathogenese de Pferdes (Haemoglobinaemia paralytica). Scand Archiv Physiol 1931;61:161–224.

89. Carlström B. Uber die atiologie und pathogenese der kreuzlahme des pferdes (Haemaglobinaemia paralytica). Scand Archiv 1932;62:1–62.

90. McLean JG. Equine paralytic myoglobinuria ("azoturia"): a review. Aust Vet J 1973;49:41–43.

91. Baird JD, Valberg SJ, Anderson SM, et al. Presence of the glycogen synthase 1 (GYS1) mutation causing type 1 polysaccharide storage myopathy in continental European draught horse breeds. Vet Rec 2010;167:781–784.

92. McCue ME, Anderson SM, Valberg SJ, et al. Estimated prevalence of the type 1 polysaccharide storage myopathy mutation in selected North American and European breeds. Anim Genet Suppl 2010;2(41):145–149.

93. McCue ME, Valberg SJ. Estimated prevalence of polysaccharide storage myopathy among overtly healthy Quarter Horses in the United States. Am J Vet Res 2007;231:746–750.

94. Tryon RC, Penedo MC, McCue ME, et al. Evaluation of allele frequencies of inherited disease genes in subgroups of American Quarter Horses. J Am Vet Med Assoc 2009;234:120–125.

95. Annandale EJ, Valberg SJ, Mickelson JR, et al. Insulin sensitivity and skeletal muscle glucose transport in horses with equine polysaccharide storage myopathy. Neuromuscul Disord 2004;14:666–674.

96. Annandale EJ, Valberg SJ, Essen-Gustavsson B. Effects of submaximal exercise on adenine nucleotide concentrations in skeletal muscle fibers of horses with polysaccharide storage myopathy. Am J Vet Res 2005;66:839–845.

97. Ribeiro WP, Valberg SJ, Pagan JD, et al. The effect of varying dietary starch and fat content on serum creatine kinase activity and substrate availability in equine polysaccharide storage myopathy. J Vet Intern Med 2004;18:887–894.

98. Borgia LA, Valberg SJ, McCue ME, et al. Effect of dietary fats with odd or even numbers of carbon atoms on metabolic response and muscle damage with exercise in Quarter Horse-type horses with type 1 polysaccharide storage myopathy. Am J Vet Res 2010;71 326–336.

99. McCue ME, Valberg SJ, Jackson M, et al. Polysaccharide storage myopathy phenotype in Quarter Horse-related breeds is modified by the presence of an RYR1 mutation. Neuromuscl Disord 2009;19:37–43.

100. Sprayberry KA, Madigan J, Lecouteur RA, et al. Renal failure, laminitis, and colitis following severe rhabdomyolysis in a draft horse-cross with polysaccharide storage myopathy. Can Vet J 1998;39:500–503.

101. Valberg SJ, Dyson S. Skeletal muscle and lameness. In: Ross M, Dyson S, eds. Lameness in the horse. Philadelphia: Saunders, 2003;723–743.

102. Valberg SJ, MacLeay JM, Mickelson JR. Polysaccharide storage myopathy associated with exertional rhabdomyolysis in horses. Comp Cont Educ Pract Vet 1997;19:1077–1086.

103. Valberg SJ, McCue ME, Mickelson JR. The interplay of genetics, exercise and nutrition in polysaccharide storage myopathy. J Equine Vet Sci 2011;31:205–210.

104. Rudolph JA, Spier SJ, Byrns G, et al. Periodic paralysis in quarter horses: a sodium channel mutation disseminated by selective breeding. Nat Genet 1992;2:144–147.

105. Reynolds AJ. Equine hyperkalemic periodic paralysis (HYPP): overview & management strategies. Available at: www.admani.com/horse/Equine%20Library/Horse%20Equine%20HYPP.htm 2004. Accessed [October 24, 2016].

106. Reynolds JA, Potter GD, Greene LW. Genetic-diet interactions in the hyperkalemic periodic paralysis syndrome in Quarter Horses fed varying amounts of potassium: III. The relationship between plasma potassium concentration and HYPP Symptoms. J Equine Vet Sci 1998;18:731–735.

107. Spier SJ, Carlson GP, Holliday TA, et al. Hyperkalemic periodic paralysis in horses. J Am Vet Med Assoc 1990;197:1009–1017.

108. Carr EA, Spier SJ, Kortz GD, et al. Laryngeal and pharyngeal dysfunction in horses homozygous for hyperkalemic periodic paralysis. J Am Vet Med Assoc 1996;209:798–803.

5 Endocrine system

Iveta Becvarova, DVM, MS, DACVN

5.1 Equine Metabolic Syndrome

5.1.1 Definition of Equine Metabolic Syndrome

Equine metabolic syndrome (EMS) is not a specific disease but a group of clinical and laboratory symptoms that include: (1) obesity (generalized or regional), (2) hyperinsulinemia and insulin resistance, and (3) clinical or subclinical laminitis. Horses and ponies with EMS are predisposed to laminitis. The presence of an increasing number of these clinical and laboratory abnormalities can predict likelihood of development of laminitis with chronic or acute nature.

5.1.1.1 Synonyms

Peripheral Cushing's syndrome; Prelaminitic metabolic syndrome.

5.1.2 Epidemiology

Epidemiology of EMS is limited to few published studies on prevalence of obesity and hyperinsulinemia. In one recent study, the prevalence of hyperinsulinemia in a population of 300 healthy horses from central Ohio was 22.3%.[1] Another study of 300 randomly selected horses from southwest Virginia revealed that 51% of horses were overweight and obese and 10% were hyperinsulinemic.[2] The concept of EMS was first proposed in 2002 and evolved into the characterization of EMS in a consensus statement released by the American College of Veterinary Internal Medicine (ACVIM).[3]

Metabolic syndrome was first described in humans and characterized by a group of symptoms (i.e., glucose intolerance, insulin resistance, dyslipidemia, microalbuminuria, and hypertension) that increase the risk of cardiovascular disease.[4] Equine metabolic syndrome has several close similarities with human metabolic syndrome, including obesity, insulin resistance, and hyperlipidemia but instead of an increased the risk of cardiovascular

disease, the major outcome in horses is development of laminitis. Laminitis has been historically associated with onset of gastrointestinal disorders, retained placenta, metritis, and severe infections. However, results of recent studies suggest that insulin resistance, a component of EMS, represents the leading endocrine disorder responsible for equine laminitis.

5.1.3 Species, Age, and Sex Predisposition

Equine metabolic syndrome can affect all classes of equids, including ponies, horses, miniature horses, and donkeys. Obesity can develop when animals reach maturity and consequent laminitis is most often diagnosed between 5–15 years of age.[3] In one study, the prevalence of pasture associated laminitis in ponies was eight-fold lower in mature stallions than females and was associated with high body condition score and decreased insulin sensitivity.[5]

5.1.4 Genetics and Breed Predisposition

Equids belong to a species that evolved in nutritionally sparse environments and their survival likely depended on thrifty genes and insulin resistance.[6] The advantage of tissue resistance to insulin resides in glucose sparing and its utilization for energy. It is possible that grazers like equids thrived on this evolutionary advantage until establishment of new and modern management practices. In humans, a dominant mode of inheritance has been suggested for metabolic syndrome.[7] Genetic make-up of horses predisposed to EMS is not known, but familial patterns have been identified in ponies.[5] Most ponies and horses affected by EMS have a typical phenotype described as an "easy keeper." In one study in ponies, a mode of inheritance of laminitis was consistent with segregation of a major dominant gene or genes, which were especially evident in females.[5] In this study, nearly all ponies with history of laminitis were immediate descendants of laminitic females and all

Nutritional Management of Equine Diseases and Special Cases, First Edition. Edited by Bryan M. Waldridge.
© 2017 John Wiley & Sons, Inc. Published 2017 by John Wiley & Sons, Inc.

female offspring of one stallion with history of laminitis developed laminitis. Molecular characterization of such a major gene could provide a screening tool for predisposition to laminitis.

Equine metabolic syndrome occurs most frequently in pony breeds, Morgan Horses, Paso Finos, Arabians, Saddlebreds, Spanish Mustangs, warmblood breeds, Quarter horses, and Tennessee Walking horses. Breeds with rare occurrence of EMS include Thoroughbreds and Standardbreds.

5.1.5 Risk Factors

There are two major environmental risk factors for development of EMS: (1) overfeeding calories (energy) and (2) lack of exercise, both leading to obesity. The EMS phenotype may either remain latent or be expressed under certain conditions such as positive energy balance, increased intake of non-structural carbohydrates (NSC), or an overweight or obese body condition.

5.1.6 Geography and Seasonality

Seasonality has been recognized in occurrence of laminitis in populations of equids in the United States and United Kingdom. The highest incidence of pasture laminitis in US is during the late spring and early summer (May–June) and during the summer months (June, July) in the UK.[5,8,9] This seasonal occurrence of laminitis closely correlates with pasture NSC content. Fructan, which represents a major portion of the NSC in certain types of grasses under specific conditions, has been implicated in the etiology of pasture associated laminitis. Carbohydrates, including fructans, are synthesized in forages during periods of high sunshine through photosynthesis and are used for plant growth and development. Carbohydrates not utilized for growth are stored within the plant as fructans and starches. Factors that limit pasture growth can be responsible for decreased usage and increased accumulation of storage carbohydrates within the plant.

5.1.7 Associated Conditions and Disorders

In addition to the three major components of EMS, such as obesity, insulin resistance, and laminitis, there are several additional components to consider. These include hypertriglyceridemia,[5,10,11] altered reproductive cycling in mares,[12,13] hyperleptinemia,[14] seasonal

alterations in arterial blood pressure,[15] and increased systemic markers of inflammation associated with obesity.[16]

5.1.8 Clinical Presentation

5.1.8.1 Equine Metabolic Syndrome Forms and Subtypes

The majority of horses affected by EMS have generalized obesity or regional adiposity (increased adiposity in specific locations), such as "cresty neck" appearance, fat pads close to the tail head, behind the shoulder, and in the prepuce or mammary gland (see Figures 5.1 and 5.2). Furthermore, insulin resistance characterized by hyperinsulinemia and clinical or subclinical laminitis develop in the absence of grain overload, colic, colitis, or metritis. Some cases also present with hyperlipidemia or dyslipidemia, hyperleptinemia, arterial hypertension, and altered reproductive cycling.

5.1.8.2 History and Principal Complaint

Horses affected by EMS have a history of obesity, lack of exercise, and recurrent episodes of mild bilateral laminitis. Horses with EMS are described as easy to keep their body weight on a low plane of nutrition (easy keeper or EMS phenotype).

Dietary history is extremely important for the diagnosis and for the management of the EMS. Prolonged excessive caloric intake and consequent obesity can result from overfeeding grains and concentrates, but also from overconsumption of pasture or hay. Laminitis that develops after the animal has been grazing on a lush pasture is referred to as pasture associated laminitis. Therefore, information should be obtained on the quantity (by weight) and frequency of all feeds and supplements fed, frequency and duration of grazing, recent move to a new lush pasture, inspection of the pasture area, and quality of the forage.

In order to obtain good dietary history, labels with nutrient profiles from bagged concentrates should be collected for further evaluation. A representative sample of the forage should be submitted for nutritional analysis. The hay sample should be taken with a hay corer and the pasture should be sampled by collecting clippings of fresh grass. The forage sample should be sent to a laboratory that specializes in horse feed analyses (e.g., Equi-analytical Laboratories, Ithaca, NY). When evaluating forages,

Figure 5.1 A pony with generalized obesity, body condition score of 9, and the Equine Metabolic Syndrome phenotype.

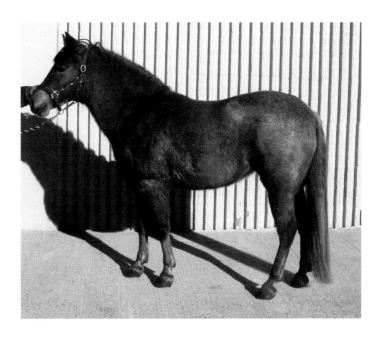

Figure 5.2 A pony exhibiting enlargement of adipose tissue within the neck region ("cresty neck"). Cresty neck score 4 (crest grossly enlarged and thickened and can no longer be cupped in one hand or easily bent from side to side. The crest may have wrinkles perpendicular to topline). Source: Carter 2009[10]. Reproduced with permission of Elsevier.

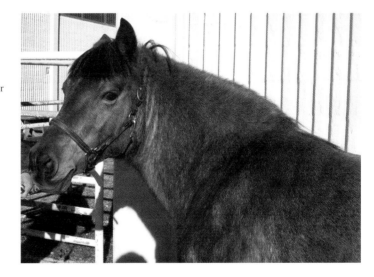

special attention should be paid to selected parameters from the nutritional analysis, such as digestible energy (DE; Mcal/kg), water soluble carbohydrates (WSC), starch content, and NSC content (NSC = WSC + starch). High values may reveal nutritional factors exacerbating EMS and these values can be used as a benchmark for dietary modification. Conversely, low values of neutral detergent fiber (NDF) and acid detergent fiber (ADF) are

signs of increased energy density, improved digestibility, and higher daily intake by horses.

5.1.8.3 Physical Examination Findings

Clinical signs associated with EMS include generalized obesity, regional adiposity, bilateral forelimb lameness, and divergent growth rings (founder lines) on the hooves as evidence of previous laminitis. Initial clinical signs of laminitis include reluctance to move, bounding digital pulses, and increased temperature of the hoof surface. Obese geldings affected by EMS may develop preputial swelling and edema as a result of adipose tissue accumulation and reduced lymphatic return. Adipose expansion into the udder can also be observed in mares with EMS.[17]

5.1.8.4 Etiology and Pathophysiology
Hyperinsulinemia and Insulin Resistance
The driving force of EMS appears to be the development of persistent hyperinsulinemia. Insulin is an anabolic hormone that stimulates liver glycogen synthesis and lipogenesis and inhibits gluconeogenesis and lipolysis. Insulin receptors are highly expressed in the liver, muscle, pancreas, adipose tissue, and vascular cells.[18] Hyperinsulinemia is a compensatory mechanism to overcome decreasing effectiveness of peripheral tissues to metabolize glucose (i.e., insulin resistance). As a result of insulin resistance in peripheral tissues, pancreatic beta-cells secrete more insulin, which can be measured as an elevated resting plasma or serum insulin concentration. Hyperinsulinemia can result from increased pancreatic insulin secretion in response to reduced insulin sensitivity[9] but also from reduced hepatic insulin clearance[19] (see Figure 5.3).

Two major hypotheses describing the mechanism of insulin resistance exist and both are associated with increased adiposity. The first hypothesis describes insulin resistance as the result of lipid overload in the liver and muscle cells leading to defects in insulin signaling. The second theory emphasizes the role of lipid accumulation in adipose tissue, which leads to the release of adipokines and development of chronic local inflammation that modulates the response of adipose to insulin (lipotoxicity).[20]

Insulin is cleared from plasma by the liver and any alteration in liver function can reduce insulin clearance. Lipid accumulation in the liver as well as higher plasma gamma-glutamyl transferase (GGT) and aspartate aminotransferase (AST) activities were detected in certain horses with EMS, which might represent a risk factor for development of hyperinsulinemia.[17]

Insulin sensitivity in equids is not only driven by adiposity, but seasonal fluctuations may also occur. In one study, obese mares had higher resting serum insulin concentrations in December compared to September, October, and November.[13]

5.1.8.5 Obesity
Obesity and overweight body condition are the result of an imbalance between energy intake and energy expenditure and are caused by environmental factors such as

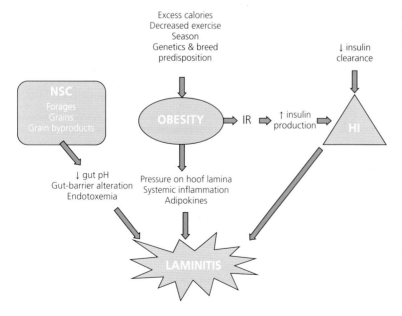

Figure 5.3 Factors suggested in pathogenesis of laminitis in equids with equine metabolic syndrome.

diet, decreased exercise, season, and genetic factors (see Figure 5.3). Horses and ponies with EMS phenotype appear to have high metabolic efficiency, which increases capability to accumulate adipose tissue. Studies clearly demonstrate that obesity is associated with reduced insulin sensitivity in horses and ponies.[1,11–13,21] However, not every obese horse is resistant to insulin. Furthermore, obese animals are more likely to develop pasture associated laminitis if they are insulin resistant.[10,11] The mechanism(s) by which insulin resistance increases susceptibility to pasture associated laminitis has not yet been clarified.

Other effects of obesity in equids include increased pressure on the hoof lamina, production of hormones (adipokines) by adipocytes, and release of inflammatory cytokines by macrophages residing in adipose tissue (see Figure 5.3). Leptin is an adipokine released by adipose cells and inhibits appetite through receptors on neurons within the arcuate nucleus of the hypothalamus. Hyperleptinemia is associated with obesity[11,22] and represents a mechanism by which the body sends signals to lower the feed intake. Hyperleptinemia has been detected in insulin resistant horses and ponies[10,11] and this might represent a state of leptin resistance. Conversely, adiponectin is an adipokine with appetite stimulating properties and blood concentrations are positively correlated with insulin sensitivity in animals.[23]

Growing evidence has pointed to a correlative and causative relationship between obesity-induced systemic inflammation and insulin resistance. The proinflammatory cytokine tumor necrosis factor-α (TNF-α) has been demonstrated to mediate insulin resistance in many rodent obesity models.[24,25] It is hypothesized that when adiposity reaches a certain threshold, factors derived from adipocytes induce macrophage activation and infiltration (chemotaxis). Activated macrophages secrete cytokines that can impair adipocyte insulin sensitivity and stimulate further activation and infiltration of peripheral monocytes and macrophages into fat. In one study, obese horses had increased expression of TNF-α and interleukin-1β in the blood, which provided evidence of systemic inflammation associated with obesity.[16] However, no differences in inflammatory cytokine expression were found when comparing adipose tissue of insulin resistant horses and their controls.[26] More research is needed to elucidate relationship of obesity induced systemic inflammation and insulin resistance in horses.

The prevalence of obesity is growing in the general equine population. A recent study of 300 randomly selected horses from southwest Virginia[2] found that 19% of the horses were obese, an additional 32% were overconditioned, and 10% had elevated blood insulin levels. A strong positive association between hyperinsulinemia and adiposity was determined, as 18% of the overconditioned or obese horses were hyperinsulinemic versus only 1.4% of optimally conditioned or underconditioned horses.[2] Of interest was that most of the horses in the study were kept at pasture and were not fed grain or other concentrate feeds as part of their diet. As well, the majority of horses were classified as receiving little or no exercise.

Pastures offer the most natural and healthy way of living for equids; they provide feed and space for exercise. However, unrestricted grazing may lead to excess body condition in some equids, particularly when the horses do not undergo any type of forced exercise. For example, in one study, mature horses on pasture for 24 h a day consumed 0.41 kg DM/h of fescue or 0.38 kg DM/h of orchardgrass.[27] An average grass pasture has approximately 2 Mcal of DE/kg DM, but the DE may be as high as 2.7 Mcal/kg DM in some forages. Therefore, depending on the energy density of the pasture, a 500-kg horse with predicted maintenance energy requirement of 16.4 Mcal/day that has opportunity to graze fescue pasture for 24 h would consume calories at the average rate of 0.8–1.1 Mcal/h, which would provide an excess of calories in the range of 1.2–1.6 times above maintenance. The rate of pasture consumption will vary somewhat based on pasture quality and palatability, but it is dramatically affected by length (of time) of access. In the same study, when mature horses had time-restricted access to pasture for only 3 h per day, their consumption rate increased to 1.5 kg DM/h of tall fescue grass. This indicates that when access to pasture is time restricted, horses will consume calories at a higher rate of 3.0–4.1 Mcal/h and could meet their daily maintenance energy requirement in just 4.0–5.5 h of intensive grazing. Energy in the feed (calories) can be either expended or used for anabolism and storage. This is why an adult horse with unrestricted pasture access that does not exercise will be predisposed to excess weight gain and obesity. In general, whenever a horse has unrestricted access to quality pasture, light exercise is the minimum level of physical activity needed to prevent becoming overweight or obese. Light exercise in a 500-kg horse will increase the daily energy requirement to about 20.5 Mcal/day (1.25 times maintenance requirements), which would expend the surplus of energy from the unlimited pasture intake.

5.1.8.6 Non-Structural Carbohydrates

Carbohydrates are a major source of energy for horses. Primary carbohydrate sources in a horse's diet include forages, grains, and grain byproducts. Plants consist of lignin and a number of major plant carbohydrates, such as cellulose, hemicelluloses, pectin, starch, oligosaccharides, and mono- and disaccharides. Analytically, plant carbohydrates are fractionated into neutral detergent fiber (NDF: cellulose, hemicelluloses, lignin); nonfiber carbohydrates (NFC: calculated value determined by subtracting the amount of NDF, protein, fat, and ash from total DM); and non-structural carbohydrates (NSC: chemically analyzed fraction of feed including mono-, and disaccharides, oligosaccharides [including fructans] and starch). The amount of NSC is approximated by summing the amount of starch and amount of water soluble carbohydrates (WSC) obtained from chemical analysis. The difference between NFC and NSC is small in feeds such as cereal grains but can be large in feeds with high content of pectin (e.g., beet pulp, soy hulls, soybean meal).[28]

A system that classifies carbohydrates based on their value as an energy source for horses was proposed by Hoffman et al.[29] This system classifies carbohydrates into three fractions: (1) hydrolyzable carbohydrates (CHO-H) measured by direct analysis; (2) rapidly fermented carbohydrates (CHO-F_R) calculated as the difference between NFC and CHO-H; and (3) slowly fermentable carbohydrates (CHO-F_S), equated with NDF values. The hydrolyzable fraction can be digested in the small intestine by the horse's digestive enzymes and includes hexoses, disaccharides, some oligosaccharides, and non-resistant starches. Consumption of hydrolysable carbohydrates increases blood glucose and releases insulin to enhance glucose uptake by many tissues, including muscle and adipose. Rapidly fermented carbohydrates such as pectin, gums, mucilages, fructan polysaccharides, fructooligosaccharides, and other oligosaccharides are not digested in the small intestine, but are readily fermented in the cecum and large intestine. The slowly fermentable carbohydrate fraction is also available for microbial fermentation and includes cellulose, hemicelluloses, and lignocellulose. The products of microbial fermentation are acetate, propionate, butyrate (volatile fatty acids), and lactate and their proportion and rate of production is driven by the gut microbial population. Conversely, diet composition influences microbial population and the proportion of fatty acids produced in the gastrointestinal tract. Volatile fatty acids are a direct source of energy for equids, can be used for fatty acid synthesis or glucose production by the liver, or provide energy for enterocytes.[28]

Clinical studies showed that excessive ingestion of starch, sugar, or fructans is capable of inducing laminitis and failure of attachment between the dermoepidermal junction in the hoof. Garner et al.[30] induced laminitis by administration of 15 g starch/kg of a cornstarch-wood flour gruel, Rowe et al.[31] by feeding 3.75–6.8 g starch/kg twice a day from corn, and French and Pollitt[33] by 7.5–12.5 g/kg of oral fructan. Fructan inulin from chicory root fed at 1 g or 3 g/kg resulted in significant decrease in fecal pH in ponies.[33] Although induction of laminitis by feeding grass forage has not been demonstrated in a randomized controlled clinical trial, the United States Department of Agriculture National Animal Health Monitoring System survey revealed that laminitis is common in equids kept on pasture.[34]

It is reported that under specific conditions, grass and hay may have concentrations of NSC (sugar, starch, fructan), up to 35% of DM.[35] This amount is concerning when compared to the NSC of content of beet pulp (5.2% DM) or grains such as whole oats (48.7% DM) or corn (73.1% DM).[36] Several years of accumulative nutritional analysis data showed that grass hay averaged 12.9% NSC of DM (range 8.0–17.7% DM) and grass pasture averaged 13% NSC of DM (range 6.1–20.1% DM).[36] Carbohydrates in plants are synthesized from carbon dioxide and water during the process of photosynthesis. The rate of photosynthesis is correlated with light intensity and carbon dioxide concentration, but is independent of temperature[35] and continues even near to freezing temperatures. Sugars produced during the day are utilized at night during plant respiration and to form components of the plant.

Common forage grasses are divided into cool season or warm season grasses. Examples of cool season grasses include fescue, brome, orchardgrass, timothy, perennial rye, and small grain hays (oat, wheat, rye, triticale). Examples of warm season grasses are bermudagrass, bahiagrass, bluestem, crabgrass, switch grass, gramma, and Teff grass. Cool season grasses preferentially use fructans as their storage carbohydrate, while warm season grasses utilize starch. Utilization of fructans as storage carbohydrate allows better winter hardiness and plant growth under cool conditions, while starch accumulation in warm season grasses shuts down under cold stress. This means that cool season grasses are in general higher in NSC than warm season grasses and the concentration is even higher under cool conditions.[35] In the cool season grasses, NSC is generally higher in grass stems than in leaves and concentration increases toward the ground, thus the stem base is considered a storage organ. In the warm season grasses, NSC in the form of starch is stored in the leaf tissue and seed heads.[35]

The NSC accumulation in grass is stimulated by environmental stress conditions (e.g., cold stress, light intensity, drought stress, low fertility, salty soil, and anaerobic conditions). In the spring and fall under cold night temperatures, cold season grasses accumulate fructans instead of utilizing them for respiration and growth. Production of sugar by the plant is directly correlated with light intensity and duration. Concentration of NSC will be lowest in early morning if the night was warm (>5°C) and sugars were utilized for respiration and growth overnight.[81] Sunny conditions during the day will increase NSC concentration when compared to cloudy days or shaded pasture areas. Drought stress also induces accumulation of NSC in the grass, since respiration is limited by low water availability to the plant. Several studies demonstrated that low fertility of the pasture, defined as nitrogen and phosphorus deficiency, increases concentration of NSC in grasses and legumes.[37–39] High salts in the soil or irrigation water can interfere with osmotic gradients and reduce plant water absorption, leading to conditions similar to drought. This may result in increased accumulation of NSC.[40] Another plant stress that can increase NSC accumulation is oxygen deficiency caused by standing water or ice.[41]

The concentration of NSC in cured hay depends on the NSC content of the grass at the time of cutting. The NSC content can be lower if the hay was cut in the morning and let dry slowly under cloudy conditions. This is because the cut forage will continue respiration and sugar utilization until the moisture content drops below approximately 40%.[35] Since NSC content is influenced by multiple factors, it is impossible to estimate its concentration by visual characteristics of the forage and nutritional analysis of the forage is warranted.

5.1.8.7 Laminitis

There are several factors implicated in the etiology of laminitis in equids. These include excessive ingestion of rapidly fermentable carbohydrate (starch, fructans),[30–32] endotoxemia,[30,31] exposure to black walnut shavings,[42] excessive concussion, glucocorticoid administration,[44] endocrine disturbances,[43] and obesity and insulin resistance.[5]

Insulin is released from the β-cells of the pancreas in response to an elevation in blood glucose, which is an expected normal physiological response. However, increased magnitude, frequency, or duration of hyperinsulinemia is likely detrimental. Indeed, Asplin et al.[45] were able to induce clinical laminitis and typical histopathologic lesions in all four hooves of healthy ponies by maintaining supraphysiologic hyperinsulinemia with euglycemia for 72h. This *in-vivo* laminitis induction model was replicated by Nourian et al. in another study.[46] Of interest was that plasma insulin concentrations in both studies markedly exceeded concentrations in ponies and horses with EMS. The relationship between elevated insulin and laminitis was further demonstrated by Bailey et al.[4–6,15,45,47–49] who provided evidence that serum insulin and triglyceride concentrations were significantly greater in pastured ponies (receiving no concentrate) with a history of laminitis compared to non-laminitic ponies in the summer. Carter et al.[10] observed laminitic episodes in ponies that were highly associated with obesity and elevated insulin and leptin concentrations.

Many theories on the pathogenesis of hyperinsulinemic laminitis have been proposed, but the exact contribution of each individual pathogenic mechanism has yet to be revealed. It has been suggested that hyperinsulinemia can cause laminitis through induction of hemodynamic changes within the lamellar vasculature. Insulin is an important vasomediator and the principal action of insulin is probably vasodilation through modulation of nitric oxide (endothelium-derived relaxing factor) release under physiological conditions. In insulin resistant horses, vasodilation in response to insulin action may be impaired that could contribute to vasoconstriction with platelet and leukocyte adhesion to endothelial surfaces.[50] Vasoconstriction likely contributes to the hypertension that was reported in ponies with EMS.[15] Another proposed mechanism for pathogenesis of hyperinsulinemic laminitis is alteration in glucose metabolism. Theories exist on development of dermo-epidermal separation as a result of a failure of glucose uptake by lamellar tissue through reduction of non-insulin dependent glucose transporter type 1 (GLUT-1) transporters or as a result of lamellar failure due to glucotoxicity in response to dietary glucose load.[51]

Based on clinical observations and epidemiological surveys, the risk of pasture-associated laminitis occurs at the time of rapid grass growth (spring, early summer, after heavy rains) or by grazing stressed pastures when accumulation of NSC in forages occurs.[34,52,53] However, very little data is available on the possible association between insulin resistance and pasture associated laminitis in horses. Evidence shows that diets rich in NSC decrease insulin sensitivity and impair glucose tolerance in horses.[54] Additionally, insulin-resistance ponies that graze lush pasture are most likely to develop laminitis.[5]

It is hypothesized that excessive quantities of rapidly fermentable carbohydrates enter the cecum and large colon and initiate intestinal disturbances that can lead to the development of laminitis.[48] Observations with the oligofructose model of laminitis revealed changes in hind gut microbes favoring proliferation of bacteria that ferment oligofructose and produce lactic acid (e.g., equine hindgut streptococcal species).[55,56] These changes lead to luminal pH values as low as 4, death and lysis of bacteria, release of endotoxin and exotoxins, damage to the hindgut epithelial barrier, and increased intestinal permeability.[55] Furthermore, carbohydrate overload increases synthesis of vasoactive amines.[57] Endotoxin absorbed from the intestinal tract is associated with systemic inflammation and clinical signs of endotoxemia (e.g., fever, tachycardia, tachypnea) and may play a role in development of laminitis.[52] It is likely that systemic inflammation induces lamellar inflammatory changes, leading to destruction of lamellar epithelium and extracellular matrix.[58] Furthermore, alterations in digital vascular hemodynamics, platelet activation, and vasoactive amines may also take part in lamellar injury.[47,57,59]

Although more work is needed to identify the pathophysiology of hyperinsulinemic laminitis, the practical implication is to develop methods for early detection of hyperinsulinemia to identify horses at risk.

5.1.9 Diagnosis
5.1.9.1 Overview
The practical importance of early EMS diagnosis is that appropriate management and treatment can reverse progression and prevent morbidity and mortality associated with EMS. The diagnosis of EMS is based on findings in the history, including dietary history, results of physical examination, radiographs of the feet, and laboratory tests.

5.1.9.2 Differential Diagnoses
The major differential diagnosis for EMS is Pituitary Pars Intermedia Dysfunction (PPID), also known as equine Cushing's disease. Equine Metabolic Syndrome and PPID are both endocrine diseases that increase risk for the development of insulin resistance and laminitis.[51] While the clinical outcome of both diseases is similar, both endocrinopathies have fundamentally different pathophysiology and epidemiology. While EMS is an endocrinopathy of young to middle-aged horses and ponies (5–15 years old), PPID is common in aged animals with recognition of clinical signs at age 18–20 years old, with only rare reports in horses younger than 10 years.[60,61] Equine metabolic syndrome exists independently from PPID, although EMS can occur concurrently with PPID in middle-aged horses.[62]

5.1.9.3 Initial Database
Horses and ponies affected by EMS present with generalized or regional obesity with a history of being easy keepers and recurrent laminitis or they originally present with laminitis. Generalized obesity is diagnosed by assignment of a body condition score (BCS) using visual assessment and palpation. A number of body condition scoring systems have been developed for horses. A system developed by Henneke et al.[63] has been widely used for many years and is appropriate for use by veterinarians, horse owners, and caregivers. This system scores horses on fat cover both visually and by palpation at several locations on the horse's body, with a low score of 1 being applied to an emaciated horse and a high score of 9 being applied to a very fat horse. Generally, BCS scores of 1–3 are considered under conditioned, BCS 4–6 optimal condition, BCS 7 over conditioned, and BCS 8–9 obese. Body weight can be determined using a scale or estimated using a weight tape calibrated for horses. When using weight tapes, it is important that the same brand of tape is used for each measurement and that the tape is applied in a consistent manner. For consistent results, the tape should be positioned immediately behind the elbows and at the highest point of the withers. Horses and ponies severely affected by EMS have BSC 8 or 9 and have a markedly enlarged neck crest.[17]

Regional adiposity, including a cresty neck, fat pads behind the scapula and around the rib cage, at the tail head, prepuce, and mammary gland, can be apparent in obese horses and even in horses with visible ribs. Regional adiposity is a common manifestation of EMS phenotype and the body regions with increased adiposity are often resistant to weight loss. The degree of adipose tissue accumulation within the neck region can be assessed with a cresty neck score, which ranges from 0–5. The cresty neck score was developed by Carter and colleagues[64] and the majority of EMS horses and ponies exhibit a cresty neck score of 3 and higher.[3,17] Another technique to measure adipose tissue accumulation is measurement of neck circumference at the midpoint of the neck by a tape measure. This measurement is taken halfway between the poll and the withers when the neck is in a normal elevated position.[11]

5.1.9.4 Advanced or Confirmatory Testing

In addition to detection of generalized and regional adiposity, horses should be screened for hyperinsulinemia as an indicator of insulin resistance. Insulin resistance is difficult to diagnose, mainly because of practical limitations to the use of the gold standard hyperinsulinemic euglycemic clamp technique for screening. Hyperglycemia is an uncommon finding in horses with EMS since most animals maintain normoglycemia with a compensatory increase of insulin. However, blood glucose concentrations can be in the upper reference range indicating some degree of loss of glycemic control. Horses with EMS have persistently elevated blood glucose concentrations that cannot be attributed to stress, recent feeding, administration of α-2 agonist sedatives, an inflammatory process, or the rare case of diabetes mellitus.[65] Middle-aged or old horses suspected to have PPID should also have an ACTH measurement performed.

There are certain conditions when measuring resting insulin concentration is not helpful in the diagnosis of EMS. These conditions include pain and stress as a result of active laminitis, times when insulin resistance is mild and insulin concentration is still within reference range, and pancreatic insufficiency resulting from prolonged insulin resistance.[62]

Hyperinsulinemia is defined as an insulin concentration above a laboratory's established reference range. Reference ranges for serum or plasma insulin concentrations differ between laboratories and different assays, which should be taken into consideration. Research studies also differ in determination of cut-off values for hyperinsulinemia. As an example, the University of Tennessee endocrine laboratory defines hyperinsulinemia as plasma or serum insulin concentration above 20 μU/mL (mU/L), which is approximately equivalent to 140 pmol/L (conversion factor of 7).[3,62] Muno defined hyperinsulinemia as plasma insulin exceeding 15 mU/L.[1] Carter et al.[10] used a cut-off value of 32 μU/mL to predict the occurrence of laminitis in ponies and Walsh et al.[66] defined EMS by an insulin concentration of 70 μU/mL. Published cutoff values (the upper limit of serum/plasma insulin concentration in normal horses and ponies) for hyperglycemia are 110 mg/dL or approximately 6.0 mmol/L (conversion factor of 18). The American College of Veterinary Internal Medicine EMS consensus statement suggested an insulin cutoff value of 20 μU/mL (mU/L), using radioimmunoassay (Coat-A-Count insulin radioimmunoassay, Siemens Medical Solutions Diagnostics, Los Angeles, CA).[3] When other types of assays are used by the laboratory, respective reference ranges for that specific laboratory should be used.

The sampling conditions to determine serum or plasma baseline insulin concentration also play a role in diagnosis, therefore, preparation of the horse prior to sampling is necessary. After collection, the blood tubes should be kept on ice and centrifuged, ideally within 30 min of collection at 1,500–3,000 times gravity. Plasma or serum should be separated before shipment and analysis. Conditions that increase blood insulin concentration include feeding (forages or concentrates), pain, or stress. Pain or stress lower tissue insulin sensitivity and increase blood glucose through the release of cortisol and epinephrine. Therefore, sampling should be delayed in all patients suffering from stress, including the horses with laminitis, until the stress has resolved. All types of feeds, including grains with a high concentration of hydrolysable carbohydrates increase blood insulin.[67] Evidence exists that insulin-resistant ponies exhibit insulin response to dietary fructans, indicating that there could be some degree of hydrolysis of fructans before they reach the large intestine.[49,67] Therefore, it is recommended to withhold access to pasture, concentrates, and grain for a minimum of 6 h before blood collection. Since not feeding the horse can itself induce a stress response, a small amount of hay (1 flake or approximately 1–1.5 kg of a low-NSC hay per 500 kg) can be fed no later than 10:00 pm the night before sampling[3] and the blood samples should be collected between 8:00–10:00 am the next morning. Horses and ponies that exhibit EMS phenotype but have insulin concentration within reference range under these conditions require a dynamic test to evaluate insulin sensitivity.

There are a number of tests described in the literature, however, the ideal test for diagnosis of insulin resistance has yet to be established. These tests are also performed after at least a 6-h fast and when the horse is free of pain or stress. Dynamic tests are described elsewhere and include oral or IV glucose tolerance tests and the combined glucose-insulin test.[17] The oral sugar test is the most practical on-farm dynamic test of insulin sensitivity currently available. Inappropriately increased insulin concentration after an oral dose of corn syrup supports insulin dysregulation.

The glucose to insulin ratio (glucose concentration in mg/dL divided by the insulin concentration in µU/mL) is not recommended for diagnosis of insulin resistance because blood glucose concentration is influenced by the stress response and by the utilization of glucose by erythrocytes if the sample is not processed correctly. Furthermore, individual laboratories use different assays to measure insulin.

Other laboratory tests to consider are measurement of leptin and serum triglyceride concentrations. Elevated leptin concentrations have been measured in horses and ponies with insulin resistance, as well as in obese horses. Leptin assay is currently not available from diagnostic laboratories but might be available in the future (Multi-species leptin radioimmunoassay, Millipore Inc., St Charles, MO). In one study,[10] a fasting leptin concentration cutoff value of 7.3 ng/mL predicted occurrence of laminitis in ponies. A leptin concentration of <5 ng/mL was considered normoleptinemic and a concentration >12 ng/mL was considered hyperleptinemic in another study.[68] Plasma triglycerides are available from most clinical pathology laboratories and triglycerides may be elevated in both ponies and horses with EMS.[5,10,11]

Some horses with EMS have low serum T4 concentration and a weak negative correlation between insulin and T4 has been detected in horses with EMS.[66] However, this finding should be interpreted as a consequence rather than a causative factor of EMS.[62]

5.1.10 Treatment

5.1.10.1 Overview

Equine metabolic syndrome should be managed by dietary, housing, and exercise modifications. Obese and overweight horses should be placed on a weight reduction program by restricting energy intake and the diet should be modified to eliminate nutrients that are implicated in the development of obesity and aggravation of blood glucose control. Decisions about housing conditions and exercise are driven by the severity of laminitis at the time of presentation and by the farm setting. The goal of treatment is to achieve and maintain long-term optimal BCS, normoinsulinemia, and improve laminitis. Medical treatments are sometimes necessary for patients that are resistant to dietary, housing, and exercise modifications.

5.1.10.2 Nutritional and Dietary Therapeutics

The key aspects of nutritional management of patients with EMS include reversal of obesity, reduction of NSC intake, and feeding a balanced ration to provide nutrients for tissue and hoof healing. The goal of any weight loss program is not only to achieve optimal BCS but also to introduce a behavioral shift that will sustain maintenance of a life-long optimal body condition.

The weight loss program should be practical and simple to achieve success within the first month, as this will encourage the owner to continue with weight reduction efforts. Following nutritional assessment and screening for hyperinsulinemia, further steps involve setting goals for weight loss, reducing caloric (DE) intake, increasing exercise when possible, and regular monitoring of progress. The presence of hyperinsulinemia does not change the protocol, but emphasizes the consequences of obesity and risk of laminitis to the owner. Most horses respond to weight loss by decreasing and normalizing insulin concentration.

Setting goals for weight loss consists of determining optimal BCS and body weight. In mature light-breed horses, each change in BCS represents approximately 18–27 kg (40–59 lb) in body weight. Predicted optimal body weight (POBW) is determined by the following formula:

POBW (kg) = SBW (kg) − [(SBCS − DBCS) × 22.5 kg]
SBW = the horse's starting body weight
SBCS = the horse's starting BCS
DBCS = desired BCS

For example, an obese horse with a starting BCS of 9, a starting body weight of 550 kg, and a desired BCS of 5, would have a predicted optimal body weight of 460 kg:

$$550 - \left[(9-5) \times 22.5 \right] = 460\,\text{kg}$$

Horses and ponies that are managed in a stall or dry lot without the access to pasture should be fed a precisely measured amount of hay with an appropriate vitamin-mineral supplement or balancer pellet. Balancer pellets supplement vitamins and minerals to meet requirements when equids graze inadequate pastures or are fed a restricted intake. All grains and concentrates that contain starches should be completely eliminated from the diet. It is generally recommended to feed an amount of hay equivalent to 1.5% of the predicted optimal body weight per day (i.e., 6.9 kg for a 460 kg horse)[17,69] or DE equivalent to approximately 70% of the maintenance energy requirement calculated for the obese or overweight body condition (e.g., 20 kcal DE/kg for an obese or overweight 250 kg pony).[70] However, the amount of hay needs to be evaluated in the face of the current hay and DE intake obtained from the dietary history as some horses are already consuming this amount or less without measurable weight loss. If the initial reduced allocation of hay does not result in weight loss within 4 weeks, then the amount should be further lowered by another 10–20% and body weight rechecked in 4 weeks. However, it is not recommended to lower the amount of hay below 1% of estimated ideal body weight per day,[72] because starving obese horses for weight loss can increase risk of hyperlipidemia, hepatic lipidosis, and reduction of metabolism.[21,72] Based on published studies, the safe and appropriate mean weight loss rate in obese horses should be approximately 1% of the starting obese body weight per week throughout the entire weight loss period.[21,70] This corresponds to a weight loss of 4.6 kg per week and 18.4 kg per month for a light-breed horse, which translates into loss of 1 BCS per month. Weight loss studies in pony breeds show that in order to achieve 1% body weight loss per week, more aggressive energy restriction of 50–70% maintenance energy requirement has to be applied.[21,70] However, feeding 50% of maintenance calories equates to feeding hay at less than 1% of body weight per day, which is not optimal. Therefore, achieving weight loss rate of 0.5–1.0% body weight per week in ponies is acceptable.

Selecting the appropriate hay for weight reduction is important to ensure successful weight loss and minimize insulin response without the need to lower the amount of hay fed below 1% body weight per day. Hays differ in energy density, fiber content, and NSC content. The NSC content cannot be visually assessed and is unpredictable; therefore, a forage nutritional analysis should be obtained for any hay that is intended to be fed to an equid with EMS. A general recommendation is to find hay with low energy density (DE/kg), moderately increased fiber content (measured as NDF and ADF), and restricted NSC content. As the fiber content in the hay increases, the DE decreases and feed intake decreases. Such hay will allow energy intake restriction without severely limiting amount of the hay fed. The importance of NSC content of the hay increases with severity of hyperinsulinemia at the time of presentation. It is recommended to feed a hay with less than 10% NSC on a DM basis to equids with marked fasting hyperinsulinemia (>100 µU/mL) to avoid spikes in glucose and insulin concentrations.[3,17] However, hays with low NSC concentration can be beneficial to any horse on a weight loss plan since NSC contribute to energy density of the forage.

The NSC content of hay can be reduced by soaking in water prior to feeding; however, this method is not always reliable to achieve ≤10% NSC DM in hays with very high NSC content. In one study, soaking hay in cold water for 20 min, 40 min, or 3 h resulted in a mean loss of 5, 9, and 16% of total WSC content. After being soaked for 16 h, the mean loss of WSC was 27% (with a broad range of 6–54%).[73]

The total daily ration should be complete and balanced to support metabolism during weight loss and to promote healing of hoof structures. Rations based on forage alone are not complete and balanced, therefore an appropriate vitamin and mineral supplement or balancer pellet should always be recommended. Hays also differ in crude protein content. Protein is needed for maintenance of muscle mass during weight loss and tissue healing. Commercial vitamin and mineral supplements with added protein (up to 30% crude protein on an as-fed basis) can complement nutrient deficits in forage. Supplements that contain purely vitamins and minerals do not add calories to the ration. However, supplements that are fortified with a protein source or flavored with molasses contain calories that must be subtracted from the total daily caloric allocation. Besides hay, commercial feeds fortified with vitamins and minerals and restricted in NSC have been formulated for management of EMS and for weight loss. Those feeds may be fed as a part of a weight reduction program or for EMS horses. Plain (white) salt and free choice water should be available at all times.

Owners should be counseled on the importance of weighing hay or feed with a scale at each feeding (see Figure 5.4) to ensure that the precisely allocated amount of hay and energy is fed. Scales to weigh fish are inexpensive and work well to weigh feed. At least two meals per day should be fed to minimize periods of hunger between feedings and to reduce boredom.

Feed and the accompanying calorie intake can markedly exceed the daily maintenance requirement when horses are turned out onto pasture. Grazing muzzles are

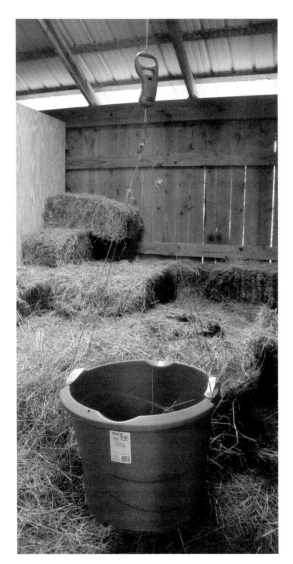

Figure 5.4 The amount of hay should be measured at each feeding using a scale for the most precise allotment and for successful weight loss.

a safe and effective means of reducing caloric intake in overweight or obese pastured horses. The grazing muzzle should be worn whenever the horse is on pasture. All grains and concentrates containing starches should be eliminated from the diet. Since fresh forage-based rations are not complete or balanced, it is necessary to feed a measured amount of a vitamin-mineral supplement or balancer pellet. White salt and free choice water should be available at all times.

There are other options for limiting forage intake that combine pasture turn out with confinement. However, under these conditions control over caloric intake is less reliable. Strategies include short periods of pasture turn out (<1 h twice a day), confinement in a small paddock or round pen, or in an area limited with an electrical fence or pen. Depending on the amount of forage biomass in the confinement area, a measured amount of supplemental hay may be needed.

After the desired BCS is achieved and insulin resistance has resolved, an appropriate weight maintenance program should be established. In many instances, horses will plateau and maintain the targeted body condition while wearing a grazing muzzle whenever on pasture. In other instances, horses will continue to lose condition and will require short periods (usually 1–2 h/day) of grazing without a muzzle to maintain appropriate body condition.[17] Care should be taken to limit grazing time to the early morning when the grass is undergoing rapid growth in the spring, late summer, or at the onset of cold weather in the fall, or on drought-stressed or frost affected pastures. If possible, grazing should be limited to time of the day when NSC content is lowest (between 3:00–9:00 am).[69] If a horse splits time between pasture and confinement, a calculated amount of hay can be fed during the time of confinement. Typically, a horse at maintenance (neither gaining nor losing weight) requires 2% of its optimal body weight in average quality hay daily to maintain an appropriate body condition. The amount of hay fed during a period of confinement can be prorated based on the amount of time that the horse is confined. For example, if a horse is on pasture for 12 h with a grazing muzzle and in a stall for 12 h, it should be fed half of its calculated daily requirement of hay during its confinement period.

5.1.10.3 Medical Management

Most horses with EMS will favorably respond to dietary control, increased physical activity, and restricted pasture access. However, there are two instances when pharmacologic treatment is indicated: (1) short-term levothyroxine treatment while the patient is undergoing weight loss program and (2) cases refractory to dietary management and increased exercise. In these instances, levothyroxine sodium can be administered to accelerate weight loss and improve insulin sensitivity. Levothyroxine sodium is administered by mouth or with a small amount of feed at a dosage of 0.1 mg/kg, PO, q24h (48 mg/day for a mature light breed horse [450–525 kg]).[17,74,75] Levothyroxine can be administered for 3–6 months to accelerate weight loss in obese horses while other treatment modalities are also instituted.[17] Long term administration of 48 mg levothytoxine/day to healthy mares for 48 weeks did not have any adverse effects and treated mares significantly lost weight from baseline.[74] Levothyroxine raises circulating thyroxine concentrations and increases basal metabolic rate. Horses are weaned off levothyroxine sodium once an ideal body condition has been attained by reducing the dosage to 24 mg PO, q24h, for 2 weeks and then to 12 mg PO, q24h, for another 2 weeks.[74]

There are only few studies reported on use of metformin hydrochloride, a drug that is administered to control hyperglycemia through suppression of hepatic glucose production and increased tissue insulin sensitivity in humans with diabetes mellitus[19,42,76,77] Metformin administration (30 mg/kg, PO) significantly decreased glucose absorption and its corresponding insulin response in horses fed a glucose-containing meal.[78] Currently, metformin is recommended for the management of insulin resistance in horses, but further research is needed to derive the effective dose for horses. Another human insulin-sensitizing drug is pioglitazone and more research is needed before this drug can be recommended for horses.[79]

5.1.10.4 Behavioral/Physical Activity Recommendations

Physical activity increases energy expenditure, promotes weight loss, maintains lean muscle mass, and thus increases basal metabolic rate. Therefore, obese horses and ponies that do not suffer from laminitis should be encouraged to exercise throughout the weight loss program and for maintenance of their desired weight. The recommended exercise should be as frequent as 4–7 days a week for a minimum of 30 min at a trot or canter under saddle or on a longe line.[17] The 30-min minimum exercise time excludes the warm up and cool down.

5.1.11 Possible Complications of Treatment or of the Disease Process

Horses and ponies that are refractory to nutritional and medical management or develop recurrent pasture-associated laminitis must be kept off pasture forever. Horses that remain insulin resistant after achieving optimal BCS and those that present in ideal BCS are challenging and may require medical therapy.

Multiple supplements and nutraceuticals are marketed for management of EMS in equids, including chromium, magnesium, cinnamon, and chasteberry (*Vitex agnus-castus*); however, scientific evidence to convincingly support recommendation of these products is lacking.

5.1.12 Recommended Monitoring

Regardless of the weight reduction plan used for each individual patient, it is important to frequently monitor body weight to ensure weight loss success within the first month of the program. Periodic assessment of BCS and body weight is critical to ensure that the feeding program remains appropriate. Owners should assess body condition and body weight regularly (at least every 2–4 weeks) so that progress can be monitored and the program is amended as needed. With the described protocol, most horses will achieve the desired BCS in 3–4 months. Follow-up insulin evaluations should be performed if initial values were abnormal and results should follow weight loss trends.

5.1.13 Prognosis and Outcome

Equine metabolic syndrome is usually a manageable condition and the risk of laminitis can be lowered by maintenance of ideal BCS with dietary changes and regular exercise. Prognosis depends on the ability to successfully identify insulin resistant horses prior to the development of debilitating laminitis, reduce obesity, and treat clinical or subclinical laminitis. Prognosis is favorable for obese horses with insulin resistance without severe laminitis once successful weight loss and normoinsulinemia are achieved. Subclinical laminitis is manageable with therapeutic farriery, dietary change, and medical management. Horses with severe acute laminitis have a poor prognosis.

5.1.14 Prevention

Feeding to prevent obesity decreases the risk of hyperinsulinemia and laminitis (see Figure 5.5). Equids with the EMS phenotype and EMS diagnosis prior to the

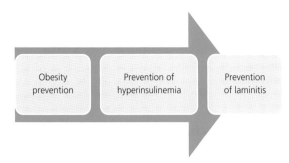

Figure 5.5 Prevention of obesity or overweight body condition normalizes insulin sensitivity and represents the most effective protection from EMS associated laminitis.

development of clinical laminitis should be kept at optimal BCS and their weight should be closely monitored. The ration should restrict NSC content, grazing should be limited or a grazing muzzle worn during pasture turnout, and the level of physical activity should be increased. Special attention should be paid to hoof care and monitoring of any hoof lesions with hoof examinations and radiographs as needed.

If EMS is diagnosed after development of painful laminitis, then laminitis treatment should be based on the clinical evaluation. Additionally, weight management, dietary changes, reduction of NSC content of the ration, and avoidance of grazing should be instituted. Since increased activity is not possible, medical management with levothyroxin should be strongly considered.

5.2 Feeding Horses with Pituitary Pars Intermedia Dysfunction

Feeding horses with PPID can sometimes be difficult because horses affected with PPID are often older, underweight, and may have insulin resistance with or without recurrent laminitis. To make the best nutritional recommendations for horses with PPID, veterinarians must first consider these questions: (1) Does the horse need to gain or lose weight? (2) Is insulin resistance present? Regardless of the answers to these questions, horses with PPID should be fed a primarily forage diet that will maintain (or regain) ideal body condition and to avoid obesity, which will worsen insulin resistance.

Not all horses affected with PPID also have insulin resistance.[80] Concentrates should be fed only as needed to maintain desired body condition, preferably BCS

4–6/9. Feeding small (<0.5% of body weight) frequent concentrate meals produces less deviation in insulin and glucose concentrations and is less likely to complicate insulin resistance. Textured or sweet feed containing greater than 3% molasses and 15–20% NSC should be avoided if there is evidence of insulin resistance. Pellets or extruded feeds that are higher in fiber (>10%) and fat (>5%) can be fed instead of sweet feed to provide additional dietary energy. Whenever possible, horses with PPID should be allowed turn out time, as exercise improves insulin sensitivity.[81] Forced exercise or work should be reserved for horses that do not have active laminitis and are free of musculoskeletal disorders.

Owners should be advised to be aware during times of the year when pasture grasses can be high in NSC because PPID can worsen insulin insensitivity in susceptible horses and result in laminitis.[80,81] Adrenocorticotrophic hormone concentrations have been shown to have seasonal variation and be highest in September.[82] Blood insulin concentration is positively associated with increased carbohydrates in pasture grass.[83] Frank et al.[83] measured ACTH concentrations over a 1-year period in mature to aged horses kept at pasture. Mean ACTH concentration was highest from August through October. Horses affected with PPID had higher ACTH concentrations than unaffected horses. Glucose and insulin concentrations peaked in September, which combined with the seasonal peak in ACTH concentration, may contribute to an increased risk of pasture-associated laminitis risk in the fall.

Vitamin C (ascorbic acid; 0.011–0.022 g/kg, PO, q12h) may be supplemented to improve immune function in PPID horses with recurring or chronic infections. However, long term high-dose ascorbic acid supplementation may impair endogenous synthesis of ascorbic acid and can result in deficiency if it is suddenly discontinued.[81]

5.2.1 Horses with Pituitary Pars Intermedia Dysfunction and Adequate Body Condition

Many horses affected with PPID are healthy and relatively asymptomatic other than hypertrichosis and mild to moderate polyuria and polydipsia. Horses with PPID and good BCS score without evidence of insulin resistance can be fed as a normal horse to maintain body condition and prevent obesity.[80] Senior-type feeds, sweet feed, or oats with hay can be fed if additional dietary energy is needed.

5.2.2 Obese Horses with Pituitary Pars Intermedia Dysfunction

Obese horses with PPID should be fed the same as previously described in this chapter for horses with EMS to encourage weight loss, improve insulin sensitivity, and reduce the risk of laminitis. A forage or fiber (beet pulp) based diet is ideal for obese horses with PPID to provide gut fill and supply energy in the form of volatile fatty acids, rather than carbohydrates.

5.2.3 Horses with Pituitary Pars Intermedia Dysfunction and Thin Body Condition or Horses with PPID that are in Work

Pituitary pars intermedia dysfunction is a disease of older horses and many are underweight as a consequence of senescence or dental problems. Nutritional recommendations for horses with PPID that need to gain weight are more difficult because the need for more calories must be balanced against the adverse effects of worsening insulin resistance.

Increased energy requirements can be provided by feeding more hay, a low starch and sugar (low NSC) pellet, and rice bran pellets or 1/2–1 cup (120–240 ml) of vegetable oil twice daily. Pasture intake should be controlled to avoid sudden increases in carbohydrate intake.[80] Feeds that are high in fat (>7%) can also be fed to supplement calories.[81] High fat diets have the potential to worsen or create insulin resistance. Pagan et al.[84] reported that a high fat (30% of DE supplied as fat) diet significantly impaired glucose tolerance in aged nonobese Thoroughbred geldings compared to a more traditional diet. Moderate carbohydrate intake (31% of DE supplied as NSC) improved glucose clearance during intravenous glucose tolerance tests compared to both a high fat and an all grass hay diet. Because a high fat diet may worsen glucose tolerance and moderate carbohydrate intake improves insulin response, it is advisable to use a combination of fats and carbohydrates along with additional forage to promote weight gain in thin horses with PPID.

5.3 Pearls and Considerations

- Obesity or overweight body condition in horses increases the risk for developing insulin resistance and laminitis.

- Resolution of obesity or overweight body condition normalizes insulin sensitivity and prevents EMS associated laminitis in almost all cases.
- Efficient weight loss in pasture-based horses can be achieved using grazing muzzles and/or by increasing exercise.
- Weight loss in horses confined to a stall or dry lot can be achieved by feeding a measured amount of hay with low NSC content.
- Forage-based rations should be balanced with essential vitamins and minerals (balancer pellets).
- A horse's dietary weight loss plan can be facilitated with oral administration of levothyroxine sodium.

5.3.1 Client Education

- Clients should understand that obesity and insulin resistance warrants intervention because it is associated with an increased risk for debilitating laminitis.
- Clients should be trained to use BCS and weight tapes for a proper monitoring and recognition of early signs of weight gain.
- Treating obesity is relatively simple and generally involves reducing caloric intake by feeding a measured amount of appropriate forage and/or using grazing muzzles and/or increasing caloric expenditure through exercise.
- Laminitic horses need optimum intake of protein, energy, minerals, and vitamins to maximize hoof growth, but a high concentration of NSC in the diet should be avoided.
- To prevent recurrence of obesity after weight loss, clients should be educated on how to monitor body condition and to adjust feeding and management programs to maintain proper body condition.
- Some horses with EMS can never be returned to pasture because they cannot tolerate seasonal changes in grass nutrient content. A horse that develops hyperinsulinemia again when reintroduced to pasture must be permanently housed in a dry lot and fed measured amount of appropriate forage.
- Medical treatment with drugs should be limited to more severely affected animals and should always be used concurrently with dietary modification.
- Feed, including hay, should be fed on a weight, rather than volume basis. Feeds can be weighed using an inexpensive fish scale that can be purchased in the sporting goods department.

5.3.2 Veterinary Technician Tips

- Diagnosis of obesity is simple. Several BCS charts have been published for horses. When description of each BCS point and illustrations are consistently and repeatedly followed, assignment of the BCS can be very accurate.
- The management program for horses with EMS is practical and simple and involves obtaining health, diet, and exercise history; performing a complete physical examination; determining the horse's starting body condition and weight; screening for hyperinsulinemia; setting goals for weight loss; collecting a representative sample of forage; selecting an appropriate forage based on results of chemical analysis; using a grazing muzzle to reduce pasture intake; increasing exercise when possible; and regularly monitoring progress.
- Rations consisting of 100% forage are not complete and balanced and an appropriate vitamin-mineral supplement or low-NSC balancer pellets should be recommended. Balancer pellets can also be used as a vehicle for medications and to placate clients who feel guilty about not feeding the horse something in its feed bucket.
- The presence of hyperinsulinemia does not change the protocol but emphasizes, for the client, the consequences of excessive weight and obesity including the risk of laminitis.

References

1. Muno JD. Prevalence, risk factors and seasonality of plasma insulin concentrations in normal horses in central Ohio. Master of Science Thesis, The Ohio State University, 2009.
2. Thatcher CD, Pleasant RS, Geor RJ, et al. Prevalence of obesity in mature horses: an equine body condition study. J Anim Physiol Anim Nutr (Berl) 2008;92:222.
3. Frank N, Geor RJ, Bailey SR, et al. Equine metabolic syndrome. J Vet Intern Med 2010;24:467–475.
4. Alberti KG, Zimmet P, Shaw J. Metabolic syndrome – a new world-wide definition. A consensus statement from the International Diabetes Federation. Diabet Med 2006;23: 469–480.
5. Treiber KH, Kronfeld DS, Hess TM, et al. Evaluation of genetic and metabolic predispositions and nutritional risk factors for pasture-associated laminitis in ponies. J Am Vet Med Assoc 2006b;228:1538–1545.
6. Neel JV. Diabetes mellitus: a "thrifty" genotype rendered detrimental by "progress"? Am J Hum Genet 1962;14: 353–362.
7. Kerem N, Guttman H, Hochberg Z. The autosomal dominant trait of obesity, acanthosis nigricans, hypertension, ischemic heart disease and diabetes type 2. Horm Res 2001;55:298–304.
8. Katz L, Debrauwere N, Elliott J. A retrospective epidemiological study of laminitis in one region of the UK. Proc 40th British Equine Veterinary Association Congress, 2001;199.
9. Treiber KH, Kronfeld DS, Geor RJ. Insulin resistance in equids: possible role in laminitis. J Nutr 2006;136:2094S–2098S.
10. Carter RA, Treiber KH, Geor RJ, et al. Prediction of incipient pasture-associated laminitis from hyperinsulinaemia, hyperleptinaemia and generalised and localised obesity in a cohort of ponies. Equine Vet J 2009;41:171–178.
11. Frank N, Elliott SB, Brandt LE, et al. Physical characteristics, blood hormone concentrations, and plasma lipid concentrations in obese horses with insulin resistance. J Am Vet Med Assoc 2006;228:1383–1390.
12. Gentry LR, Thompson DL, Gentry GT, et al. The relationship between body condition, leptin, and reproductive and hormonal characteristics of mares during the seasonal anovulatory period. J Anim Sci 2002;80:2695–2703.
13. Vick MM, Sessions DR, Murphy BA, et al. Obesity is associated with altered metabolic and reproductive activity in the mare: effects of metformin on insulin sensitivity and reproductive cyclicity. Reprod Fertil Dev 2006;18:609–617.
14. Cartmill JA, Thompson DL, Storer WA, et al. Endocrine responses in mares and geldings with high body condition scores grouped by high vs. low resting leptin concentrations. J Anim Sci 2003;81:2311–2321.
15. Bailey SR, Habershon-Butcher JL, Ransom KJ, et al. Hypertension and insulin resistance in a mixed-breed population of ponies predisposed to laminitis. Am J Vet Res 2008;69:122–129.
16. Vick MM, Adams AA, Murphy BA, et al. Relationships among inflammatory cytokines, obesity, and insulin sensitivity in the horse. J Anim Sci 2007;85:1144–1155.
17. Frank N. Equine metabolic syndrome. Vet Clin North Am Equine Pract 2011;27:73–92.
18. Pansuria M, Xi H, Li L, et al. Insulin resistance, metabolic stress, and atherosclerosis. Front Biosci (Schol Ed) 2012;4:916–931.
19. Toth F, Frank N, Martin-Jimenez T, et al. Measurement of C-peptide concentrations and responses to somatostatin, glucose infusion, and insulin resistance in horses. Equine Vet J 2010;42:149–155.
20. Pawlak J, Derlacz RA. [The mechanism of insulin resistance in peripheral tissues]. Postepy Biochem 2011;57:200–206.
21. Van Weyenberg S, Hesta M, Buyse J, et al. The effect of weight loss by energy restriction on metabolic profile and glucose tolerance in ponies. J Anim Physiol Anim Nutr (Berl) 2008;92:538–545.
22. Kearns CF, McKeever KH, Roegner V, et al. Adiponectin and leptin are related to fat mass in horses. Vet J 2006; 172:460–465.
23. Radin MJ, Sharkey LC, Holycross BJ. Adipokines: a review of biological and analytical principles and an update in dogs, cats, and horses. Vet Clin Pathol 2009;38:136–156.

24. Hotamisligl GS, Shargill NS, Spiegelman BM. Adipose expression of tumor necrosis factor-alpha: direct role in obesity-linked insulin resistance. Science 1993;259:87–91.

25. Hotamisligl GS, Spiegelman BM. Tumor necrosis factor alpha: a key component of the obesity-diabetes link. Diabetes 1994;43:1271–1278.

26. Burns TA, Geor RJ, Mudge MC, et al. Proinflammatory cytokine and chemokine gene expression profiles in subcutaneous and visceral adipose tissue depots of insulin-resistant and insulin-sensitive light breed horses. J Vet Intern Med 2010;24:932–939.

27. Jackson S, Pagan JD. Equine nutrition evaluation. Large Anim Vet 1993;48:20–24.

28. National Research Council: Nutrient Requirements of Horses. Washington, DC, National Academies Press, 2007.

29. Hoffman RM, Wilson JA, Kronfeld DS, et al. Hydrolyzable carbohydrates in pasture, hay, and horse feeds: direct assay and seasonal variation. J Anim Sci 2001;79:500–506.

30. Garner HE, Moore JN, Johnson JH, et al. Changes in the caecal flora associated with the onset of laminitis. Equine Vet J 1978;10:249–252.

31. Rowe JB, Lees MJ, Pethick DW. Prevention of acidosis and laminitis associated with grain feeding in horses. J Nutr 1994;124:2742S–2744S.

32. French KR, Pollitt CC. Equine laminitis: loss of hemidesmosomes in hoof secondary epidermal lamellae correlates to dose in an oligofructose induction model: an ultrastructural study. Equine Vet J 2004;36:230–235.

33. Crawford C, Dobson A, Bailey SR, et al. Changes in hindgut pH of ponies following feeding with fructan carbohydrate in the form of inulin. Pferdeheilkunde 2005;21:71–72.

34. United States Department of Agriculture, Animal and Plant Health Inspection Service, Veterinary Sciences, Centers for Epidemiology and Animal Health, National Animal Health Monitoring System, Fort Collins, CO: Lameness and Laminitis in U.S. Horses, 2000.

35. Watts KA. Forage and pasture management for laminitis horses. Clin Tech Equine Pract 2004;3:88–95.

36. Equi-Analytical Laboratories. Accumulated crop years: 05/01/2000 through 04/30/2011 [Online]. www.equi-analytical.com. [Accessed February 5 2012].

37. Batten GD, Blakeney AB, McGrath VB, et al. Non structural carbohydrate: analysis by near infrared reflectance spectroscopy and its importance as an indicator of plant growth. Plant Soil 1993;155/156:243–246.

38. Belesky DP, Wilkinson SR, Stuedemann JA. The influence of nitrogen fertilizer and Acremonium coenophialum on soluble carbohydrate content of grazed and non-grased Festuca arundinace. Grass Forage Sci 1991;46:159–166.

39. Wilman D, Gao Y, Altimimi MA. Differences between related grasses, times of year and plant parts in digestibility and chemical composition. J Ag Sci 1996;127:311–318.

40. Kafi M, Stewart WS, Borland AM. Carbohydrate and proline contents in leaves, roots, and apices of salt-tolerant and salt-sensitive wheat cultivars. Russ J Plant Physiol, 2003;50:155–160.

41. Bertrand A, Castonguay Y, Nadeau P, et al. Oxygen deficiency affects carbohydrate reserves in overwintering forage crops. J Exp Bot 2003;54:1721–1730.

42. Minnick PD, Brown CM, Braselton WE, et al. The induction of equine laminitis with an aqueous extract of the heartwood of black walnut (Juglans nigra). Vet Hum Toxicol 1987;29:230–233.

43. Johnson PJ, Messer NT, Bowles DK, et al. Glucocorticoids and laminitis in horses. Compend Contin Educ Pract Vet 2004;26:547–557.

44. Johnson PJ, Messer NT, Ganjam VK. Cushing's syndromes, insulin resistance and endocrinopathic laminitis. Equine Vet J 2004;36:194–198.

45. Asplin KE, Sillence MN, Pollitt CC, et al. Induction of laminitis by prolonged hyperinsulinemia in clinically normal ponies. Vet J 2007;174:530–535.

46. Nourian AR, Asplin KE, McGowan CM, et al. Equine laminitis: ultrastructural lesions detected in ponies following hyperinsulinaemia. Equine Vet J 2009;41:671–677.

47. Bailey SR, Adair HS, Reinemeyer CR, et al. Plasma concentrations of endotoxin and platelet activation in the developmental stage of oligofructose-induced laminitis. Vet Immunol Immunopathol 2009;129:167–173.

48. Bailey SR, Marr CM, Elliott J. Current research and theories on the pathogenesis of acute laminitis in the horse. Vet J 2004;167:129–142.

49. Bailey SR, Menzies-Gow NJ, Harris PA, et al. Effect of dietary fructans and dexamethasone administration on the insulin response of ponies predisposed to laminitis. J Am Vet Med Assoc 2007;231:1365–1373.

50. Geor R, Frank N. Metabolic syndrome-From human organ disease to laminar failure in equids. Vet Immunol Immunopathol 2009;129:151–154.

51. deLaat MA, McGowan CM, Sillence MN, et al. Hyperinsulinemic laminitis. Vet Clin North Am Equine Pract 2010;26:257–264.

52. Geor RJ. Current concepts on the pathophysiology of pasture-associated laminitis. Vet Clin North Am Equine Pract 2010;26:265–276.

53. Longland AC, Byrd BM. Pasture nonstructural carbohydrates and equine laminitis. J Nutr 2006;136:2099S–2102S.

54. Pratt SE, Geor RJ, McCutcheon LJ. Effects of dietary energy source and physical conditioning on insulin sensitivity and glucose tolerance in standardbred horses. Equine Vet J Suppl 2006;36:579–584.

55. Milinovich GJ, Klieve AV, Pollitt CC, et al. Microbial events in the hindgut during carbohydrate-induced equine laminitis. Vet Clin North Am Equine Pract 2010;26:79–94.

56. Pollitt CC, Visser MB. Carbohydrate alimentary overload laminitis. Vet Clin North Am Equine Pract 2010;26:65–78.

57. Elliott J, Bailey SR: Gastrointestinal derived factors are potential triggers for the development of acute equine laminitis. J Nutr 2006;136:2103S–2107S.

58. Eades SC. Overview of current laminitis research. Vet Clin North Am Equine Pract, 2010;26:51–63.

59. Eades SC, Stokes AM, Johnson PJ, et al. Serial alterations in digital hemodynamics and endothelin-1 immunoreactivity, platelet-neutrophil aggregation, and concentrations of nitric oxide, insulin, and glucose in blood obtained from horses following carbohydrate overload. Am J Vet Res 2007;68:87–94.

60. Orth DN, Holscher MA, Wilson MG, et al. Equine Cushing's disease: plasma immunoreactive proopiolipomelanocortin peptide and cortisol levels basally and in response to diagnostic tests. Endocrinology 1982;110:1430–1441.

61. Schott HC. Pituitary pars intermedia dysfunction: equine Cushing's disease. Vet Clin North Am Equine Pract 2002;18:237–270.

62. Frank N. Equine metabolic syndrome. J Equine Vet Sci 2009;29:259–267.

63. Henneke DR, Potter GD, Kreider JL, et al. Relationship between condition score, physical measurements and body fat percentage in mares. Equine Vet J 1983;15:371–372.

64. Carter RA, Geor RJ, Burton-Staniar W, et al. Apparent adiposity assessed by standardised scoring systems and morphometric measurements in horses and ponies. Vet J 2009;179:204–210.

65. Durham AE, Hughes KJ, Cottle HJ, et al. Type 2 diabetes mellitus with pancreatic beta cell dysfunction in 3 horses confirmed with minimal model analysis. Equine Vet J 2009;41:924–929.

66. Walsh DM, McGowan CM, McGowan T, et al. Correlation of plasma insulin concentration with laminitis score in a field study of equine Cushing's disease and equine metabolic syndrome. J Equine Vet Sci 2009;29:87–94.

67. Shepherd ML, Pleasant RS, Chrisman MV, et al. Effects of high and moderate non-structural carbohydrate hay on insulin, glucose, triglyceride, and leptin concentrations in overweight Arabian geldings. J Anim Physiol Anim Nutr (Berl) 2012;96:428–435.

68. Caltabilota TJ, Earl LR, Thompson DL, et al. Hyperleptinemia in mares and geldings: assessment of insulin sensitivity from glucose responses to insulin injection. J Anim Sci 2010;88:2940–2949.

69. Johnson PJ, Wiedmeyer CE, LaCarrubba A, et al. Laminitis and the equine metabolic syndrome. Vet Clin North Am Equine Pract 2010;26:239–255.

70. Dugdale AH, Curtis GC, Cripps P, et al. Effect of dietary restriction on body condition, composition and welfare of overweight and obese pony mares. Equine Vet J 2010;42:600–610.

71. Geor RJ, Harris P. Dietary management of obesity and insulin resistance: countering risk for laminitis. Vet Clin North Am Equine Pract 2009;25:51–65,vi.

72. Waitt LH, Cebra CK. Characterization of hypertriglyceridemia and response to treatment with insulin in horses, ponies, and donkeys: 44 cases (1995–2005). J Am Vet Med Assoc 2009;234:915–919.

73. Longland AC, Barfoot C, Harris PA. Effects of soaking on the water-soluble carbohydrate and crude protein content of hay. Vet Rec 2011;168:618.

74. Frank N, Buchanan BR, Elliott SB. Effects of long-term oral administration of levothyroxine sodium on serum thyroid hormone concentrations, clinicopathologic variables, and echocardiographic measurements in healthy adult horses. Am J Vet Res 2008;69:68–75.

75. Toth F, Frank N, Geor RJ, et al. Effects of pretreatment with dexamethasone or levothyroxine sodium on endotoxin-induced alterations in glucose and insulin dynamics in horses. Am J Vet Res 2010;71:60–68.

76. Durham AE, Rendle DI, Newton JE. The effect of metformin on measurements of insulin sensitivity and beta cell response in 18 horses and ponies with insulin resistance. Equine Vet J 2008;40:493–500.

77. Hustace JL, Firshman AM, Mata JE. Pharmacokinetics and bioavailability of metformin in horses. Am J Vet Res 2009;70:665–668.

78. Durham AE, Rendle DI, Rutledge F, et al. The effects of metformin hydrochloride on intestinal glucose absorption and use of tests for hyperinsulinaemia. Proc Am Coll Vet Intern Med 2012; 281.

79. Wearn JG, Suagee JK, Chrisman MV. Effects of the insulin sensitizing drug pioglitazone on indices of insulin homeostasis in horses following endotoxin administration. J Vet Intern Med 2010;24: 709.

80. Frank N. Management of pituitary pars intermedia dysfunction (PPID). Proc 16th Annual North Carolina Vet Conf, 2011.

81. Ralston SL. Nutrition of horses with pituitary dysfunction. Proc 3rd Mid-Atlantic Nutrition Conf 2005;171–176.

82. Donaldson MT, McDonnell SM, Schanbacher BJ, et al. Variation in plasma adrenocorticotrophic hormone concentration and dexamethasone suppression test results with season, age, and sex in healthy ponies and horses. J Vet Intern Med 2005;19:217–222.

83. Frank N, Elliott SB, Chameroy KA, et al. Association of season and pasture grazing with blood hormone and metabolite concentrations in horses with presumed pituitary pars intermedia dysfunction. J Vet Intern Med 2010;24: 1167–1175.

84. Pagan JD, Waldridge BM, Lange J. Moderate dietary carbohydrate improves glucose tolerance and high dietary fat impairs glucose tolerance in aged Thoroughbred geldings. Proc Am Assoc Equine Pract 2011;57:192.

6 Respiratory system

Bryan M. Waldridge, DVM, MS, DABVP, DACVIM

Stabled horses are constantly exposed to large amounts of airborne irritants. This is especially true when horses are kept in stalls, fed hay, and bedded on straw. Environmental management is critical to reduce aeroallergen exposure for reactive airway diseases such as heaves and inflammatory airway disease. Horses with infectious respiratory tract infections also likely benefit from reduced inhaled dust levels because they have damaged respiratory epithelium and impaired mucociliary clearance.

6.1 Effects of Inhaled Dust and Potential Aeroallergens on Equine Respiratory Disease

Equine respiratory tract infections may be exacerbated and prolonged by concomitant airborne dust exposure.[1,2] Horses with infectious respiratory tract infections that are kept in dusty environments have prolonged recovery due to increased coughing, hypersecretion of mucus, and brochoconstriction. Some authors speculate that respiratory tract infection coupled with stabling in a dusty environment may cause horses to become sensitized to inhaled environmental aeroallergens and contribute to the development of heaves later in life. It is important to minimize dust exposure for horses recovering from respiratory tract infections.

Heaves (recurrent airway obstruction) is a reactive airway disease of horses characterized by bronchoconstriction, excessive mucus production, and pathologic changes of the bronchioles.[3] Affected horses are hypersensitive to inhaled environmental dust. Hay has been shown to be an important source of many of the inhaled allergens that induce clinical signs of heaves. Environmental changes to reduce inhaled dust exposure are essential for the successful treatment of heaves, regardless of pharmacologic therapy.

6.2 Respirable Dust Deposition in the Airways

Particles in inhaled air will be deposited onto the respiratory epithelium depending on their diameter, shape, and hydrophobic or hydrophilic properties.[1] Elongated particles can penetrate deeper into the lungs than spherical particles. Most large particles ($\geq 5 \mu m$ in diameter) settle in the nasal turbinates, pharynx, or bifurcation of large airways by inertial impaction when airflow changes in direction or velocity. For size comparison, an equine erythrocyte is approximately $5 \mu m$ in diameter. Small particles (0.5–$5.0 \mu m$ in diameter) can settle in the lungs as deep as the respiratory bronchioles. Small particles deposit by gravitational sedimentation which is proportional to the particle's density and square of its diameter. Particles $< 0.5 \mu m$ in diameter are usually exhaled back out of the respiratory tract. Very small particles ($< 0.1 \mu m$ in diameter) can be cleared by diffusion in the small airways and alveoli.

Respiratory rate and depth, tidal volume, and lung volume all impact the deposition of particles in the lung. Deep breaths increase the proportion of particles that are deposited farther into the lungs. Important clearance mechanisms of inhaled particles include coughing, the mucociliary escalator, and phagocytosis by pulmonary macrophages. Alveolar clearance is much slower than tracheobronchial clearance.

The respirable dust concentration (RDC) is defined as the small particles ($< 5 \mu m$ in diameter) that are able to enter the peripheral, small diameter airways and potentially cause pulmonary inflammation.[4,5] The RDC is considered a good indicator of the health hazard created by inhalation of an airborne dust.[4–6] The breathing zone is defined as the region surrounding the horse's nostrils (Figure 6.1).[6] Dust exposure in the horse's breathing zone more accurately reflects its respiratory challenge

Nutritional Management of Equine Diseases and Special Cases, First Edition. Edited by Bryan M. Waldridge.
© 2017 John Wiley & Sons, Inc. Published 2017 by John Wiley & Sons, Inc.

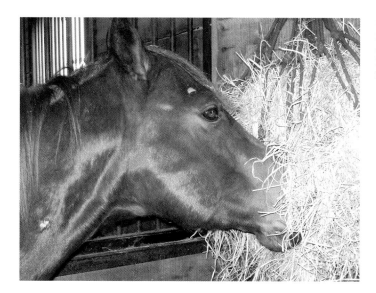

Figure 6.1 A horse eating from a haynet with its nostrils buried into the hay. This illustrates the close contact that a horse has with its forage and how respirable dust from forage enters the breathing zone.

because horses spend much of their time with their muzzles in close contact with hay and bedding.[1] Hay and bedding are the primary sources of airborne dust for horses.[1,2] The highest exposure of airborne irritants comes from mold contaminated forages and bedding sources.

Even in well-ventilated stables, airborne dust concentrations (ADC) in the horse's breathing zone are still high when the horse eats and nuzzles its forage.[2] Stable ventilation alone does not remove particles from the horse's breathing zone.[1] The amount of respirable dust in the horse's breathing zone can be much higher than the overall stall or stable environment.[1,6] The only effective way to reduce inhaled particles in the horse's breathing zone is to feed a less dusty forage.[6,7] Several studies have found that total ADC is highest during the day when stall cleaning and barn activity are greatest.[1,5,6]

Researchers have developed several methods to measure airborne particles in the horse's breathing zone and in the stable or stall environment. Many air samplers draw a continuous stream of air through a filter over a given period of time. The filter is then weighed to determine dust concentration. Other air samplers can measure changes in real time ADC data using a laser photometer or piezoelectric balances. The specific microbiologic population of respirable dust that is collected can be identified by microscopic examination, culture, or use of polymerase chain reaction methods.

Good quality hay that passes visual inspection still contains large numbers of particles that can reach the terminal airways and irritate the respiratory tract.[1,2,8–10] Hay is the primary source of inhaled respiratory irritants in the horse's environment, especially if it was baled under less favorable conditions.[11] Clements and Pirie[4] reported that feed had a greater influence on mean and maximum RDC in the horse's breathing zone than stall bedding. Inhaled particles in hay that can act as respiratory irritants include mold spores, bacteria, endotoxin, and plant and insect fragments.[1,8,11]

If hay is baled with a high moisture content, then it produces heat and promotes growth of thermotolerant fungi (*Aspergillus fumigatus*) and bacteria, such as the actinomycetes (*Saccharopolyspora rectivurgula* and *Thermoactinomyces vulgaris*).[1,8] Ideally, hay is baled at 15–20% moisture content because it will heat very little and contain small amounts of dust and mold spores.[8] Hay baled at 20–30% moisture can heat to 35–45 °C (95–113 °F), favoring the growth of fungi and actinomycetes. The heaviest growth of thermotolerant fungi and actinomycetes occurs when hay is baled at 35–50% moisture. High moisture hay can contain large amounts of fungal and actinomycete spores. These spores range from 1–5 μm in diameter and can be inhaled into the lower airways and cause inflammation. Dust mites feed on fungal spores. Consequently, if hay is moldy, then it may also contain large numbers of dust mites and their feces which are another respiratory irritant.

6.3 Effects of Soaking Hay

Soaking hay in water has been the traditional method to reduce RDC. However, soaking hay is difficult and not always a practical management recommendation for horse owners. The nutritional impact of soaking hay can be significant, especially if the hay is of marginal quality, and is often overlooked. Recommended soaking times to reduce respirable dust range from simply dunking the hay in water and feeding immediately afterwards to soaking overnight for hours. Researchers have also investigated whether flakes of hay can be soaked in a haynet or as the entire bale with the baling twine cut. The ideal soak time will maximize the benefit of reduced aeroallergen challenge with minimal loss of nutritional value. The results of several studies investigating the effects of soaking hay on its respirable dust content and/or nutritional value are summarized in Table 6.1.

Clements and Pirie[5] found that only immersing 5 kg of hay in a haynet in a bucket of water and feeding immediately afterwards significantly reduced both mean breathing zone dust and RDC compared to dry hay. There was no significant difference in mean breathing zone RDC between hay that was only immersed (dunked in a bucket of water until completely submerged) or soaked for 16 h. Blackman and Moore-Colyer[7] reported no significant difference in the decrease of respiratory dust particles when 2.5 kg of hay in a haynet was soaked for either 10 or 30 min. Both treatments reduced respiratory dust by at least 93%, compared to unsoaked hay.

Soaking hay affects its nutritional value in a time-dependent manner.[7,10,11] Even soaking hay for as short as 30 min or less can reduce sodium, potassium, phosphorous, magnesium, and copper concentrations.[7,11] Studies differ on soaking hay and the decrease in water-soluble carbohydrates and crude protein.[7,10] Prolonged soaking reduces the nutritional value of hay and soaking hay for longer than 30 min has a considerable negative impact on nutrient composition.[7,10,11] Two studies[7,11] reported that there was little to gain regarding reduced respiratory challenge and much nutritional value to lose if hay was soaked for longer than 30 min. Soaking hay for 30 min effectively minimized its respirable challenge and maintained maximal nutritional value.[11]

6.4 Effects of Steam Treating Hay

Steam treatment reduces airborne dust and preserves the nutritional content of hay. Both steaming and soaking hay have been shown to reduce respiratory particles by at least 93%.[7] There was no significant difference in respirable particles between hay that was soaked for 10 or 30 min and hay that was steamed for 80 min. When compared with dry hay, steam treatment resulted in no loss of nutrients. Soaking hay for 10 or 30 min significantly reduced phosphorus, potassium, magnesium, sodium, and copper. Using a commercially available hay steamer (Figure 6.2; Haygain hay steamer, Haygain North America, Union City, TN), James and Moore-Colyer[9] reduced fungal elements by 100% and bacterial growth by 98.84%, compared to dry hay. The palatability of steamed hay was reported to be good.

6.5 Feeding Forage Alternatives

6.5.1 Haylage
Haylage is fermented forage that has higher moisture content than hay and is lower in dust and mold spores, if properly processed. Clements and Pirie[5] investigated the effects on RDC when feeding hay or haylage and bedding horses on straw or wood shavings. The results of their study indicated that feed has a greater impact on RDC than bedding and haylage is preferable to hay to improve equine respiratory health. Feeding haylage instead of hay reduced mean RDC by 60–70% and maximum RDC by 76–93%. Changing bedding from straw to wood shavings also reduced RDC, especially maximum RDC, but the results showed that RDC in the horse's breathing zone is more influenced by close contact with feed rather than bedding.

6.5.2 Hay Cubes
Feeding hay cubes instead of hay significantly lowers a horse's respirable dust exposure. Raymond et al.[2] investigated the respirable dust levels that horses were exposed to when fed alfalfa cubes and good or poor quality hay. Feeding hay cubes significantly reduced the amount of dust in the horses' breathing zone as compared to when the horses were fed hay. Interestingly, there was no difference in dust levels in the horses' breathing zone or in the center aisle of the barn when

Table 6.1 Summary of results from studies investigating the effects of soaking hay on respirable dust and nutrient composition.

Duration of Hay Soaking	Decrease in Respirable Dust* (%)	Effects of Soaking on Nutritional Content, Compared to Hay Before Soaking	Conclusions	Reference
• 10 min	• 93	• K, Mg, and Cu reduced by 30, 14, and 27%, respectively	• No significant difference in the decrease of respirable particles between 10 and 30 min soak	7
• 30 min	• 96	• K, Mg, Cu, and Na reduced by 40, 15, 30, and 36%, respectively	• Soaked hay with a high mineral content will still meet maintenance requirements • Supplementation of minerals may be necessary after soaking hay that has poor mineral content	
• 30 min • 3 h • 12 h	• 88 • 89 • 93	• After 30 min of soaking, Na, K, and P reduced by 43, 27, and 14%, respectively • ≥180 min of soaking reduced Na, K, P, and Mg by 60, 58, 35, and 19%, respectively	• Soaking hay for 30 min effectively minimizes respirable particles and maintains nutritional value • Soaking hay for >30 min significantly increases losses of Na, K, P, and Mg • Working horses may need supplemental Na to meet losses in sweat if fed soaked hay	11
• Immersed‡ • 16 h	• 60 • 71		No significant difference in respirable dust between hay that was only immersed or soaked for 16 h	5
• 5 min • 10 min • 30 min • 2 h • 8 h • 12 h		• 12-h soak reduced water-soluble carbohydrates by 2–4% and crude protein by 1.5–2.0%	• Soaking hay for 30 min or less reduced losses of water-soluble carbohydrates and crude protein • Soaking hay for 5–10 min minimizes nutrient losses while significantly reducing respiratory challenge	10

* Decrease in respirable dust significantly different (p ≤ 0.05) from unsoaked hay
‡ Hay immersed in a bucket of water only until completely submerged

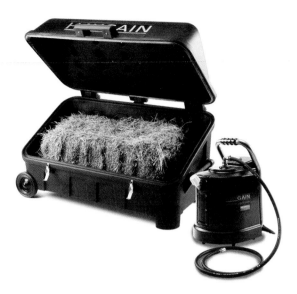

Figure 6.2 A commercially available hay steamer. Photograph courtesy of Haygain North America, Union City, TN. Courtesy of Haygain, North America.

fed either good or poor quality hay. Compared to alfalfa cubes, good and poor quality hay contained increasingly more potential aeroallergens, such as plant material, fungal spores, pollen grains, dust mites, and their feces. In contrast to hay, alfalfa cubes contained negligible fungal spores and no pollen grains.

6.5.3 Pellets

Woods et al.[6] reduced dust in the breathing zone of ponies to only 3% of previous levels when feed was changed from dusty hay to pellets and bedding was changed from straw to wood shavings. Airborne dust concentration in the stall was significantly affected by environmental change as well; ADC was approximately doubled when ponies were fed dusty hay and bedded on straw, compared to feeding pellets and bedding on wood shavings. Aeroallergens such as *S. rectivurgula*, *A. fumigatus*, and dust mite allergens, were significantly higher when hay and straw were in the ponies' environment.

6.6 Exercise-Induced Pulmonary Hemorrhage

Erythrocyte numbers in bronchoalveolar fluid were reduced when horses were supplemented with the long chain omega-3 fatty acids docasahexaenoic acid (DHA)

and eicosapentaenoic acid (EPA) for 83 and 145 days and exercised on a high-speed treadmill.[12] There was no effect when horses were supplemented with only DHA. Fish oils are an excellent source of omega-3 fatty acids such as DHA and EPA. Supplementation of DHA and EPA may improve erythrocyte membrane fluidity and their movement through capillaries, which could reduce the likelihood for pulmonary capillary bleeding. Omega-3 fatty acids have inherent anti-inflammatory effects that may also reduce airway inflammation and, consequently, the predisposition for capillary rupture.

6.7 Acute Interstitial Pneumonia

Horses do not develop acute atypical interstitial pneumonia (AIP; pulmonary edema and emphysema) after eating lush green pastures, moldy sweet potatoes, or other plants associated with AIP in cattle. For example, horses do not have a rumen and L-tryptophan in lush pasture is not converted to pulmonary toxic metabolites such as 3-methyl indole. It is still prudent to avoid feeding moldy sweet potatoes, kale, rape, and turnip tops to horses to avoid any possible pulmonary problems.

References

1. Art T, McGorum BC, Lekeux P. Environmental control of respiratory disease. In: Lekeux P, ed. Equine respiratory diseases. Ithaca, NY: International Veterinary Information Service (www.ivis.org), Document No. B0334.0302, 2002.
2. Raymond SL, Curtis EF, Clarke AF. Comparative dust challenges faced by horses when fed alfalfa cubes or hay. Eq Pract 1994;16(10):42–47.
3. Lavoie JP. Heaves (recurrent airway obstruction): practical management of acute episodes and prevention of exacerbations. In: Robinson NE, Ed. Current therapy in equine medicine, 5. Philadelphia: Saunders, 2003;417–421.
4. Clements JM, Pirie RS. Respirable dust concentrations in equine stables. Part 1: validation of equipment and effect of various management systems. Res Vet Sci 2007;83: 256–262.
5. Clements JM, Pirie RS. Respirable dust concentrations in equine stables. Part 2: the benefits of soaking hay and optimising the environment in a neighbouring stable. Res Vet Sci 2007;83:263–268.
6. Woods PSA, Robinson NE, Swanson MC, et al. Airborne dust and aeroallergen concentration in a horse stable under two different management systems. Eq Vet J 1993;25:208–213.

7. Blackman M, Moore-Colyer MJS. Hay for horses: the effects of three different wetting treatments on dust and nutrient content. Anim Sci 1998;66: 745–750.

8. Clarke AF, Madelin T. Technique for assessing respiratory health hazards from hay and other source materials. Eq Vet J 1987;19:442–447.

9. James R, Moore-Colyer M. The effect of steam treatment on the total viable count, mould and yeast numbers in hay using the Haygain hay steamer. In: Ellis AD, Longland AC, Coenen M, et al., eds. The impact of nutrition on the health and welfare of horses. Wageningen Academic Pub, 2010;128–132.

10. Warr EM, Petch JL. Effects of soaking hay on its nutritional quality. Eq Vet Educ 1992;5:169–171.

11. Moore-Colyer MJS. Effects of soaking hay fodder for horses on dust and mineral content. Anim Sci 1996;63:337–342.

12. Erickson HH, Epp TS, Poole DC. Review of alternative therapies for EIPH, in Proceedings. Am Assoc Equine Pract, 2007;68–71.

7 Neurologic system

Peter Huntington, BVSc (Hons), MANZCVS

The horse does not suffer the same number of neurologic diseases related to nutritional deficiency, excess, or feed related toxicity as other domestic animals. However, there are some neurologic diseases where modified feeding and nutritional support plays a key part in the treatment and management of affected horses.

7.1 Cervical Vertebral Malformation

Cervical vertebral malformation (CVM or wobbler) causes ataxia and weakness related to stenosis or instability of the vertebral canal. This is caused by malformation or malalignment of vertebrae. There is an association with osteochondrosis in affected horses; suggesting a general failure in development of the skeletal system.[1] The disorder usually affects fast growing, young, large breed horses and feeding programs that promote rapid growth may increase the risk of CVM. In a classic study, Wagner et al.[2] bred radiographically confirmed wobbler mares and stallions. Only one resulting foal had cervical vertebral subluxation, but the other offspring had a high incidence of osteochondrosis, physitis, and flexural limb deformities. This study emphasized that CVM is strongly associated with developmental orthopedic disease. Therefore, the same management and nutritional strategies to prevent developmental orthopedic disease are recommended to reduce the incidence of CVM in young horses.

Management changes may correct CVM in horses less than 1 year of age that have neurologic deficits and/or radiographic signs of CVM. A 5-year field study was performed on a Thoroughbred breeding farm with a high incidence of CVM.[3,4] Foals that had radiographic changes with or without neurologic deficits were weaned and treated with dietary and exercise restriction. Foals were examined every 3–4 months from birth until they entered race training. Examinations included physical and neurologic examinations, standing cervical radiographs, and weekly body condition scoring and measurement of height and body weight. Horses older than 1 year of age and showing severe ataxia were less likely to improve with dietary and exercise restriction because they already had significant spinal cord damage and there was insufficient time for skeletal growth to correct bony remodeling of the vertebral column.[3]

Confinement to a stall or small paddock and a reduction in energy intake to only 65–75% of total digestible nutrient and crude protein requirements for a horse's given age and expected growth rate has been used as a successful treatment in some horses less than 12 months of age (Table 7.1).[4-6] This diet aims to supply recommended daily allowances of protein, amino acids, minerals, and vitamins, but restricted energy intake leads to a reduction in growth rate and a loss in body condition. Treated horses became very thin with dietary restriction. The diet was adjusted on an individual basis every 3–4 months, based on the rate of growth compared to other foals, body condition, and improvement in neurologic signs or radiographic changes. Affected horses were confined to a stall or small paddock to reduce the risk of neurologic injury and better control dietary intake. Feeding was not increased for horses that did not improve or lose body condition, which effectively reduced dietary intake to 65% of National Research Council (NRC) recommendations.[7] Horses that improved neurologically (ataxia score less than 1/5) or radiographically (no stenosis) had their dietary intake slowly increased to 75% of NRC recommendations. Normal diet and activity was gradually increased over a 4-week period.

All horses treated with dietary restriction and reduced exercise went into race training.[4] Eighty-three percent (15/18) of treated foals made at least one race start and won 18% (32/179) of starts and 87% at least placed in a race.

Nutritional Management of Equine Diseases and Special Cases, First Edition. Edited by Bryan M. Waldridge.
© 2017 John Wiley & Sons, Inc. Published 2017 by John Wiley & Sons, Inc.

Table 7.1 Restricted diet for young horses with cervical vertebral malformation.[3,4]

Energy (total digestible nutrients) and protein	65–75% of National Research Council (NRC) recommendations[7]
Vitamins and minerals	≥100% of NRC recommendations
Vitamins A and E	300% of NRC recommendations
Calcium and phosphorous	100% of NRC recommendations, as dicalcium phosphate and limestone
Zinc*	200% of NRC recommendations, as $ZnSO_4$
Copper*	350% of NRC recommendations, as $CuSO_4$
Selenium	0.3 ppm (mg/kg) in total diet
Grass or low quality timothy hay	6–9% crude protein
Plain white salt	Free choice

* Copper and zinc were supplemented for less than 2 out of the 5 total years of the study.

Hoffman and Clark reported that only 30% of young Thoroughbreds in race training diagnosed with CVM based on neurologic examination and standing cervical radiographs and treated conservatively started at least one race.[8] Horses in this retrospective study were treated with dietary and exercise restriction, anti-inflammatories, and/or vitamin E supplementation. Neither dietary changes nor vitamin E supplementation had a significant effect for affected horses to return to racing. Horses that raced had lesser neurologic deficits and less severe radiographic changes than horses that were euthanatized or never started a race. It should be noted that horses in race training are 2–3 years of age and older than those in the studies by Donawick et al.[3,4]

7.2 Botulism

Botulism is a disorder caused by neurotoxins produced by *Clostridium botulinum* bacteria. Clinical signs result from irreversible binding of a neurotoxin at the presynaptic neuron cell membrane that inhibits release of acetylcholine, leading to muscle weakness that can progress to generalized flaccid paralysis. The classic signs are poor tongue and eyelid tone and dysphagia, but general muscle weakness, stiff gait, and increased periods of recumbency are also observed. An early clinical sign of botulism is feed left in the bottom of the feed bin, as weakness of the muscles controlling the lips makes it difficult to pick up feed.[9] One simple diagnostic test for suspected cases of botulism is the "grain test" where the horse is offered 8 oz of grain. A normal horse should consume the grain within 2 min; horses with botulism cannot eat the grain normally or swallow. Affected horses will often try to eat the grain without using their lips and difficulty swallowing can be exhibited by saliva, occasionally mixed with grain, draining from the nostrils.[10]

Most cases of botulism in adult horses are called forage poisoning as preformed toxin is ingested from hay, haylage, silage, or chaff. Grain has also been reported as a source, but forage is the more likely culprit. The contamination often comes when small field animals are trapped in forage and the bacteria multiply in anaerobic conditions inside baled hay or haylage. Horses can also ingest soil-borne botulism toxin from hay that has been trampled into the ground. Botulism is often associated with improperly ensiled silage or haylage that was not maintained at a sufficiently acidic pH and then fed to horses. Toxin can rarely be detected in feed samples, but spores can be isolated in affected feed. Toxicoinfectious botulism (shaker foal syndrome) is observed in foals, when clostridial spores germinate in the gastrointestinal tract. A third and less common cause relates to wound or surgical site contamination by botulism spores (wound botulism).[5]

Diagnosis is based on clinical signs and detection of toxin in feed, gastrointestinal contents, serum, or wounds. Horses are so sensitive to low levels of toxin that it is not always detected by mouse inoculation or other assays. The most important treatment is intravenous administration of antitoxin, which binds circulating toxin and prevents further neuromuscular impairment. The prognosis depends upon the amount of bound and circulating toxin when antitoxin is administered. Antitoxin can bind only free botulinum toxin, not the toxin already affecting the neuromuscular junction. If given whilst the horse is still standing, approximately 70% of horses can recover once the damaged neurons regenerate.[11]

If horses affected with botulism are unable to swallow, then supportive care includes administration of fluids and feed by nasogastric tube or parenteral nutrition. Dysphagia creates a risk of aspiration pneumonia and ileus may be present, which necessitates a switch to parenteral nutrition. There are a number of enteral nutrition formulas that have been used successfully, but consideration needs to be given to electrolyte intake, digestible energy, and protein sources, as well as fiber for large intestinal function. The use of high quality digestible protein sources can supply amino acid needs in spite of a feeding program that does not meet all the daily crude protein requirements. Milk-based protein sources such as casein or whey are valuable in these situations. Alfalfa meal or soaked and ground alfalfa pellets or cubes are good sources of high quality protein, fiber, calcium and potassium. Complete pelleted feeds can be ground and mixed with water. For a further discussion on enteral and parenteral nutrition, refer to Chapter 3 on the gastrointestinal system.

Prevention of botulism involves avoiding feeding suspect or spoiled haylage or silage to horses. Any hay that contains animal carcasses should not be fed and disposed of where livestock will not consume it. Feeding hay off the ground or on pads, especially in muddy areas or where horses congregate reduces horses' exposure to botulism spores where hay can be trodden in the soil. Vaccination against botulism type B is recommended in endemic areas and before foaling in pregnant mares. However, there are several different types of botulism and vaccination will not be cross-protective against all types.

7.3 Ryegrass Staggers

Ryegrass staggers occurs in horses and other animals grazing perennial ryegrass (*Lolium perenne*) pasture or hay infected with the endophyte *Neotyphodium lolii* (ex *Acremonium loliae*), which produces the toxic alkaloid lolitrem B. There is a seasonal pattern to the disease with late summer and autumn being the period of highest risk.

Affected horses should be removed from the toxic source of ryegrass and will recover quickly. A reduction in the intake of infected ryegrass is recommended for unaffected horses by paddock change or supplementary feeding. Oral mycotoxin binders are used in the prevention of this disorder, but there is no data in horses or other animals to support their use.[12] Low endophyte varieties of ryegrass seed are available for planting in pasture where the disorder presents a major problem.

7.4 Equine Degenerative Myelopathy and Neuroaxonal Dystrophy

Equine degenerative myelopathy (EDM) and neuroaxonal dystrophy (NAD) are degenerative diseases of the central nervous system (CNS). Differences between clinical signs and classification depend on what area of the CNS is affected, but ataxia and weakness are common signs. EDM occurs in many light horse breeds and clinical signs are usually observed before 6 months of age. NAD affects growing horses less than 2 years of age and affected horses often appear dull and depressed. Both disorders have breed predispositions and a heritable component linked with dietary vitamin E deficiency.[13,14] NAD is associated with neurologic disease in humans, sheep, cats, and dogs as well as horses. A familial tendency has been found in Appaloosas, Morgans, and Quarter Horses.[15] EDM and NAD cannot be clinically distinguished from each other and share many histopathologic lesions.[16] EDM involves additional white matter tracts and is speculated to be a more severe form of NAD.

Clinical signs of NAD include mild to severe ataxia, obtundation, decreased to absent menace reflex, proprioceptive deficits, and a wide-based stance.[15,16] Diagnosis of NAD can only be made with histopathologic examination of the nervous system. Lesions involve the brain stem and thoracic spinal cord and are characterized by bilaterally symmetrical neuroaxonal degeneration with axonal spheroids. Horses affected with NAD have low serum vitamin E concentration, but vitamin E supplementation does not improve neurologic deficits. Vitamin E supplementation will reduce the prevalence of new NAD cases on affected breeding farms.

Low to very low serum vitamin E concentrations are found in affected horses and the pathologic features are in common with experimental vitamin E deficiency in other animals. Normal serum vitamin E concentrations are greater than 2 µg/ml and deficiency can be diagnosed if levels are 1 µg/ml or less. However, low serum vitamin E concentration can be seen in normal horses without any signs of neurologic disease.

EDM has been reported in many domestic breeds and in some wild equids.[13,17,18] Clinical signs of EDM usually begin in the first year of life and include bilaterally symmetrical ataxia (which may be worse in the hind limbs), weakness, and proprioceptive deficits. Histopathologic lesions of EDM consist of neuroaxonal dystrophy and variable lipofuscinosis in brain stem nuclei and diffusely throughout the spinal cord.

Treatment of severe chronic EDM cases with 2,000 IU of synthetic vitamin E has not been effective, but high doses (6,000 IU, PO, q24h) of synthetic vitamin E have halted the progression of clinical signs in some foals. Supplementation with 1,000–3,000 IU per day to all horses on farms where EDM cases have occurred has led to increased serum vitamin E concentrations and reduced incidence of the disease.[17,19] As well as specific vitamin E supplements, the provision of fresh green forage will substantially improve vitamin E status.

7.5 Equine Motor Neuron Disease

Equine motor neuron disease (EMND) is a rare neuro-degenerative disorder of the somatic lower motor neurons within the spinal cord, affecting horses from 2–25 years of age. EMND was first reported in 1990 by Cornell University veterinarians. EMND is very similar to human motor neuron disease (amyotrophic lateral sclerosis or Lou Gehrig's disease). EMND is an oxidative disorder that preferentially affects motor neurons in the spinal cord that have a high oxidative activity. Neuronal cell death results in preferential neurogenic atrophy of type I muscle fibers. Horses that are deprived of pasture or green, high-quality hay and not supplemented with vitamin E for more than 18 months are at greatest risk for EMND.

Subacute and chronic forms of EMND are observed. Chronic weight loss related to muscle atrophy is often the first sign. Signs for the subacute form include acute onset trembling, muscle fasciculations, lying down, shifting of weight onto the hind legs, low head carriage, inability to lock the stifles, and symmetrical loss of muscle mass throughout the body. Affected horses are not ataxic and walking is easier than standing. In chronic cases, trembling and muscle fasciculations decrease and the horse may stabilize with varying degrees of muscle atrophy or clinical signs can progress to emaciation.[9,20]

There is no definitive antemortem diagnosis for EMND, but it is usually based on history, clinical signs, biopsy of the sacrocaudalis dorsalis medialis muscle, and measurement of serum vitamin E concentration and muscle enzyme activities. Previous cases of EMND on a premise or history that the horse has been without green forage or supplementary vitamin E for an extended period of time increase the level of suspicion of EMND. Many, but not all, cases of EMND will have serum vitamin E concentrations lower than 1 µg/ml and vitamin E concentration is also low in other tissues. High copper concentration in the spinal cord and elevated iron concentration in the liver are also noted in some affected horses. Muscle biopsy of the sacrocaudalis dorsalis medialis muscle and histopathologic evidence of neurogenic atrophy are often diagnostic for EMND. This muscle is used because it has a high proportion of oxidative type I muscle fibers that are preferentially damaged.

The role of low vitamin E intake and high copper and iron in the diet was investigated by Divers et al.[21] Eight horses were confined to a dry lot and fed a diet low in vitamin E from old grass hay and a concentrate, which supplied approximately 20 IU/kg vitamin E. The experimental concentrate also contained high levels of copper (4,000 ppm) and iron (2,000 ppm). Control horses were allowed seasonal access to pasture or fed grass hay and concentrate, which contained recommended amounts of vitamin E, copper, and iron. Four of eight experimental horses developed clinical signs of EMND after 21–28 months on this diet, but no control horses developed EMND. All experimental horses had low serum concentrations of vitamin E. The clinically affected cases had a mean serum vitamin E concentration of 0.25 µg/ml, compared to the unaffected horses with a mean concentration of 0.39 µg/ml. The affected horses showed classic histologic changes in spinal cord, nerves, and muscles. Control horses had some histopathologic changes in nerves. The eight horses fed the experimental diet had low hepatic vitamin E concentrations and very high concentrations of copper compared to control horses and expected normal ranges. This study provided evidence that the lack of access to pasture, dietary deficiency of vitamin E, and excessive copper intake are risk factors for EMND. As vitamin E is a fat soluble vitamin, it takes some months before tissue stores are depleted, even when horses are fed a very deficient diet.

Adult horses with clinical signs of EMND should be treated with 5,000–10,000 IU of vitamin E/500 kg, PO, q24h. Stabilization of clinical signs and gradual improvement may occur if horses are not too debilitated prior to treatment. Natural vitamin E provides higher blood and cerebrospinal fluid (CSF) concentrations of vitamin E for affected horses. Horses on the same premises without access to green pasture should receive at least 1,000 IU of supplementary vitamin E per day. However, there have been no clinical trials showing that treatment with vitamin E can stop or reverse the disease process in EMND cases. With treatment, about 40% of cases improve or stabilize, but often the long-term prognosis is poor.[9]

7.6 Effect of Form and Dose of Vitamin E on Serum and Cerebrospinal Fluid Concentrations

The α-tocopherol molecule has eight possible stereoisomers. Several studies have shown that the RRR-α-tocopherol or d-α-tocopherol isomer (natural vitamin E) has a higher biologic antioxidant activity and better absorption than others. Synthetic vitamin E is a racemic α-tocopherol mixture (all-rac-α-tocopherol or d,l-α-tocopherol).

Higgins et al.[22] supplemented horses with either 1,000 IU or 10,000 IU of water-soluble, natural, micellized vitamin E for 10 days. Serum vitamin E concentrations were measured every three days and CSF was obtained from the atlantooccipital space on the first and tenth day. Serum vitamin E concentrations significantly increased with either dose of vitamin E. Vitamin E concentrations in CSF were highest in horses that received 10,000 IU of supplemental vitamin E, but the difference in CSF α-tocopherol was not statistically significant. The results of the study showed that supplemental vitamin E, at either dose, could raise CSF α-tocopherol concentrations by 1.3–3.4 times within 10 days. This research confirmed that a micellized natural form of vitamin E could penetrate the blood-brain barrier and enter the CSF.

In another study by Pusteria et al.,[23] horses were supplemented with either 5,000 or 10,000 IU of water-soluble natural, micellized vitamin E or 10,000 IU of synthetic vitamin E for 14 days. Serum vitamin E concentrations were measured every 3 days and CSF was sampled on the first and fourteenth day. Serum and CSF vitamin E concentrations were significantly correlated. The highest serum α-tocopherol concentrations were found after 7 days of supplementation in the horses given 10,000 IU of d-α-tocopherol. This dose also produced higher serum and CSF α-tocopherol concentrations than the 5,000 IU dose of d-α-tocopherol.

Treatment with d,l-α-tocopherol acetate led to a small increase in serum α-tocopherol concentration, but did not change CSF concentration, a finding that has also been seen in humans. Natural vitamin E was better absorbed and passed through the blood-brain barrier more effectively than synthetic vitamin E. The results of this study showed that natural micellized vitamin E was more bioavailable and resulted in greater serum and CSF vitamin E concentrations.

Pagan et al.[24] compared the bioavailability of a single 5,000 IU dose of 2 preparations of d-α-tocopherol and synthetic vitamin E. The d-α-tocopherol administered was either a water soluble micellized form or a nanodispersed natural form. The natural vitamin E preparations had a significantly greater area under the curve (AUC) than the synthetic form, but there was no significant difference in AUC between the two natural forms. The bioavailability of the natural vitamin E preparations was 559 and 613%, respectively, compared to synthetic vitamin E. Other work with a nanodispersed natural vitamin E liquid has shown that a 5,000 IU dose will increase serum concentrations by 1.5–2.0 times over baseline within 6 h, whereas a similar dose of synthetic vitamin E produces little change in serum concentration.[19]

Horses suffering from neurologic disease may require more vitamin E than normal, healthy horses. Vitamin E supplementation and increased CSF vitamin E concentration can enhance the antioxidant defenses of the CNS when neurologic disease is present. Daily supplementation of 5,000–10,000 IU of natural vitamin E has been recommended over synthetic vitamin E for the treatment of neurologic disease to maintain normal neurologic function and to reduce inflammation and degeneration of the CNS.

In a review of vitamin E associated disorders in horses, Finno and Valberg[25] state that there is no evidence to support supplementing with more than the NRC recommendations (1–2 IU/kg/day) unless the horse is at risk for NAD/EDM or affected with a specific vitamin E responsive condition such as EMND or vitamin E deficient myopathy. Because of its higher biologic activity and superior absorption, natural vitamin E is approximately twice as potent as synthetic α-tocopherol. Therefore, if supplementing with natural vitamin E, then half as much can be administered (ex. if 500 IU vitamin E is required, then 250 IU of natural vitamin E can be given for an equivalent amount).

References

1. Stewart R, Reed SM, Kohn CW, et al. The frequency and severity of osteochondrosis in horses with cervical stenotic myelopathy. Am J Vet Res 1991;52:873–879.
2. Wagner PC, Grant BD, Watrous BJ, et al. A study of the heritability of cervical vertebral malformation in horses. Proc Am Assoc Equine Pract 1985;31:43–50.
3. Donawick WJ, Mayhew IG, Galligan DT, et al. Early diagnosis of cervical vertebral malformation in young Thoroughbred horses and successful treatment with restricted, paced diet and confinement. Proc Am Assoc Equine Pract 1989;35:525–528.
4. Donawick WJ, Mayhew IG, Galligan DT, et al. Results of a low-protein, low-energy diet and confinement on young horses with wobbles. Proc Am Assoc Equine Pract 1993;39:125–127.
5. Mayhew IG. Large animal neurology – a handbook for veterinary clinicians. Philadelphia: Lea and Febiger, 1989.
6. Reed SM, Saville WJA, Schneider RK. Neurologic disease: current topics in depth. Proc Am Assoc Equine Pract 2003;49:243–258.
7. National Research Council: Nutrient requirements of horses, 6th ed. National Academies Press, Washington, DC, 2007.
8. Hoffman CJ, Clark CK. Prognosis for racing with conservative management of cervical vertebral malformation in Thoroughbreds: 103 cases (2002–2010). J Vet Intern Med 2013;27:317–323.
9. Norton JL, Johnson AL. How to diagnose and treat neuromuscular diseases: the weak trembling horse. Proc Am Assoc Equine Pract 2009;55:167–171.
10. Whitlock R, personal observation, 1999.
11. McKay R. Neurodegenerative disorders. In: Furr M, Reed SM, ed. Equine neurology, Ames, IA: Blackwell University Press, 2008;235–255.
12. Mayhew IG. How on earth can we diagnose perennial ryegrass staggers? In Proceedings. Ann Semin Equine Branch N Z Vet Assoc, 2007;177–182.
13. Blythe LL, Craig AM. Equine degenerative myeloencephalopthy. Part I. Clinical signs and pathogenesis. Compend Contin Educ Pract Vet 1992;14:1215–1221.
14. Mayhew IG, Brown CM, Stowe HD, et al. Equine degenerative myeloencephalopathy: a vitamin E deficiency that may be familial. J Vet Intern Med 1987;1:45–50.
15. Aleman M, Finno CJ, Higgins RJ, et al. Neuraxonal dystrophy in Quarter Horses. Proc Am Assoc Equine Pract 2010;56:348.
16. Aleman M, Finno CJ, Higgins RJ, et al. Evaluation of epidemiological, clinical, and pathological features of neuroaxonal dystrophy in Quarter Horses. J Am Vet Med Assoc 2011;239:823–833.
17. Blythe LL, Craig AM. Equine degenerative myeloencephalopthy. Part II. Diagnosis and treatment. Compend Contin Educ Pract Vet 1992;14:1633–1636.
18. Blythe LL, Craig AM, Lassen ED, et al. Serially determined plasma α-tocopherol concentrations and results of the oral vitamin E absorption test in clinically normal horses and in horses with degenerative myelopathy. Am J Vet Res 1991;52:908–911.
19. Pagan JD, personal communication, 2010.
20. Divers TJ, Mohammed HO, Cummings JF, et al. Equine motor neurone disease: findings in 26 horses and a proposal for a pathologic mechanism for the disease. Equine Vet J 1994;26:409–415.
21. Divers TJ, Cummings JE, de Lahunta A, et al. Evaluation of the risk of motor neuron disease in horses fed a diet low in vitamin E and high in copper and iron. Am J Vet Res 2006;67:120–126.
22. Higgins JK, Puschner B, Kass PH, et al. Assessment of vitamin E concentrations in serum and cerebrospinal fluid of horses following oral administration of vitamin E. Am J Vet Res 2008;69:785–790.
23. Pusteria N, Puschner B, Steidl S, et al. Alpha tocopherol concentrations in equine serum and CSF after vitamin E supplementation. Vet Rec 2010;166:366–368.
24. Pagan JD, Lennox MA, Perry LA, et al. Form of alpha tocopherol affects vitamin E bioavailability in Thoroughbred horses. Proc Australasian Equine Sci Symp 2010;3:17.
25. Finno CJ, Valberg SJ. A comparative review of vitamin E and associated equine disorders. J Vet Intern Med 2012;26:1251–1266.

8 Mycotoxins

Ramesh C. Gupta, DVM, MVSc, PhD, DABT, FACT, FACN, FATS

Mycotoxins are secondary metabolites produced by a variety of pathogenic fungi. Common mycotoxins of human and veterinary interest are produced by species in the genera *Aspergillus, Claviceps, Fusarium*, and *Penicillium*. There are over 100 known species of fungi that produce mycotoxins. Some species of fungi produce single mycotoxins, while others produce multiple toxins. It is important to mention that contamination of food or feed with fungi and their mycotoxins can occur at any stage of the food production chain, that is, from the time of planting through harvesting, transportation, storage, and until the food or feed is consumed.

Animal poisonings by mycotoxins, commonly referred to as "mycotoxicosis," have been recorded for centuries. The oldest known mycotoxicosis involving mass poisoning in both man and animals are associated with ergot and ergot-related alkaloids produced from *Claviceps purpurea*. From time to time, several large outbreaks of mycotoxicoses have occurred in many countries. Alimentary toxic aleukia was reported in eastern Siberia from 1942 to 1947 and it was caused by a species of *Fusarium* growing on grain that had over-wintered on the ground. In the 1930s, horses were poisoned in Russia by eating straw infected with *Stachybotrys chartarum* known to produce the mycotoxin, satratoxin H. Over 5,000 horses died between 1934–1935 from Equine Leukoencephalomalacia in central Illinois and some other parts of the midwest United States after consuming corn infected with *Fusarium verticillioides* (formerly *Fusarium moniliforme*) and *Fusarium proliferatum*. In 1989, these fungi were shown to produce mycotoxins identified and confirmed as fumonisins. During 1989–1992 in the United States, a significant number of horses died from consuming corn contaminated with fumonisins. Horses were also intoxicated in 1966 in the US by consuming barley contaminated with *Fusarium graminearum* (barley scab). Yearly losses in livestock, particularly in horses, due to mycotoxicosis are enormous throughout the world. Unlike ruminants, horses are monogastrics and more sensitive to mycotoxins because of their limited detoxication capability in the gastrointestinal tract.

There are hundreds of fungal metabolites that are potentially toxic to animals. This chapter describes the toxicity of some commonly occurring mycotoxins (such as aflatoxins, fumonisins, slaframine, trichothecenes, and zearalenone) in equine species.

8.1 Aflatoxins

Aflatoxins were discovered as a result of massive losses of turkeys in Great Britain in 1960. Over 100,000 turkeys died in the outbreak, which was called "turkey X disease." The cause of death was identified as aflatoxin, found in moldy groundnut meal imported from Brazil. Since then, sporadic incidences of aflatoxicosis have occurred in many species around the world. Almost all livestock animals are sensitive to the toxicity of aflatoxins, but a great variability exists in that sensitivity.

There are four major aflatoxins of toxicological importance: aflatoxin B_1 (AFB_1), aflatoxin B_2 (AFB_2), aflatoxin G_1 (AFG_1), and aflatoxin G_2 (AFG_2). These four aflatoxins are named according to their fluorescent properties under long wavelength ultraviolet light on thin-layer chromatography (TLC) plates. Aflatoxins B_1 and B_2 fluoresce blue, whereas aflatoxins G_1 and G_2 fluoresce green. The subscript numbers 1 and 2 indicate major and minor compounds, respectively. AFB_1 and AFB_2 are hydroxylated and excreted in the milk as AFM_1 and AFM_2, which are less toxic than the parental aflatoxins. There are more than 14 metabolites of the four major aflatoxins that have been chemically characterized. Certain environmental factors and insects damage corn, small grains, peanuts, cottonseed, and so on, and thereby promote the growth of fungi and the production of aflatoxins. Structural formulas of aflatoxins are shown in Figure 8.1.

Nutritional Management of Equine Diseases and Special Cases, First Edition. Edited by Bryan M. Waldridge.

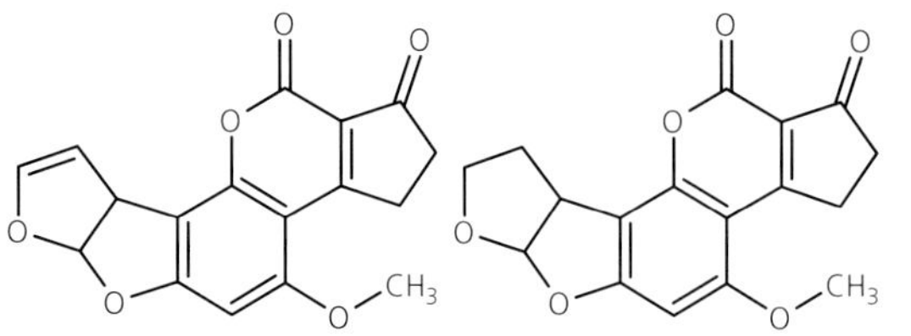

AFLATOXIN B$_1$ AFLATOXIN B$_2$

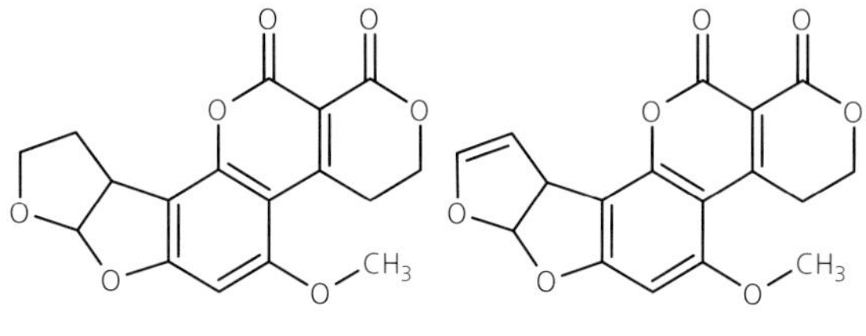

AFLATOXIN G$_1$ AFLATOXIN G$_2$

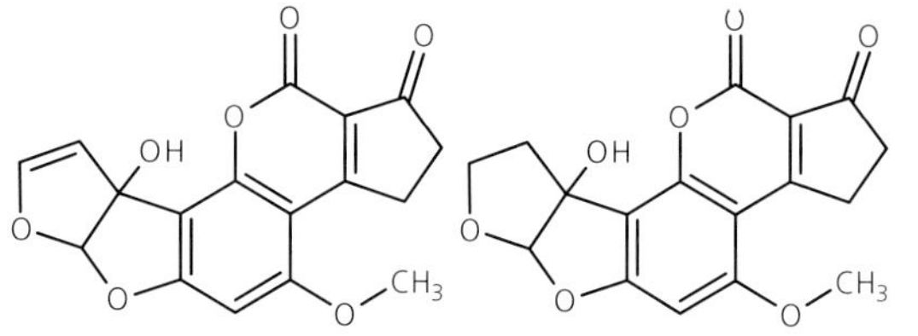

AFLATOXIN M$_1$ AFLATOXIN M$_2$

Figure 8.1 Chemical structures of aflatoxins.

Aflatoxins are mainly produced by *Aspergillus flavus*, *A. parasiticus*, and *A. nomius*. Other fungi known to produce aflatoxins are *A. bombycis, A. fumigatus, A. ochraceus*, and *A. pseudotamarii*. Details of aflatoxigenic species of *Aspergillus* and their worldwide distribution has been described in recent publications.[1,2] Among these fungi, *A. flavus* has been most extensively studied for the production of aflatoxins. The production of aflatoxins is associated with spore production by species of *Aspergillus*.[3] Strains of *A. flavus* can vary in aflatoxin capability from nontoxic to highly toxigenic and are more likely to produce more AFB$_1$ than AFG$_1$. *A. flavus* and other species can also produce cyclopiazonic acid (CPA). Strains of *A. parasiticus* generally have less variation in toxigenicity and generally produce AFB$_1$ and varying amounts of AFB$_2$, AFG$_1$, and AFG$_2$. The aflatoxin profile produced by *A. nomius* is considered to be similar to *A. parasiticus*, and like *A. parasiticus*, *A. nomius*

does not produce CPA. Recent studies have shown that *A. nomius* is more important as a producer of aflatoxins than previously suspected.[4] Aflatoxigenic strains of *Aspergillus* can also produce sterigmatocystin.

8.1.1 Toxicokinetics

Aflatoxins are rapidly absorbed from the gastrointestinal tract by passive diffusion and are primarily transferred to the hepatic portal system. Young animals absorb aflatoxins more efficiently than older animals. Metabolism of aflatoxins primarily takes place in the liver. With the exception of the AFB$_1$-8,9-epoxide, the metabolites are less toxic than AFB$_1$. Cytochrome P450 (AFB$_1$ hydroxylase) plays a key role in the biotransformation of AFB$_1$ to AFB$_1$-8,9-epoxide. The formation of AFB$_1$-8,9-epoxide is considered to be the most significant biotransformation pathway because the AFB$_1$-8,9-epoxide forms adducts with DNA, RNA, and proteins. Conjugation of AFB$_1$-8,9-epoxide with glutathione is considered to be an important detoxification pathway. Another biotransformation product of AFB$_1$ is AFQ$_1$, which can be metabolized to AFH$_1$. AFB$_1$ is also metabolized to AFP$_1$, AFM$_1$, aflatoxicol, and other metabolites. AFP$_1$, AFM$_1$, AFQ$_1$, and aflatoxicol form glucuronide and sulfate conjugates. Aflatoxins and their metabolites are excreted in urine, bile, feces, milk, and semen.

8.1.2 Mechanism of Action

In general, aflatoxins are mutagenic, carcinogenic, teratogenic, and immunosuppressive. Aflatoxins cause oxidative stress by increasing lipid peroxidation and decreasing enzymatic and nonenzymatic antioxidants.[5] Depending on the concentration of aflatoxins, many metabolic processes are affected. Reduced synthesis of nucleic acids and proteins is very characteristic. AFB$_1$ is metabolized in a cytochrome P450-dependent reaction to AFB$_1$-8,9-epoxide, which forms adducts with macromolecules in the cell. The affinity of AFB$_1$-8,9-epoxide in decreasing order for macromolecules is DNA > RNA > protein. The formation of these adducts is a critical step for aflatoxicosis. The DNA adduct is formed with N^7-guanine[6] and this adduct is relatively resistant to the DNA repair process. Both AFB$_1$ and AFM$_1$ induce carcinogenesis in many animal species and in humans.

AFB$_1$ is reported to exhibit immunosuppressive effects, therefore ingestion of AFB$_1$ contaminated feed increases susceptibility to infections.[7,8] AFB$_1$ mainly affects cell-mediated immunity.[9,10] It decreases lymphoid cell populations, especially circulating activated lymphocytes, suppresses lymphoblastogenesis, and impairs both cutaneous delayed type hypersensitivity and graft versus host response. AFB$_1$ also decreases natural killer cell mediated cytolysis and several macrophage functions, such as phagocytic activity and intracellular killing or production of oxidative radicals.[11] Effects of AFB$_1$ are primarily on cell mediated immunity; however, T cell dependent humoral responses are also adversely affected. Recent evidence suggests that AFB$_1$ may depress many aspects of humoral and cellular immunities.[12] For further details on aflatoxin-induced immunosuppression, readers are referred to a publication by Mishra and Sopori.[13]

8.1.3 Toxicity and Clinical Signs

The primary aflatoxins of toxicologic concern in feedstuffs are AFB$_1$, AFB$_2$, AFG$_1$, and AFG$_2$. On a functional basis, analyses for aflatoxins generally are the sum of the concentrations of these four toxins.[1] Among all aflatoxins, AFB$_1$ occurs with the greatest frequency in feedstuffs and is found to be the most toxic in all laboratory, companion and livestock animals. In general, the order of toxicity is AFB$_1$ > AFG$_1$ > AFB$_2$ > AFG$_2$. The LD$_{50}$ of aflatoxin B$_1$ in ducklings, rabbits, dogs, and guinea pigs is about 1 mg/kg. This value is about 10 mg/kg in monkeys, cattle, pigs, rats and hamsters. Mice and sheep are less sensitive to aflatoxin B$_1$, as the LD$_{50}$ values are 63 and 500 mg/kg, respectively.

Toxicity due to aflatoxins under natural conditions is usually subacute or chronic, depending on the level of exposure. Occasionally, acute cases are also seen. In general, affected animals show reduced growth rate, weight loss, immune suppression, icterus, hemorrhagic enteritis, reduced performance, and ultimately death.

The major target for the toxicity of aflatoxins is the liver. AFB$_1$ is known to cause hepatocellular carcinomas (HCC) in many animal species and in humans. The occurrence of HCC can vary with age of exposure. For example, brief exposures to large doses of AFB$_1$ during the neonatal period result in a high incidence of HCC in adulthood, whereas adult mice exposed to the same doses fail to develop HCC at any age. Aflatoxins produce necrosis of liver cells, damage to mitochondria, and proliferation of bile ducts. The clinical pathology of aflatoxicosis has been studied in several animal species, including horses. Weanling ponies were administered AFB$_1$ at 0.0 (control), 0.5, 1.0, and 2.0 mg/kg.[14]

Serum activity of gamma-glutamyl transpeptidase (GGT) was increased in all ponies receiving AFB$_1$. The GGT activity remained increased until day 3 and then decreased. Serum activity of alanine aminotransferase (ALT) remained unchanged. Ponies given 4, 5, 6, and 7.4 mg AFB$_1$/kg had an increase in serum ALT and the activity of ALT remained increased until the ponies died at 33–46 h after dosing.

Animals poisoned with aflatoxins may show hemorrhage into the gastrointestinal tract, body cavities, and on body organs due to decreased production of clotting factors by the liver.[14,15] At necropsy, common findings include firm and pale liver, clear yellow ascites, and pleural fluid accumulation. Histopathological lesions are commonly reported in liver and kidney. Angsubhakorn et al.[16] reported hemosiderin deposition in tubule cells, cardiac myofiber degeneration, and edema of the brain in horses. Hepatic encephalopathy could occur as a result of liver damage.

8.1.4 Reproductive and Developmental Effects

There are many reports that describe deleterious effects of aflatoxins on development and the reproductive system, such as sexual maturation, growth and maturation of the follicles, levels of hormones, gestation, and growth of the fetus.[17–19]

In many *in vivo* and *in vitro* studies, aflatoxins have been investigated for male reproductive toxicity and the principle target organ is the testes, and of course, various aspects of spermatogenesis. Aflatoxins are known to cause testicular degeneration, sloughing of germ cells, and concomitant reduction in the rate and efficiency of sperm production. Recently, Shuaib et al.[20] demonstrated that AFB$_1$ caused regression of the testes, impairment of spermatogenesis, and premature loss of germ cells. An intraperitoneal injection of 50 μg of AFB$_1$/kg/day (estimated to be equivalent to ~330 ppm in diet) was given to male mice at various intervals.[21] At day 35, fertility testing showed a decrease in litter size and tissue examination showed a decrease in spermatozoa numbers in the caudal epididymis. When the numbers of spermatozoa decreased, progressive motility of spermatozoa was decreased and abnormal spermatozoa were observed. It is important to mention that toxicants targeting spermatogenesis and spermiogenesis may not become apparent for 3–6 weeks, depending on the species, due to the time required for spermiogenesis.

AFB$_1$ has also been shown to impair the reproductive performance of female animals.[22,23] Female rats (Druckery Strain) receiving AFB$_1$ (7.5 mg/kg, PO, for 21 days) showed significant dose-dependent reductions in the number of oocytes and large follicles. Blood hormone levels and sex organ weights were significantly altered. There were reductions in ovarian and uterine sizes, increases in fetal resorption, implantation loss, and intra-uterine death in aflatoxin-exposed female rats.

It is important to mention that AFB$_1$ in animals and humans crosses the placental barrier and thereby reaches the fetus.[17,24] High AFB$_1$ concentrations in umbilical cord have been associated with low birth weight, kernicterus, and in some cases also with death of the fetus.[25] Chronic exposure to AFB$_1$ may cause endocrine disruption in the fetoplacental unit, as it has been shown to affect the expression of the aromatase enzyme.[26] These authors demonstrated that AFB$_1$ affects genes important to endocrine regulation in placental cells. The developmental toxicity of AFB$_1$ has been studied in various laboratory animal models and this mycotoxin has been found to be embryotoxic and/or teratogenic in rats, mice, hamsters, chick embryos, tadpoles, and Japanese medaka eggs. Evidence suggests that aflatoxins are teratogenic to most animal species.[17,27,28]

8.1.5 Treatment

There is no specific antidote for toxicity of aflatoxins. Timely administration of L-methionine (200 mg/kg, PO, q8h) and sodium thiosulfate (50 mg/kg, PO, q8h) is proven to be of therapeutic value. Supplementation with increased protein, vitamins, and antioxidants can also be rewarding.

Immediate removal of contaminated feed is the single most important step in avoiding any further loss in productivity and/or death. The United States Food and Drug Administration's goal for aflatoxins has been to minimize contamination by implementing regulations that focus special attention on management of the problem. Currently, less than 20 ppb aflatoxin B$_1$ in feed is considered to be safe.

Biological exposure of aflatoxins can be minimized by chemoprotection and/or enterosorption. Chemoprevention against aflatoxins has been demonstrated with a number of compounds (such as esterified glucomanoses and other yeast extracts) that either increase detoxification of aflatoxins or prevent the production of the aflatoxin epoxide, thereby reducing or blocking AFB$_1$-induced hepatocarcinogenesis. Compounds such as oltipraz and chlorophyll are available to decrease the biologically effective dose. Enterosorptive food additives are recommended because they bind aflatoxins and render them biologically unavailable to humans and animals.[29] Dietary supplementation with a feed anti-caking agent or adsorbents, such as 0.5% hydrated sodium calcium aluminosilicate, has been demonstrated to minimize aflatoxicosis in a number of species. Selective calcium montmorillonites have proven to be the most selective and effective of these enterosorbents. Following absorption, some zeolites can be effective reactive oxygen species scavengers.[30] The efficiency of mycotoxin binders differs considerably, depending mainly on the chemical structure of both the adsorbent and the toxin.[31] It is important to mention that by no means should these binders be considered mycotoxin eliminators. One disadvantage with binders is that there can be some interference in the absorption of essential nutrients. This should definitely be taken into consideration, especially during pregnancy and the fetal developmental period.

8.2 Fumonisins

The discovery of the fumonisins (FB$_1$, FB$_2$, and others) was a major breakthrough in the identification of mycotoxin(s) involved in moldy corn poisoning in equine species associated with corn or feeds contaminated with *Fusarium verticillioides* (formerly *F. moniliforme* Sheldon) or *F. proliferatum*.[32–34] Some fumonisins and related mycotoxins are also produced in minor amounts by other *Fusarium* spp., such as *F. subglutinans, F. anthophilum,* and *Aspergillus niger*.[35] More than 30 fumonisins have been identified and still new stereoisomers such as *epi*-FB$_3$ and *epi*-FB$_4$ and novel congeners, such as fumonisin B$_6$, continue to be discovered and structural confirmation of more toxins is likely.[35,36] Fumonisin B$_1$ is the predominant isomer and usually accounts for 60% or more of the fumonisins in corn. The chemical structure of FB$_1$ is shown in Figure 8.2. FB$_2$ and FB$_3$ occur in small amounts with FB$_2$ being more prevalent.

Problems related to fumonisins are common throughout the world. Fumonisins are known to cause Equine Leukoencephalomalacia (ELEM), commonly referred to as "moldy corn poisoning." Fumonisins have

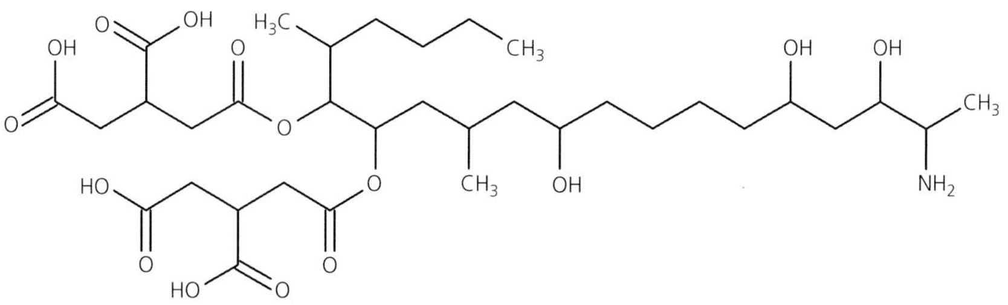

Figure 8.2 Chemical structure of fumonisin B$_1$.

been implicated in the production of pulmonary edema or "hydrothorax" in pigs, esophageal cancer in humans, liver cancer in rats and mice, and immunosuppression in chickens.

8.2.1 Toxicokinetics

The pharmacokinetics of FB$_1$ have been studied in several species, including rats, pigs, cattle, poultry, and primates.[37] In general, fumonisin is rapidly absorbed following intravenous or intraperitoneal administration and is eliminated in both urine and feces. Residues are undetectable by 24 h after dosing in virtually all species and significant residues have not been detected in muscle, milk, or eggs. Following oral dosing, very little FB$_1$ is found in the serum of animals, suggesting a low bioavailability. No pharmacokinetic data is available for fumonisin in horses.

8.2.2 Mechanism of Action

The exact mechanism of action involved in fumonisin-induced intoxication is not yet fully understood. Although it is well established that fumonisins, especially B$_1$ and B$_2$, specifically inhibit *de novo* sphingolipid biosynthesis, it is not clear why fumonisins attack the brain in horses, lungs in pigs, liver in rats and mice, esophagus in humans, and the immune system in poultry.

Fumonisins are structurally related to sphingosine and sphinganine, the major long chain base backbone of cellular sphingolipids. Fumonisins are competitive inhibitors of sphinganine and sphingosine N-acetyltransferase (also known as ceramide synthase), key enzymes in the *de novo* sphingolipid biosynthetic pathway.[37] These N-acetyltransferase enzymes are responsible for catalyzing the acylation of sphinganine and the reutilization of sphingosine derived from sphingolipid turnover.

Sphingolipids are located in cellular membranes, lipoproteins (especially low-density lipoproteins), and other lipid-rich structures. Sphingolipids are involved in the regulation of cell growth, cell to cell communication, differentiation, and neoplastic transformation. Inhibition of ceramide synthase by fumonisins disrupts sphingolipid metabolism, resulting in increased sphinganine and sphingosine, along with a decrease in complex sphingolipids in the serum and tissues of animals. This disruption of sphingolipid metabolism is generally accepted as the probable mechanism of fumonisin toxicity.[37]

The mechanism of ELEM may also be a direct result of fumonisin-induced increases in sphingosine concentrations. Smith et al.[38] demonstrated that fumonisin administration induced cardiovascular dysfunction in horses. These authors established an association between neurologic signs, increased serum and myocardial sphingosine concentrations, and cardiovascular depression in fumonisin-treated horses. At necropsy, horses with leukoencephalomalacia have histologic evidence of cerebral edema. Another study revealed that fumonisin-treated horses also have elevated levels of protein, albumin, and IgG in cerebrospinal fluid samples.[39] In essence, these findings indicate that fumonisin toxicity in horses is associated with the development of vasogenic cerebral edema, as a direct result of increased blood-brain barrier permeability.

8.2.3 Toxicity and Clinical Signs

Fumonisins have been known to adversely affect the brain, lungs, liver, esophagus, kidneys, pancreas, testes, thymus, gastrointestinal tract, and blood cells. Depending upon the species, some tissues are more affected than others.

Horses are the most sensitive species for fumonisins.[40] As little as 5 ppm fumonisin B$_1$ in corn can cause ELEM in 7–35 days. Symptoms reflect neurologic injury and include ataxia, head pressing, paralysis of the lips and

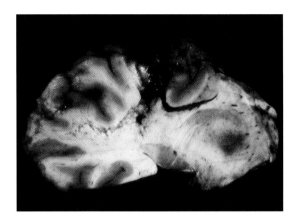

Figure 8.3 Fumonisin induced ELEM in horse brain. Courtesy of Dr. Geoff W. Smith 2012.

tongue, and convulsions. The disease progresses rapidly and the mortality rate is near 100%. At necropsy, one or more foci of hemorrhagic liquefactive necrosis are characteristically present in the white matter of the brain, predominantly in the cerebrum (Figure 8.3).

A hepatotoxic syndrome also occurs in horses, characterized by icterus, elevated concentrations of serum bilirubin and liver enzymes, and swelling of the face and head. Necropsy usually reveals a small, firm liver and upon microscopic examination, centrilobular necrosis, and periportal fibrosis. Neurotoxic signs may also develop before death.[41] In general, high doses of fumonisins induce fatal hepatotoxicity with mild brain lesions, whereas low doses cause mild hepatotoxicity and severe brain lesions characteristic of ELEM. Fumonisin-induced liver damage also occurs in other species, including pigs, cattle, rabbits, and primates.

In horses, FB_1 also causes cardiotoxicity.[38] Decreased heart rate and cardiac contractility and increased systemic vascular resistance were found in horses exposed to 0.2 mg/kg FB_1 administered intravenously. Repeated daily doses of 0.01 mg/kg FB_1 over 28 days caused no cardiovascular impairment, but affected sphingolipid profiles of cardiac tissue.[39]

Accumulation of sphinganine, sphingosine, and their 1-phosphates in tissues, blood or urine are useful biomarkers of fumonisin exposure. A close correlation between increased sphingoid base concentrations, especially those of sphinganine, and toxicity have been shown in many species, including horses.

Fumonisins are also known to adversely affect the immune system. Several studies have demonstrated that fumonisin B_1 affects innate immunity, as well as humoral and cellular responses of acquired immunity.[9,13,42,43] Exposure to FB_1 was reported to cause localized activation of cytokines, suggesting that toxin-induced changes in innate immune responses may be important in its immunotoxicity.[42]

Recently, Voss et al.[41] described in detail the reproductive and developmental effects of fumonisins in various animal species. Abdel-Wahhab et al.[44] reported that FB_1 proved to be teratogenic and induced severe fetal growth retardation and skeletal malformation. In many studies, fumonisin exposure has been linked to neural tube defects.[40,45]

Diagnosis of fumonisin toxicity can be made based on: (1) detection of fumonisins (FB_1 and FB_2) in feed or animal tissue or fluids and (2) an increase in the sphinganine to sphingosine ratio in serum and tissue.

8.2.4 Treatment

There is no specific treatment for fumonisin toxicity in horses. Immediate removal of contaminated corn or feed is the single most important step in preventing other animals from developing signs.

8.3 Slaframine

Slaframine (6-aminooctahydroindolizin-1-yl acetate), commonly referred to as "slobber factor," is produced by the fungus *Rhizoctonia leguminicola*. The fungus is ubiquitous in soil and parasitizes red clover (*Trifolium pratense*), white clover (*Trifolium repens*), alsike clover (*Trifolium hybridum*), and many other legumes. *Rhizoctonia leguminicola* causes a pasture disease called "black patch." Fungal infestation is usually associated with periods of wet and cool weather, that is, spring or fall, which are ideal for the growth of *R. leguminicola*. Slaframine is a piperidine or indolizidine alkaloid with the empirical formula $C_{10}H_{10}N_2O_2$ and a molecular weight of 198.26 (Figure 8.4). Slaframine is known to produce excessive salivation in many animal species, including sheep, swine, and guinea pigs, but more importantly in cattle and horses.[46,47] A serious outbreak of slobbers occurred in a herd of horses in the fall of 1979 near High Point, North Carolina. This was caused by a shipment of high-quality second cutting red clover-orchard grass hay from a supplier in West Virginia.[48] Since then, problems with slaframine have been noted

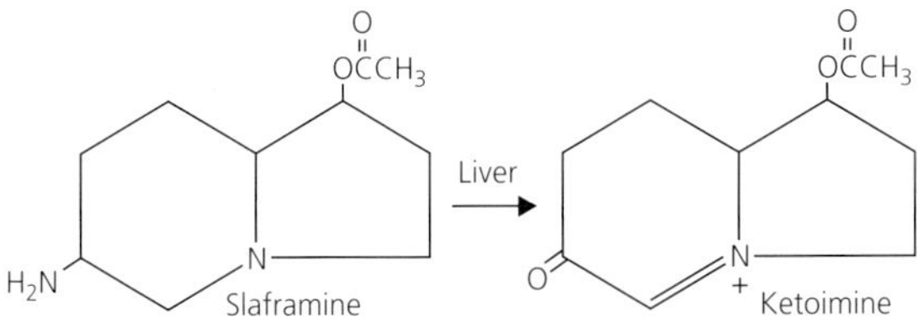

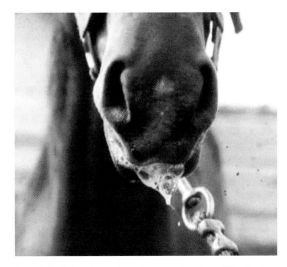

Figure 8.4 Activation of slaframine to ketoimine in liver.

Figure 8.5 Slaframine poisoned horse. Courtesy of Dr. Geoff W. Smith 2012.

in many parts of the United States, particularly in the midwest. In Kentucky and surrounding states, problems associated with slaframine are quite common in horses. In 2010, problems related to slaframine toxin were observed in central Kentucky because of the wet spring weather and abundant clover growth.[49] It is important to note that slaframine is not destroyed during drying of plants or during the process of making silage or haylage.

8.3.1 Mechanism of Action

Slaframine itself is not very toxic, but in the liver it is activated by a microsomal flavoprotein oxidase enzyme to a ketoimine metabolite (Figure 8.4) and its structure resembles that of acetylcholine.[50] Thus, the metabolite produces excessive salivation, lacrimation, and other hypersecretory effects, by stimulating the cholinergic system, especially its muscarinic (M_3 subtype) receptors. The M_3 acetylcholine receptor is important in the control of exocrine and endocrine glands.[46,51] Accordingly, slaframine is pharmacologically classified as a cholinergic agonist. Experimental studies have revealed that slaframine has no effect on the cardiovascular system nor does it inhibit blood cholinesterase activity.[52,53]

8.3.2 Toxicity and Clinical Signs

The clinical signs of slaframine toxicity are similar in all species. In experimental studies, animals exposed to a single dose of slaframine showed salivation for 6–10 h. Slaframine exposure above 10 ppm can be associated with slobbering. Naturally occurring cases of slaframine poisoning are primarily reported in horses and ruminants. Figure 8.5 depicts a horse slobbering from slaframine poisoning. Slobber syndrome usually occurs soon after consumption of hay or forage contaminated with slaframine. In addition to excessive salivation, horses may show signs of lacrimation, colic, and diarrhea. One case report described abortion in a mare.[54]

Excessive salivation may persist for several days, even after withdrawal of the contaminated source. Clinical signs in cattle, in addition to salivation, are lacrimation, bloating, frequent urination, and watery diarrhea. Other clinical signs may include anorexia and involve the gastrointestinal tract, cardiac, and respiratory systems. Weight loss, decreased milk production, uterine hemorrhage, and abortions have also been associated with slaframine toxicosis. Fatalities with slaframine toxicosis are not common. However, death may occur due to suffocation from pulmonary edema and/or emphysema.

Diagnosis of slaframine toxicity is based on clinical signs (particularly profuse salivation) in animals consuming red clover or some other legume forage, identification of *R. leguminicola*, and detection of slaframine/swainsonine in forage, plasma, or milk.[55]

8.3.3 Treatment

Therapy with atropine sulfate is quite effective in combating the clinical signs associated with parasympathomimetic action. However, it is unlikely that clinical signs will be completely resolved.[51] In laboratory animals, antihistamines such as promethazine hydrochloride, have also been found effective. Recovery of animals is usually rapid, as the prompt removal of the contaminated source generally alleviates all signs of intoxication within 2–5 days.

8.4 Trichothecenes

Trichothecene mycotoxins occur worldwide and as a result, their impact on animal and human health is of global concern. Trichothecenes were named after the fungus *Trichothecium roseum*, from which the first trichothecene was isolated in 1948. Now, approximately 190 trichothecenes have been isolated and identified from *Fusarium, Myrothecium, Verrucaria*, and other genera. The major mycotoxins of the trichothecenes group are deoxynivalenol (DON or vomitoxin), diacetoxyscirpenol (DAS), and T-2 toxin. These three closely related trichothecene mycotoxins are most commonly found in agricultural commodities infected with *Fusarium* species. The chemical structures of DON and T-2 toxin are shown in Figures 8.6 and 8.7, respectively. These fungal metabolites are a group of sesquiterpenoids characterized by a tetracyclic 12,13-epoxytrichothec-9-ene skeleton and a variable number of acetoxy or hydroxyl group substitutions. All trichothecenes share a tricyclic nucleus named trichothecene and usually contain an epoxide at C-12 and C-13, which is considered essential for toxicity. Trichothecenes can be broadly divided into two groups, macrocyclic and non-macrocyclic, based on the presence of a macrocyclic ring linking C-4 and C-15 with diesters (roridin series) and triesters (verrucarin series).[56]

Vomitoxin is produced by the fungus *Fusarium roseum*, whereas DAS and T-2 toxin are produced by several fungi, such as *F. tricinctum, F. solani, F. roseum*, and *F. nivale*. Production of these mycotoxins is usually

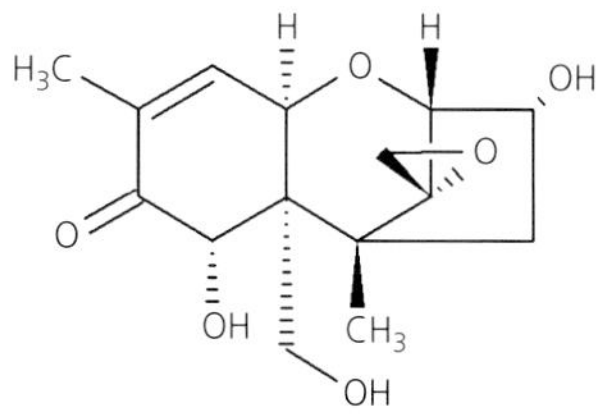

Figure 8.6 Chemical structure of Deoxynivalenol (DON).

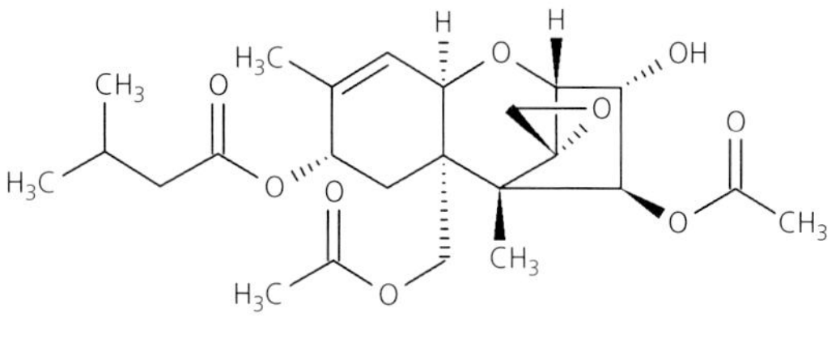

Figure 8.7 Chemical structure of T-2 toxin.

triggered by a variety of environmental conditions, such as cool and wet weather. Trichothecenes have been known to contaminate a variety of field crops including wheat, barley, rice, oats, corn, sorghum, and sunflower. During the past four decades, it has been noted that among trichothecenes, vomitoxin occurs with the greatest frequency. Humans and almost all livestock animals are sensitive to trichothecene toxicity. Dogs and pigs are more sensitive to vomitoxin than other species. Occurrence of toxicosis in domestic animals involving T-2 toxin or DAS is rare. Although DON occurs as a feed contaminant with greater frequency, T-2 toxin has been studied in greater detail because of its relevance to chemical warfare. It is important to note that trichothecenes are stable for long periods and as a result, their concentrations generally magnify during feed processing and storage.

8.4.1 Toxicokinetics

No pharmacokinetic data of trichothecenes is available for equine species. Therefore, some data available for other monogastric species are described here in brief. Much of the pharmacokinetic studies are performed with DON because this mycotoxin occurs with the greatest frequency. After oral exposure, DON is rapidly and completely absorbed in the stomach and proximal small intestine in pigs.[57] Following an intravenous dose of 1 mg/kg DON in swine, the mycotoxin distributed rapidly to all tissues and body fluids and then declined to negligible levels within 24 h, except for urine and bile.[58] Pigs chronically dosed with 5.7 mg DON/kg of diet for 4 weeks or with one single acute oral exposure (one feeding) had quick absorption of greater than 50% of the dose administered. Deoxynivalenol was highly distributed, with an apparent volume of distribution higher than total body water and serum elimination half-lives of 6.3 and 5.3 h in the chronic and acute DON-fed pigs, respectively.[59] A total of 97% of the DON dose (five elimination half-lives) was eliminated 31.5 and 26.5 h after chronic feeding or in one single, acute exposure, respectively.

Following absorption, trichothecenes may undergo all four basic reactions of xenobiotic metabolism. Phase I hydrolysis and oxidation and phase II glucuronide conjugation occur in the body tissues, while reduction of the 12,13-epoxide is thought to occur through microbial action in the gastrointestinal tract; although T-2 toxin is the only trichothecene for which all four basic reactions occur simultaneously in the same animal.[60] The ability to remove the epoxide oxygen (deepoxidation) is an important step in the detoxification of trichothecenes. Orally or parenterally administered trichothecenes do not accumulate in the body to a significant extent and are rapidly excreted within a few days in urine and feces. The majority of DON ingested from dietary exposure is eliminated in urine and feces, with urine being the main excretory route of DON in an unmetabolized form. Some trichothecenes undergo enterohepatic recirculation and are excreted in the feces.

8.5 Mechanism of Action

Trichothecenes induce toxicity through multiple mechanisms of action, including inhibition of protein, RNA, and DNA synthesis, alterations of membrane structure and mitochondrial function, stimulation of lipid peroxidation, induction of apoptosis, and activation of cytokines and chemokines.[56] It appears that the primary effect of trichothecenes is inhibition of protein synthesis, as all of the other reported effects might be secondary to decreased protein synthesis.[61,62] With trichothecenes in general and DON in particular, feed refusal is a very common toxic sign and the underlying mechanism of action is not yet known. DON could act directly via a central mechanism controlling hunger by modulating the levels of neurotransmitters, including norepinephrine, dopamine, and serotonin in discrete regions of the brain.

Trichothecenes cause immunotoxicity due to both stimulation and impairment of humoral immunity and cell-mediated immunity. T-2 toxin exposure in numerous laboratory animal models and other species is known to cause apoptosis and immunosuppression.[61] T-2 toxin given by intraperitoneal administration to mice reduced thymus weights, inhibited antibody synthesis against sheep erythrocytes, and prolonged skin graft rejection times.[63] Increased serum IgA and potential IgA dysregulation and nephropathy have been reported in rodents after high dietary DON exposure (about 25 mg/kg). Elevated serum IgA in animals exposed to oral DON does not appear to be consistent across species. Elevations in serum IgA concentrations were not observed in horses fed DON-contaminated feed (0.06–0.1 mg DON/kg/day).[64,65] Apoptosis has been proposed to explain the loss of lymphocytes and hematopoietic cells during trichothecene poisoning.[66,67] Islam et al.[68] demonstrated that T-2 toxin, given by intraperitoneal injection to mice, induced thymic atrophy, DNA fragmentation, and histopathologic changes characteristic of apoptosis in thymic tissue, including cell shrinkage and nuclear condensation. Macrophages appeared to be very sensitive to trichothecenes and could undergo trichothecene- mediated apoptosis.[69] It has been suggested that in addition to trichothecenes binding to the 60S ribosomal subunits and producing translational inhibition, another molecular pathway for trichothecene induction of apoptosis was through triggering a ribotoxic stress response activating mitogen-activated protein kinases.

8.5.1 Toxicity and Clinical Signs

Trichothecenes are toxic to all animal species that have been tested. Toxicity of trichothecenes appears to vary as verrucarins and roridin E are the most acutely toxic trichothecenes, followed by DAS and T-2 toxin, and nivalenol and crotocin are the least toxic.[61,70] Furthermore, neonatal animals are more susceptible than adults to the toxicity of trichothecenes. Their toxicity also varies from species to species. Based on toxicity, the species susceptibility to DON are ranked as pig > rodent > dog > cat > poultry > ruminants (least sensitive).[71] No information is available for equine species.

The toxic effects may depend upon the route of exposure, concentrations of trichothecenes in the diet, and the duration of exposure. Clinical signs can range from subtle effects, such as feed refusal or reduced feed consumption, decreased weight gain, skin irritation, and increased susceptibility to diseases, to the more severe effects, such as bloody diarrhea, complete anorexia, emaciation, and finally death. As little as 1 ppm vomitoxin in feed can cause feed refusal in pigs and dogs. Refusal concentrations for DAS and T-2 toxin in pigs are 10 ppm and 16 ppm, respectively. Trichothecenes are known to cause dermal necrosis, gastrointestinal effects, hemorrhage, coagulopathy, and immunosuppression. T-2 toxin is associated with a large range of toxic effects, such as weight loss, decreased red blood cell and leukocyte counts, reduction in plasma glucose concentration, pathologic changes in the liver and stomach, and alimentary toxic aleukia. Animal feeding experiments also demonstrated that trichothecenes are teratogenic, but provided no evidence that they are carcinogenic.[72]

Field cases of lethality in horses from trichothecene mycotoxicoses (*Stachybotrys*) in the Soviet Union have been recorded since the 1930s.[73–75] Stachybotryotoxicosis typically occurred during indoor feeding of horses with *S. alternans*-contaminated straw or hay. Horses are very sensitive to *Stachybotrys* toxin and 1 mg of toxin can be lethal. In the peracute form of stachybotryotoxicosis, which is associated with high concentrations of *Stachybotrys* toxin in feed, horses show signs of nervous system irritation or depression, cardiac arrhythmias, pulmonary edema, and hemorrhage of serosal and mucosal membranes and muscular tissue, muscle necrosis, and oral ulcers.[75] Hemorrhage occurs on serous and mucous membranes and in the spleen, liver, lungs, brain, spinal cord, lymph nodes, and most notably in muscle tissue. In the early 1970s, horses died in northern Japan from consuming moldy bean hulls that were commonly used as fodder and bedding, especially in the winter and spring.[76] Affected horses showed clinical signs of central nervous system disturbances, including convulsions and cyclic movements, depressed respiration, icterus, and bradycardia. Poisoning in these horses was linked to several trichothecenes (T-2 toxin, DAS, and neosolaniol).

In an experimental study conducted by Johnson et al.,[64] five horses (about 444 kg) were fed DON-contaminated barley (36–44 ppm) and they consumed approximately 1.27 kg barley/horse/day (about 0.099–0.124 mg DON/kg/day) for 40 days. No signs of feed refusal were observed in the horses and no remarkable changes were detected in any hematological or serum biochemical parameters. Both serum IgG and IgA decreased in a linear manner through the trial. The authors suggested that gastric microflora detoxified DON prior to absorption. In another trial performed by Raymond et al.,[65] mares were fed one of three treatments, a control diet, a mycotoxin diet (11.2 mg DON/kg and 0.7 mg 15-acetyldeoxynivalenol/kg diet), and a mycotoxin diet (14.15 mg DON/kg feed and 0.7 mg 15-acetyldeoxynivalenol/kg diet) with 0.2% glucomannan polymer (an adsorbent) for 21 days. Feed intake and body weight gains were depressed in horses fed the mycotoxin-contaminated diets, as compared with control mares. No effect of diet was seen on hematology or serum chemistries, including GGT activity, nor was there any difference noted in athletic ability. Feeding glucomannan polymer did not prevent a depression in feed consumption.

8.5.2 Treatment

The most effective control strategy for trichothecene toxins is prevention of fungal infection and toxin production in the field and storage. Proper agricultural practices such as avoiding late harvests, removing overwintered stubble from fields, and avoiding a corn/wheat rotation that favors *Fusarium* growth in residue, can reduce trichothecene contamination of grains. Storage of grains at less than 13–14% moisture and storage of hay and straw at less than 20% moisture are important in preventing trichothecene production.

There is no specific treatment for trichothecene mycotoxicoses. A number of binders, such as clay and zeolitic products, have been suggested for use with trichothecene-contaminated feed to prevent absorption by animals. However, the United States Food and Drug Administration has not approved any chemical for use as a trichothecene mycotoxin binder. Toxic effects can be alleviated by replacing contaminated feed with clean feed. Studies show that washing of corn for 48 h, with a change of water every 2 h, is very effective. Clinical signs of feed refusal usually disappear within a week after removal of the contaminated feed and animals return to production within 14 days.

For further details on trichothecenes, readers are referred to a publication by Mostrom and Raisbeck.[56]

8.6 Zearalenone

Zearalenone, also referred to as F-2 toxin, is chemically described as 6-(10-hydroxy-6-oxo-*trans*-1-undecenyl)-ß-resorcylic acid lactone (Figure 8.8). At least seven derivatives of zearalenone have been found that naturally occur in corn.[77] Zearalenone and its derivatives are also commonly found in barley, oats, wheat, corn silage, rice, sorghum, and occasionally in forages. The occurrence of zearalenone in grain and feed is worldwide, especially in temperate climates. Zearalenone is primarily produced by *Fusarium graminearum*, but it can also be

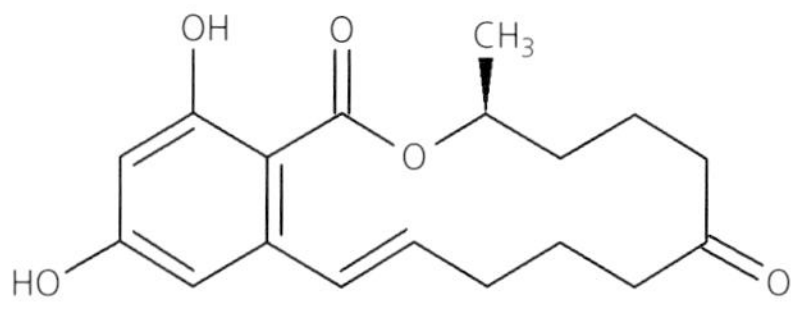

Figure 8.8 Chemical structure of zearalenone.

produced by other *Fusarium* fungi, including *F. culmorum*, *F. verticillioides* (formerly *F. moniliforme*), *F. sporotrichioides*, *F. semitectum*, *F. equiseti, and F. oxysporum.* Moisture content and the presence of oxygen are critical factors for zearalenone production. If the fungus is stressed by a cool temperature (8–15 °C) for several weeks, then zearalenone can be produced. This mycotoxin can be produced fairly quickly in the field during wet weather in the late summer or early fall weather following hail damage to corn. Very high concentrations of zearalenone can also be found in grain stored improperly at high moisture. Corn stored in a crib and exposed to winter is particularly prone to fungal invasion and production of zearalenone. It needs to be emphasized that in addition to other estrogenic metabolites, such as α- and ß-zearalenol, zearalenone is commonly detected in grain with deoxynivalenol. Zearalenone and its metabolites are heat stable.

8.6.1 Toxicokinetics

Following oral ingestion, zearalenone is rapidly absorbed from the gastrointestinal tract. In monogastric animals, bioavailability of zearalenone is estimated to be over 80%. Zearalenone and its metabolites are known to localize in reproductive tissues (ovary and uterus), adipose tissue, and interstitial cells of the testes.[78,79] Zearalenone can be metabolized in the liver and intestinal mucosa, but also by the gastrointestinal flora. The two major metabolites of zearalenone are α-zearalenol and ß-zearalenol. α-zearalenol exerts greater estrogenic activity than ß-zearalenol. Zearalenone undergoes extensive enterohepatic circulation and biliary excretion in most species. As a result, the major route of excretion for most species is through the feces. Rabbits excrete zearalenone through the urine. Excretion of an administered dose of zearalenone is complete within 3 days.

Zearalenone and its major metabolites (α-zearalenol and ß-zearalenol) have been shown to be excreted in the milk of cows, sheep, and pigs for a few days, even after cessation of contaminated feed. Hyperestrogenism has been reported in lambs and pigs nursing dams dosed with zearalenone.[80,81] No information is available for equine species.

8.6.2 Mechanism of Action

Zearalenone undergoes reduction and forms two diastereoisomeric zearalanols (α-zearalanol and ß-zearalanol) that are naturally occurring fungal metabolites.

Zearalenone and its metabolites can interact directly with the cytoplasmic receptor that binds to 17ß-estradiol and translocate receptor sites to the nucleus. In the nucleus, stimulation of RNA leads to protein synthesis and clinical signs of estrogenism. Within the resorcylic acids, α-zearalenol exhibited the greatest binding affinity for cytosolic estrogen receptors, while zearalenone and ß-zearalenol displayed much lower binding affinities.[82] The hydroxylation of zearalenone to α-zearalenol apparently is an activation process, whereas the production of ß-zearalenol is a deactivation process. Interspecies variations in sensitivity to zearalenone in the feed could be related to different metabolites produced and the relative binding affinities of zearalenone and metabolites formed.[77] Among all species tested, pigs are the most sensitive to zearalenone and its metabolites.

Zearalenone can also act on the hypothalamic-hypophysial axis. Rainey et al.[83] determined that prepubertal exposure to zearalenone in pigs affected the hypothalamic-hypophysial axis and luteinizing hormone (LH) surges that lasted for at least 44 days post-exposure. However, zearalenone consumption did not delay the onset of pubertal estrus nor impair conception rates, ovulation rates, or number of fetuses. Male rats (70 days old) treated orally with zearalenone at 20 mg/kg for 35 days had elevated serum prolactin concentrations but showed no changes in serum LH and follicle stimulating hormone concentrations, body and testes weights, or in spermatogonia, spermatocytes, and spermatids.[84] In an *in vitro* study, Fenske and Fink-Gremmels[85] demonstrated that zearalenone at high concentrations (~400 µM) appeared to act directly on interstitial cells of the testes inhibiting steroidogenesis.

8.6.3 Toxicity and Clinical Signs

In general, zearalenone has a low acute toxicity in most animal species. A wide variability also exists in species sensitivity to zearalenone toxicity. Prepubertal swine are the most sensitive and poultry appear to be the least sensitive species. Also, females are more sensitive than males and the young are more sensitive than the old. Gimeno and Quintanilla[86] reported estrogenic signs of edematous vulvas, prolapsed vaginas, oversized uteri, and internal hemorrhage in mares and severe flaccidity of genitals in two male horses fed corn screenings for 30 days in a field exposure. All sick animals collapsed with respiratory paralysis, sudden blindness, and died quickly. Feed analysis revealed zearalenone at 2–3 mg/kg.

Unfortunately, the feed was not also analyzed for fumonisin, which is known to cause blindness. In another study conducted on six cycling trotter mares, Juhász et al.[87] determined that daily oral administration of 7 mg purified zearalenone starting 10 days after ovulation until the subsequent ovulation had no adverse effect on reproduction. The dose of purified zearalenone represented a natural contamination of feed with about 1 mg zearalenone/kg feed and ranged between 0.013–0.010 mg zearalenone/kg/day for approximately 8–10 days. In this study, a short duration of zearalenone exposure produced no effect on the length of the inter-ovulatory intervals, ovarian luteal and follicular phases, and did not significantly affect uterine edema.

8.7 Treatment

There is no specific antidote for zearalenone toxicity. Symptomatic treatment is advisable. Replacement of contaminated feed with clean feed allows recovery from estrogenic signs within 1–2 weeks. Within 3–7 weeks following removal of the contaminated feed, animals will return to normal reproductive status. No zearalenone binder has been proven to be efficacious and there are none currently approved by the United States Food and Drug Administration.[77]

8.8 Concluding Remarks

Mycotoxicoses usually occur from consuming mycotoxin contaminated feed, which affects equine health worldwide and produces hundreds of millions of dollars in economic losses each year. This chapter describes the toxicity of some commonly encountered mycotoxins, such as aflatoxins, fumonisins, slaframine, trichothecenes, and zearalenone in equine species. Fumonisins and aflatoxins are the two most frequently encountered mycotoxins in feed causing mycotoxicoses in equine species. Evidently, each mycotoxin adversely affects equine health by a single or multiple mechanism of action, involving selected target organ(s). There is no specific antidotal treatment for any mycotoxin. A number of binders have been tested and they offer some beneficial effects. However, these binders can also cause a nutritional deficiency of some nutrients. Therefore, replacement of contaminated feed with clean feed appears to be the best solution. Future research is needed to understand the detailed mechanism of action of these mycotoxins so that effective antidotes can be developed.

Acknowledgment

The author would like to thank Mrs. Robin B. Doss and Ms. Michelle Lasher for their technical assistance in preparation of this chapter.

References

1. Coppock RW, Christian RG, Jacobsen BJ. Aflatoxins. In: Gupta RC, ed. Veterinary toxicology: basic and clinical principles. 2nd ed. New York: Elsevier, 2012;1181–1199.
2. Varga J, Frisvad JC, Samson RA. A reappraisal of fungi producing aflatoxins. World Mycotoxin J 2009;2:263–277.
3. Calvo AM, Wilson RA, Bok JW, et al. Relationship between secondary metabolism and fungal development. Microbiol Mol Biol Rev 2002;66:447–459.
4. Johnsson P, Lindblad M, Thim AM, et al. Growth of aflatoxigenic moulds and aflatoxin formation in Brazil nuts. World Mycotox J 2008;1:127–137.
5. Abdel-Wahhab MA, Kholif AM. Mycotoxins in animal feeds and prevention strategies. Asian J Anim Sci 2008;2:7–25.
6. Woo LL, Egner PA, Belanger CL, et al. Aflatoxin B1-DNA adduct formation and mutagenicity in livers of neonatal male and female B6C3F1 mice. Toxicol Sci 2011;122: 38–44.
7. Joens LA, Pier AC, Cutlip RC. Effects of aflatoxin consumption on the clinical course of swine dysentery. Am J Vet Res 1981;42:1170–1172.
8. Venturini MC, Quiroga MA, Risso MA, et al. Mycotoxin T-2 and aflatoxin B1 as immunosuppressors in mice chronically infected with Toxoplasma gondii. J Comp Pathol 1996;115:229–237.
9. Bondy G, Pestka JJ. Immunomodulation by fungal toxins. J Toxicol Environ Health B 2000;3:109–143.
10. Wada K, Hashiba Y, Ohtsuka H, et al. Effects of mycotoxins on mitogen-stimulated proliferation of bovine peripheral blood mononuclear cells. J Vet Med Sci 2008;70:193–196.
11. Ghosh RC, Chauhan HV, Jha GJ. Suppression of cell-mediated immunity by purified aflatoxin B1 in broiler chicks. Vet Immunol Immunopathol 1991;28:165–72.
12. Meissonnier GM, Pinton P, Laffitte J, et al. Immunotoxicity of aflatoxin B1: impairment of the cell-mediated response to vaccine antigen and modulation of cytokine expression. Toxicol Appl Pharmacol 2008;231:142–149.
13. Mishra NC, Sopori ML. Immunotoxicity. In: Gupta RC, ed. Veterinary toxicology: basic and clinical principles. 2nd ed. New York: Elsevier, 2012;364–380.

14. Boatell R, Asquith RL, Edds GT, et al. Acute experimentally induced aflatoxicosis in the weanling pony. Am J Vet Res 1983;44:2110–2114.

15. Greene HJ, Oehme FW. A possible case of equine aflatoxicosis. Clin Toxicol 1976;9:251–254.

16. Angsubhakorn S, Poomvises P, Romruen K, et al. Aflatoxicosis in horses. J Am Vet Med Assoc 1981;178:274–278.

17. Gupta RC. Aflatoxins, ochratoxins and citrinin. In: Gupta RC, ed. Reproductive and developmental toxicology. Amsterdam: Academic Press/Elsevier, 2011;753–763.

18. Kourousekos GD, Lymberopoulos AG. Occurrence of aflatoxins in milk and their effects on reproduction. J Hellenic Vet Med Soc 2007;58:306–312.

19. Turner PC, Collinson AC, Cheung YB, et al. Aflatoxin exposure in utero causes growth faltering in Gambian infants. Intl J Epidemiol 2007;36:1119–1125.

20. Shuaib FMB, Ehiri J, Abdullahi A, et al. Reproductive health effects of aflatoxins: A review of literature. Reprod Toxicol 2010;29:262–270.

21. Agnes FA, Akbarsha MA. Spermatotoxic effect of aflatoxin B(1) in the albino mouse. Food Chem Toxicol 2003;41:119–130.

22. Ibeh IN, Saxena DK. Aflatoxin B1 and reproduction. I. Reproductive performance in female rats. Afr J Reprod Health 1997;1:79–84.

23. Ibeh IN, Saxena DK. Aflatoxin B1 and reproduction. II. Gametoxicity in female rats. Afr J Reprod Health 1997;1:85–89.

24. Partanen HA, El-Nezami HS, Leppanen JM, et al. Aflatoxin B1 transfer and metabolism in human placenta. Toxicol Sci 2010;113:216–225.

25. Abdulrazzaq YM, Osman N, Yousif ZM, et al. Morbidity in neonates of mothers who have ingested aflatoxins. Ann Trop Pedtri 2004;24:145–151.

26. Storvik M, Huuskonen P, Kyllönen T, et al. Aflatoxin B1- a potential endocrine disruptor- up regulates CYP19A1 in JEG-3 cells. Toxicol Lett 2011;202:161–167.

27. Wangikar PB, Dwivedi P, Sharma AK, et al. Effects of aflatoxin B1 on embryo fetal development in rabbits. Food Chem Toxicol 2005;43:607–615.

28. World Health Organization: World Health Organization Environmental Health Criteria 105. Selected mycotoxins: ochratoxins, trichothecenes, ergot. Geneva: WHO, 1990.

29. Williams JH, Phillips TD, Jolly PE, et al. Human aflatoxicosis in developing countries: a review of toxicology, exposure, potential health consequences, and interventions. Am J Clin Nutr 2004;80:1106–1022.

30. Pellegrino P, Mallet B, Delliaux S, et al. Zeolites are effective ROS-scavengers in vitro. Biochem Biophys Res Comm 2011;410:478–483.

31. Huwig A, Freimund S, Käppeli O, et al. Mycotoxin detoxication of animal feed by different adsorbents. Toxicol Lett 2001;122:179–188.

32. Gelderblom WCA, Jaskiewicz K, Marasas WFO, et al. Fumonisins – novel mycotoxins with cancer promoting activity produced by Fusarium moniliforme. Appl Environ Microbio. 1988;54:1806–1811.

33. Marasas WFO, Kellerman TS, Gelderblom WCA, et al. Leukoencephalomalacia in a horse induced by fumonisin B1 isolated from Fusarium moniliforme. Onderstepoort J Vet Res 1988;55:197–203.

34. Marasas WFO. Discovery and occurrence of the fumonisins: a historical perspective. Environ Health Perspect (Suppl 2) 2001;109:239–243.

35. Månsson M, Klejnstrup ML, Phipps RK, et al. Isolation and NMR characterization of fumonisin B2 and a new fumonisin B6 from *Aspergillus niger*. J Agri Food Chem 2010;58:949–953.

36. Bartók T, Tolgyesi L, Szekeres A, et al. Detection and characterization of twenty-eight isomers of fumonisin B1 (FB1) mycotoxin in a solid rice culture infected with Fusarium verticillioides by reversed-phase high-performance liquid chromatography/electron spray ionization time-of-flight and ion trap mass spectrometry. Rapid Commun Mass Spectrom 2010;24:35–42.

37. Smith GW. Fumonisins. In: Gupta RC, ed. Veterinary toxicology: basic and clinical principles. 2nd ed. New York: Elsevier, 2012;1205–1219.

38. Smith GW, Constable PD, Foreman JH, et al. Cardiovascular changes associated with intravenous administration of fumonisin B1 in horses. Am J Vet Res 2002;63:538–545.

39. Foreman JH, Constable PD, Waggoner AL, et al. Neurologic abnormalities and cerebrospinal fluid changes in horses administered fumonisin B1 intravenously. J Vet Intern Med 2004;18:223–230.

40. Voss KA, Riley RT, Gelineau-van Waes JB. Fetotoxicity and neural tube defects in CD1 mice exposed to the mycotoxin fumonisin B1, Mycotoxins (Suppl) 2007;57:67–72.

41. Voss KA, Riley RT, Waes JG. Fumonisins. In: Gupta RC, ed. Reproductive and developmental toxicology. Amsterdam: Academic Press/Elsevier, 2011;725–737.

42. Bhandari N, Sharma RP. Fumonisin B(1)-induced alterations in cytokine expression and apoptosis signaling genes in mouse liver and kidney after an acute exposure. Toxicology 2002;172:81–92.

43. Theumer MG, Lopez AG, Masih DT, et al. Immunobiological effects of fumonisin B1 in experimental subchronic mycotoxicoses in rats. Clin Diagn Lab Immunol 2002;9:149–155.

44. Abdel-Wahhab MA, Hassan AM, Amer HA, et al. Prevention of fumonisin- induced maternal and developmental toxicity in rats by certain plant extracts. J Appl Toxicol 2004;24:469–474.

45. Missmer SA, Suarez L, Felkner M, et al. Exposure to fumonisins and the occurrence of neural tube defects along the Texas-Mexico border. Environ Health Perspect 2006;114:237–241.

46. Croom WJ Jr, Hagler WM Jr, Froetschel MA, et al. The involvement of slaframine and swainsonine in slobbers syndrome: a review. J Anim Sci 1995;73:1499–1505.

47. O'Dell BL, Reagan WO, Beach TJ. A study of the toxic principle in red clover. Univ of Missouri Agr Exp Sta Bull 1959;702:1–12.

48. Hagler WM, Behlow RF. Salivary syndrome in horses: Identification of slaframine in red clover hay. Appl Environm Microbiol 1981;42:1067–1073.

49. Gaskill C. Slaframine toxication. Bluegrass Equine Digest. Retrieved from www.ca.uky.edu/gluck/images/BED/BED-July10.pdf on April 12, 2011 (accessed October 13, 2016).

50. Guengerich FP, Aust SD. Activation of the parasympathomimetic alkaloid slaframine by microsomal and photochemical oxidation. Mol Pharmacol 1977;13:185–195.

51. Smith GW. Slaframine. In: Gupta RC, ed. Veterinary toxicology: basic and clinical principles. 2nd ed. New York: Elsevier, 2012;1227–1230.

52. Aust SD, Broquist HP, Rinehart KL Jr. Slaframine: A parasympathomimetic from Rhizoctonia leguminicola. Biotech Bioeng 1968;10:403–412.

53. Crump MH, Smalley EB, Nichols RE, et al. Pharmacologic properties of a slobber-inducing mycotoxin from Rhizoctonia leguminicola. Am J Vet Res 1967;28:865–874.

54. Smith JE, Henderson RS. Mycotoxins and animal foods. Boston, MA: CRC Press, 1991;683.

55. Imerman PM, Stahr HM. New, sensitive high-performance liquid chromatography method for the determination of slaframine in plasma and milk. J Chromatogr A 1998;815:141–145.

56. Mostrom MS, Raisbeck MF. Trichothecenes. In: Gupta RC, ed. Veterinary toxicology: basic and clinical principles. 2nd ed. New York: Elsevier, 2012;1239–1265.

57. Dänicke S, Valenta H, Döll S. On the toxicokinetics and the metabolism of deoxynivalenol (DON) in the pig. Arch Anim Nutri 2004;58:169–180.

58. Prelusky DB, Trenholm HL. Tissue distribution of deoxynivalenol in swine dosed intravenously. J Agric Food Chem 1991;39:748–751.

59. Goyarts T, Dänicke S. Bioavailability of the Fusarium toxin deoxynivalenol (DON) from naturally contaminated wheat for the pig. Toxicol Lett 2006;163:171–182.

60. Swanson SP, Corley RA. The distribution, metabolism, and excretion of trichothecene mycotoxins. In: Beasley VR, ed. Trichothecene mycotoxicosis: Pathophysiologic effects. Vol I. Boca Raton, FL: CRC Press Inc., 1989;37–61.

61. Li Y, Wang Z, Beier RC, et al. T-2 toxin, a trichothecene mycotoxin: review of toxicity, metabolism, and analytical methods. J Agri Food Chem 2011;59:3441–3453.

62. Rocha O, Ansari K, Doohan FM. Effects of trichothecene mycotoxins on eukaryotic cells: A review. Food Addit Contam 2005;22:369–378.

63. Rosenstein Y, Lafarge-Frayssinet C, Lespinats G, et al. Immunosuppressive activity of fusarium toxins. Effects on antibody synthesis and skin grafts of crude extracts, T-2 toxin and diacetoxyscirpenol. Immunology 1979;36:111–117.

64. Johnson PJ, Casteel SW, Messer NT. Effect of feeding deoxynivalenol (vomitoxin)-contaminated barley to horses. J Vet Diagn Invest 1997;9:219–221().

65. Raymond SL, Smith TK, Swamy HV. Effects of feeding a blend of grains naturally contaminated with Fusarium mycotoxins on feed intake, metabolism, and indices of athletic performance on exercised horses. J Anim Sci 2005;83:1267–1273.

66. Pestka JJ, Yan D, King LE. Flow cytometric analysis of the effects of in vitro exposure to vomitoxin (deoxynivalenol) on apoptosis in murine T, B and IgA+ cells. Food Chem Toxicol 1994;32:1125–1136.

67. Shinozuka S, Suzuki M, Noguchi N, et al. T-2 toxin induced apoptosis in hematopoietic tissues of mice. Toxicol Pathol 1998;26:674–681.

68. Islam W, Nagase M, Yoshizawa T, et al. T-2 toxin induces thymic apoptosis in vivo in mice. Toxicol Appl Pharmacol 1998;148:205–214.

69. Zhou H-R, Islam Z, Pestka JJ. Induction of competing apoptotic and survival signaling pathways in the macrophage by the ribotoxic trichothecene deoxynivalenol. Toxicol Sci 2005;87:113–122.

70. Ueno Y. General toxicology. In: Ueno Y, ed. Trichothecenes – Chemical, biological, and toxicological aspects. New York: Elsevier, 1983;135–146.

71. Prelusky DB, Rotter BA, Rotter RG. Toxicology of mycotoxins. In: Miller JD, Trenholm HL, eds. Mycotoxins in grain. Compounds other than a flatoxin. St. Paul: Eagan Press, 1994;359–403.

72. Anonymous. Protection against trichothecene mycotoxins. National Academy Press, Washington DC, 1983.

73. Dankø G. Stachybotryotoxicosis and immunosuppression. Intern J Environ Studies 1975;8:209–211.

74. Forgacs J. Stachybotryotoxicosis. In: Kadis S, Ciegler A, Ajl SJ, eds. Microbial toxins. Vol 8. New York, NY: Academic Press, 1972;95–128.

75. Hintikka E-L. Stachybotryotoxicosis in horses. In: Wyllie TD, Morehouse LG, eds. Mycotoxic fungi, mycotoxins, mycotoxicoses. Vol 2. Mycotoxicoses of domestic and laboratory animals, poultry, and aquatic invertebrates and vertebrates. New York, NY: Marcel Dekker, 1978;181–185.

76. Ishii K, Sakai K, Ueno Y, et al. Solaniol, a toxic metabolite of Fusarium solani. Appl Micrbiol 1971;22:718–720.

77. Mostrom MS. Zearalenone. In: Gupta RC, ed. Veterinary toxicology: basic and clinical principles. 2nd ed. New York: Elsevier, 2012;1266–1271.

78. Kuiper-Goodman T, Scott PM, Watanabe H. Risk assessment of the mycotoxin zearalenone. Regul Toxicol Pharmacol 1987;7:253–306.

79. Ueno Y, Ayaki S, Sato N, et al. Fate and mode of action of zearalenone. Ann Nutr Aliment 1977;31:935–948.

80. Hagler WM, Dankø G, Horvath L, et al. Transmission of zearalenone and its metabolite into ruminant milk. Acta Vet Acad Sci Hungar 1980;28:209–216.

81. Palyusik M, Harrach B, Mirocha CJ, et al. Transmission of zearalenone and zearalenol into porcine milk. Acta Vet Acad Sci Hungar 1980;28:217–222.

82. Fitzpatrick DW, Picken CA, Murphy LC, et al. Measurement of the relative binding affinity of zearalenone, α-zearalenol and ß-zearalenol for uterine and oviduct estrogen receptors in swine, rats and chickens: An indicator of estrogenic potencies. Comp Biochem Physiol C 1989;94:691–694.

83. Rainey MR, Tubbs RC, Bennett LW, et al. Prepubertal exposure to dietary zearalenone alters hypothalamo-hypophysial function but does not impair postpubertal reproductive function of gilts. J Anim Sci 1990;68:2015–2022.

84. Milano GD, Becu-Villalobos D, Tapia O. Effects of long-term zearalenone administration on spermatogenesis and serum luteinizing hormone, follicle-stimulating hormone, and prolactin values in male rats. Am J Vet Res 1995;56:954–958.

85. Fenske M, Fink-Gremmels J. Effects of fungal metabolites on testosterone secretion in vitro. Arch Toxicol 1990;64: 72–75.

86. Gimeno A, Quintanilla JA. Analytical and mycological study of a natural outbreak of zearalenone mycotoxicosis in horses, in Proceedings. Int Symp Mycotoxins, 1983; 387–392.

87. Juhász J, Nagy P, Kulcsár M, et al. Effect of low-dose zearalenone exposure on luteal function, follicular activity, and uterine edema in cycling mares. Acta Veter Hungar 2001;49:211–222.

9 Poisonous plants

Anthony P. Knight, BVSc, MS, DACVIM

Plant poisoning was recognized as a problem facing the horse and livestock industry in the mid-1800s. One of the earliest recognized plant poisonings was a neurologic disease of horses appropriately named locoism, a name derived from the Spanish word meaning crazy.[1] The association between locoism and the grazing of locoweeds to this day remains a major cause of economic loss to the equine industry. Although plant poisoning of horses continues to be a problem, the full economic impact on the horse industry is not known. Indirectly, poisonous plants add to the cost of raising and managing horses through fencing, herbicides, mowing, and reseeding of pastures where undesirable plants predominate. The costs of subclinical poisoning from plants and the loss of pasture due to the displacement of normal forages by noxious plants are significant. Typically, horses are at greatest risk when pastures are overgrazed and noxious weeds can proliferate. At other times, accidental poisoning may occur when horses are given access to garden clippings or when toxic plants and trees are planted in or around horse pastures as hedges, wind-breaks, or for shade. Although most plant poisonings occur in horses on pasture during the spring and summer, losses may also occur during the winter if hay contains toxic plants.

To paraphrase the famous fifteenth century alchemist Paracelsus, all things are poisons, for there is nothing without poisonous qualities. "It is the dose which makes a thing poisonous." (Paracelsus 1493–1541. <http://en.wikipedia.org/wiki/Paracelsus>.) Rarely is a horse poisoned by a few bites of a plant, with the possible exception of the most toxic of plants such as water hemlock (*Cicuta douglasii*) and yew (*Taxus* spp.). Horses generally must eat large quantities of a toxic plant in amounts equal to 5–10% of their body weight over a period of several weeks or months. It is therefore unlikely that a few toxic plants in a pasture pose a significant risk. Factors such as drought, excessive moisture, herbicides, fertilization, and soil mineral imbalances can alter the amount of toxin in plants, making them more of a problem in some years than in others. Herbicides can increase the palatability and toxicity of plants and therefore must be used cautiously where animals graze.

This chapter is intended to provide recognition of the more common toxic plants, their potential for poisoning, the clinical signs that can be expected in the event a horse consumes a toxic amount of the plant, and therapeutic and management practices that can be used to prevent poisoning. Because clinical signs are often the reason a horse is presented for veterinary care, the most common poisonous plants affecting horses in North America will be grouped by the main clinical effects of the plant toxin. Plant toxins however often exert their effects directly or indirectly on multiple organ systems, and therefore the clinical signs will reflect the variety and degree of organ involvement. For example, Tansy ragwort (*Senecio jacobaea*) poisoning in horses often presents as neurologic disease or severe photodermatitis, yet the underlying problem is severe liver disease. Plants that have only been suspected of being toxic to horses, but not confirmed, will not be included. Commonly used botanical terms helpful to describe plants, but unfamiliar to those not knowledgeable in botany, are described in a glossary at the end of this chapter.

9.1 Excessive Salivation Induced by Plants

Excessive salivation or slobbering characterized by frothing or drooling is generally an indication of traumatic or chemical mouth injury or esophageal

Nutritional Management of Equine Diseases and Special Cases, First Edition. Edited by Bryan M. Waldridge.
© 2017 John Wiley & Sons, Inc. Published 2017 by John Wiley & Sons, Inc.

obstruction (choke) that prevents normal swallowing of saliva and food. Trauma and pain resulting from sharp points of broken or diseased teeth, poorly fitting or inappropriately used bits, or infectious viral diseases such as vesicular stomatitis, which causes mouth ulcers, also cause hypersalivation. A variety of grasses and other plants may traumatize the mucous membranes of the mouth. Plants with thorns, bristles, or sharp awns can produce lesions ranging from reddening to deep granulating ulcers on the tongue and gums. Grasses such as foxtail barley (*Hordeum jubatum*, Figure 9.1), bristle grass (*Setaria* spp.), and wheat or rye awns can become embedded in the mucous membranes of the cheeks, tongue, and gums, causing painful ulcers, excessive salivation, and difficulty eating. Grass awns are often not visible in the ulcers, as they are covered by a layer of granulation tissue. A wide variety of plants (Table 9.1) has the potential to cause irritation and trauma in the mouth of horses if they are present in hay or are abundant in pasture. Occasionally, these plants can cause trauma to the skin; sometimes potentially serious injury to the eyes may result from bristles of burdock (*Arctium* spp.) and other plants that become lodged in the conjunctival sack or cornea.[2]

Numerous other plants may also cause excessive salivation in addition to their primary toxic effect. For example, laurel (*Kalmia* spp.), rhododendrons and azaleas (*Rhododendron* spp.), and buttercups (*Ranunculus* spp.) cause colic primarily with secondary salivation. Poison hemlock (*Conium maculatum*), water hemlock (*Cicuta* spp.), and death camas (*Zigadenus* spp.) primarily will most noticeably cause death. Yellow star thistle (*Centaurea solstitialis*), Russian knapweed (*Acroptilon repens*), white snakeroot (*Eupatorium rugosum*), Crofton weed (*E. adenophorum*), Jimmyweed or rayless goldenrod (*Haplopappus* spp.), and Burrow weed (*H. tenuisectus*) cause neurologic signs with salivation.

Profuse salivation without evidence of mouth irritation or injury occurs in horses and other livestock eating clover or alfalfa pasture and hay that is infected with the fungus *Rhizoctonia leguminicola* causing Black Patch disease.[3,4] The toxin responsible has been identified as slaframine, an indolizidine alkaloid mycotoxin produced most commonly by this fungus on red clover (*Trifolium pratense*), but it may also be produced on other common legumes, including alfalfa, white clover, alsike clover, lupines, cow pea, and kudzu.[5,6] *Rhizoctonia leguminicola*

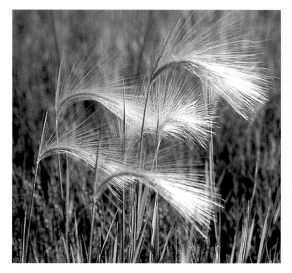

Figure 9.1 Foxtail barley (*Hordeum jubatum*) seed heads.

Table 9.1 Mechanically injurious plants.

Common Name	Scientific Name
Burdock bristles	*Arctium* spp.
Three awn grasses	*Aristida* spp.
Oat awns	*Avena sativa*
Sand burs	*Cenchrus* spp.
Thistles	*Cirsium* spp.
Foxtail barley awns	*Hordeum jubatum*
Barley awns	*Hordeum vulgare*
Prickly pear cactus, cholla	*Opuntia* spp.
Rye awns	*Secale cereale*
Bristle grasses, foxtails	*Setaria* spp.
Horse nettle	*Solanum carolinensis*
Buffalo bur	*Solanum rostratum*
Needle, spear, or porcupine grass	*Stipa* spp.
Wheat awns	*Triticum aestivum*
Puncture vine, goat head	*Tribulus terrestris*
Stinging nettle	*Urtica* spp.
Cockle burs	*Xanthium* spp.

Commonly cause oral lesions resulting in: excess salivation or slobbering, difficulty in eating, and decreased feed intake. Occasionally, some may cause skin and eye trauma (bristles of burdock adhered to eyelashes).

produces two similar indolizidine alkaloids, slaframine and swainsonine, that are synthesized from lysine through pipecolic acid. Swainsonine is also produced in locoweeds (*Astragalus* and *Oxytropis* spp.) that are covered later under neurotoxic plants.[7]

Under wet or humid conditions, the fungus grows on leaves and produces visible black or brown spotting. After eating infected legumes for several days, horses begin to salivate excessively, lose weight, and may have excessive lacrimation, diarrhea, and frequent urination.[3–5] Pregnant mares may abort if they continue to consume infected clover. Recovery occurs rapidly once horses are removed from the infected legume pasture or hay. Problem pastures can be grazed if they are mowed, the affected hay is removed, and regrowth has no brown or black spots on the leaves.

Unusual causes of increased salivation have been reported in horses at a horse show that developed blister-like lesions around the lips, nose, and eyes.[8] It was found that all 50 affected horses were bedded on a common source of wood shavings that contained some bitterwood (*Quassia simarouba*), a tree indigenous to Central and South America, where it is harvested for lumber. Similar blisters have been reported on the hands and face of people who prune these trees. Horses in this outbreak recovered completely from the vesicular dermatitis once they were removed from the wood shavings.

9.2 Colic and Diarrhea-Inducing Plants

Poisonous plants are but one of many causes of colic and diarrhea in horses. Plant toxins may either have a direct irritant effect on the gastrointestinal system, causing hyperperistalsis, colic, and diarrhea, or they may act on the parasympathetic nervous system, causing ileus, flatulence, and colic. Yet other plants may cause severe colic through obstruction or impaction of the small or large intestine, respectively. Fruits of plants such as Cockspur hawthorn (*Crataegus crusgalli*), mesquite (*Prosopis glandulosa*), and persimmon (*Diospyros virginiana*) can cause obstruction of the small or large intestine.[9,10]

Plants most frequently associated with colic and/or diarrhea in horses are listed along with their toxin and additional effects in Table 9.2. Horses eating the fruit, seeds, or leaves of avocado (*Persea americana*) trees usually die within a few days or less, depending on the amount consumed, as described later in the section on sudden death-inducing plants. Prior to death, however,

colic, diarrhea, and signs of acute congestive heart failure occur. A variety of other common plants also may be incriminated as a cause of colic and diarrhea if horses are deprived of normal forages. Invasive pasture plants such as leafy spurge (*Euphorbia esula*), wild iris (*Iris missouriensis*), horsetail or scouring rush (*Equisetum arvense*), bitter weeds (*Helenium* spp.), and a variety of mustard plants (*Brassica* spp.) have the potential to cause colic and diarrhea due to a variety of irritant compounds in the plants.

Diagnosing plant-induced causes of colic and diarrhea is difficult because generally there are no specific lesions detectable in the gastrointestinal tract at postmortem examination and it is difficult to identify plants in the gastrointestinal tract once they have been chewed and denatured by digestive enzymes. When plants are suspected of causing colic and diarrhea, a careful history and thorough examination of the horse's pasture and feed should be made in an attempt to identify the plants in Table 9.2 and described in this section.

Plants such as halogeton (*Halogeton glomeratus*), greasewood (*Sarcobatus vermiculatus*), and shamrock, soursob, or sorrel (*Oxalis* spp.) contain high amounts of oxalate, which has the potential to cause gastroenteritis and diarrhea. Prolonged consumption of low amounts of oxalate from these plants or others containing low amounts of oxalate may cause a calcium deficiency-induced hyperparathyroidism.

9.2.1 Horse Chestnut or Buckeye

Horse chestnut or buckeye (*Aesculus* spp.) are common small to medium-sized shrubs or trees with large palmate leaves, white to red flower spikes borne terminally on the branches, and characteristic spiny or smooth fruit capsules containing 1–3 shiny brown nuts when ripe (Figure 9.2). Horse chestnut species grow throughout most of the United States but are concentrated in the eastern and southern states. Those reportedly toxic to animals are: Ohio, California, red and yellow buckeyes (*A. glabra, A. californica, A. pavia,* and *A. octandra*, respectively), and the introduced species horse chestnut (*A. hippocastanum*).[11,12] Toxic chestnuts are not related to the edible chestnut (*Castanea* spp.).

The toxins in buckeyes and chestnuts are saponins (aesculin), present in new growth, leaves, and nuts. The principal action appears to be on the gastrointestinal

Table 9.2 Colic or diarrhea-inducing plants.

Common Name	Scientific Name	Clinical Effects
Foxglove	*Digitalis purpurea*	Diarrhea, regurgitation, cardiac
Oleander	*Nerium oleander*	
Yellow oleander	*Thevetia peruviana*	
Be-Still, lucky nut tree	*Thevetia thevetioides*	
Halogeton	*Halogeton glomeratus*	Diarrhea, rarely renal disease
Greasewood	*Sarcobatus vermiculatus*	Prolonged intake of low amount causes calcium deficiency
Shamrock, soursob, sorrel	*Oxalis* spp.	
Horse chestnut, buckeye	*Aesculus* spp.	
Corn cockle	*Agrostemma githago*	Muscle tremors and ataxia
Pokeweed	*Phytolacca americana*	Diarrhea
Coffee or senna weed	*Cassia* spp.	
Oaks	*Quercus* spp.	Hard, dark feces; later bloody diarrhea, anorexia, depression
Gambels oak	*Q. gambelii*	
Shinnery oak	*Q. harvardii*	May have oral ulcers and choke signs, liver and kidney damage,
	Q. breviloba	hypocalcemia, hyperphosphatemia
Field bindweed	*Convolvulus arvensis*	Bradycardia and dilated pupils
Laurel	*Kalmia* spp.	
Azaleas	*Rhododendron* spp.	
Fetterbush	*Leucothoe* spp.	Salivation, defecation, depression, and ataxia
Mountain pieris	*Pieris* spp.	
Maleberry	*Lyonia* spp.	
Privets	*Ligustrum vulgare*	
Buttercup & anemone	*Ranunculus* spp.	
Hellebore	*Helleborus* spp.	
Marsh marigold	*Caltha palustris*	Salivation and diarrhea
Clematis	*Clematis* spp.	
Castor beans	*Ricinus communis*	
Rosary peas	*Abrus precatorius*	Trembling, ataxia, and diarrhea
Black locust	*Robinia pseudoacacia*	
Nightshade and potato	*Solanum* spp.	
Jimson weed (thorn apple)	*Datura stramonium*	Excitement then depression
Tomato	*Lycopersicon* spp.	Diarrhea and weakness
Jessamine	*Cestrum* spp.	
Avocado (Guatemalan variety)	*Persea americana*	Diarrhea, congestive heart failure, edema of abdomen, head, and lungs. Death in <2 days.
Persimmon	*Diospyros virginiana*	Impaction colic
Cockspur or hawthorn	*Crataegus crusgalli*	
Mesquite	*Prosopis glandulosa*	

NB: In addition to the clinical effects listed, all plants listed cause colic, except those causing acute oxalate poisoning (*Halogeton*, *Sarcobatus*, and *Oxalis* spp.).

tract and nervous system. Colic has been the main problem reported in horses, although muscle tremors, ataxia, incoordination, and paralysis are possible. There is no specific treatment, but administering mineral oil by nasogastric tube as a laxative and supportive fluid therapy may be beneficial. Poisoning is rarely fatal.

9.2.2 Field Bindweed (Morning Glory)

Field bindweed (*Convolvulus arvensis*), found throughout North America, is an extremely persistent invasive perennial twining or creeping weed with alternate leaves and white or pink funnel-shaped flowers (Figure 9.3). The plant reproduces readily from seed and its extensive root system.

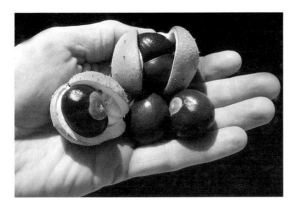

Figure 9.2 Fruits of horse chestnut or buckeye (*Aesculus* spp.).

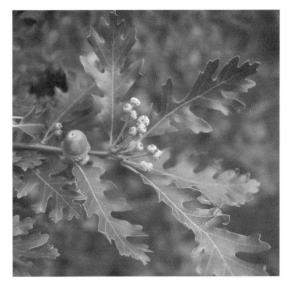

Figure 9.4 Gambel's oak (*Quercus gambelii*) showing typical leaves and acorn.

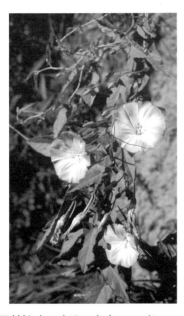

Figure 9.3 Field bindweed (*Convolvulus arvensis*).

The toxins in bindweed are tropane alkaloids (pseudotropine), which are present in all parts of the plant and have an atropine-like action. Colic is the result of intestinal stasis and flatulence. Parasympatholytic signs such as bradycardia and dilated pupils may result if toxic levels of bindweed are consumed. Chronic weight loss and colic in horses grazing predominantly bindweed was attributed to severe intestinal fibrosis and vascular sclerosis. No specific treatment is known. Symptomatic colic therapy is indicated.

9.2.3 Oak

Horses are susceptible to oak poisoning and will eat oak leaves and acorns when normal forages are scarce.[13] Poisoning is unlikely unless large quantities of the leaves and/or acorns are eaten. Although all 60 species of oak (*Quercus* spp.) that grow in North America are potentially toxic, most livestock poisoning is attributed to Gambels oak (*Quercus gambelii*), Shinnery oak (*Q. havardii*), and *Q. breviloba*.[14] Oaks range from shrubs to large trees. All have alternate, simple, toothed, or lobed, dark green glossy leaves that turn red in the fall (Figure 9.4). The plants are monoecious, with the staminate flowers occurring in long catkins and pistillate flowers occurring singly or in small clusters. The acorn fruit is a nut partially enveloped by an involucre of scales.

Tannins (gallotannic acid) are found in the leaves, bark, and acorns of most oak species and are responsible for poisoning in animals.[15–17] Tannic acid fed to rabbits produced effects similar to that produced by Shinnery oak.[17] Tannins are potent precipitators of cellular protein (astringents), which cause severe necrosis of the intestinal tract and kidney when ingested. Oaks at any stage of growth are poisonous, but are particularly toxic when the leaf and flower buds are just opening in the spring. As the leaves mature, they become less toxic. Ripe acorns are less toxic than green acorns. Cattle, sheep, horses, and pigs are susceptible to oak poisoning.[13,17–20] Ruminants frequently browse on oak without apparent problems, provided they have ample access to normal forages.

Clinical signs of oak poisoning vary according to the quantity of oak leaves, bark, or acorns consumed. Initially, animals stop eating, become depressed, and develop colic.[17,18] The feces are hard and dark, but a hemorrhagic diarrhea often occurs later in the course of poisoning. Some horses present as though they are choked and saliva passes out the nose. Mouth ulcers may also be present. Severe liver and kidney damage is detectable by elevations in serum liver enzyme activity and blood urea nitrogen.[21] Urinalysis may show low specific gravity, proteinuria, glucosuria, hemoglobinuria, and casts.[17] Hypocalcemia and hyperphosphatemia are usually present. Horses may die within 24 hours after eating large quantities of acorns or they may live for 5–7 days after the onset of clinical signs.

On postmortem examination, mucoid hemorrhagic gastroenteritis with edematous large intestinal mesentery are the predominant gross lesions in horses that die from oak poisoning.[17,19] Hemorrhages on various organs and excessive amounts of fluid in the peritoneal and pleural cavities may be present. The kidneys are usually found to be pale, swollen, and covered with small hemorrhages. Histologically, the kidneys show tubular necrosis.[17,19] Liver necrosis may also be evident.

Affected animals should be removed from oak pasture and given supportive care in the form of fresh water, hay, and intravenous fluids to promote diuresis and to maintain hydration and acid-base balance. Mineral oil (1 gal/1000 lb or 4 L/450 kg horse) should be administered by nasogastric tube to help rid the intestinal tract of tannic acid. The therapy described here and appropriate analgesics to control pain are particularly indicated for colicky horses.

9.2.4 Mountain Laurel

Laurels (*Kalmia latifolia*) are common branching shrubs or small trees with glossy, green, alternate lanceolate leaves. The characteristic white to pink flowers are produced in showy clusters (Figure 9.5). Laurels are common to the eastern and southern United States.

The principal toxins in laurels are complex diterpenes grayanotoxins (andromedotoxin) which are present in all parts of the plant including the nectar. The principal

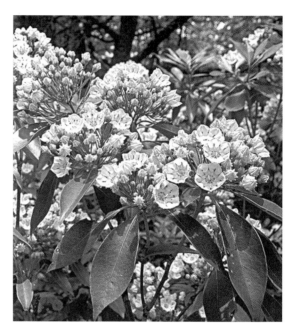

Figure 9.5 Mountain laurel (*Kalmia latifolia*).

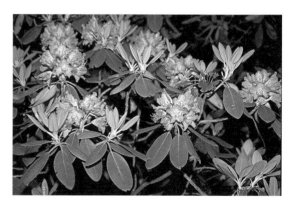

Figure 9.6 Azaleas (*Rhododendron catawbiense*).

action of the grayanotoxins is to bind to sodium channels in cell membranes, thus preventing inactivation of action potentials and causing prolonged depolarization. In low doses this has a positive inotropic effect on the heart, but at toxic levels cardiac conduction disturbances occur. Tannins cause gastrointestinal irritation. Similar toxins are also present in azaleas (*Rhododendron* spp.) (Figure 9.6), fetterbush (*Leucothoe* spp.) (Figure 9.7), mountain pieris (*Pieris* spp.) (Figure 9.8), and maleberry (*Lyonia* spp.) (Figure 9.9).[22,23]

Although all animals are susceptible to laurel and rhododendron poisoning, horses and donkeys are rarely

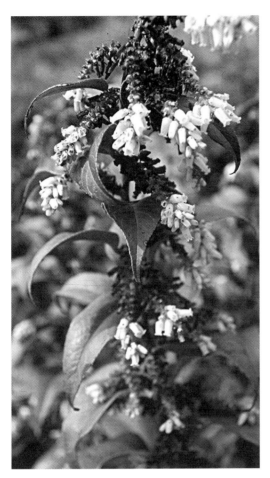

Figure 9.7 Fetterbush (*Leucothoe* spp.).

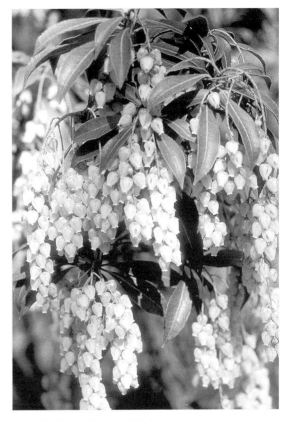

Figure 9.8 Mountain pieris (*Pieris* spp.).

poisoned. Affected animals may show excessive frothy green salivation, colic, frequent defecation, depression, weakness, and ataxia. If a sufficient quantity of laurel has been eaten, recumbency, coma, and death occur. There is no specific treatment. Mineral oil should be administered by stomach tube, and intravenous fluid therapy is administered as necessary.

9.2.5 Pokeweed

Pokeweed (*Phytolacca americana*) is a perennial branching herb 3–10 feet (1–3 m) tall, with a large taproot, green or purple stems, and large, alternate, petioled, and ovate leaves. The flowers are small, white, and without petals. The distinctive fruits are shiny purple berries (Figure 9.10). Pokeweed grows mostly in the eastern and southern United States. All parts of the plant, especially the roots, contain saponins and

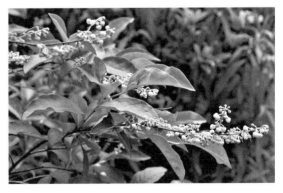

Figure 9.9 Maleberry (*Lyonia* spp.).

oxalates. Glycoproteins present in the plant may also cause hemagglutination through the activation of B and T lymphocytes (pokeweed mitogens).[24] Depending on the amount consumed, mild to severe colic and diarrhea may develop. Poisoning from pokeweed is rare in horses. Mineral oil (4 L/450 kg horse) by

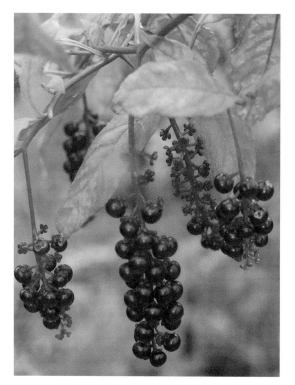

Figure 9.10 Pokeweed berries (*Phytolacca americana*).

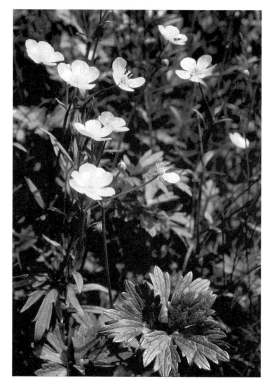

Figure 9.11 Buttercup (*Ranunculus* spp.).

nasogatric tube and intravenous fluids should be administered as needed.

9.2.6 Buttercups

Buttercups (*Ranunculus* spp.) are perennial herbaceous plants with fibrous roots, erect hairless stems, and leaves deeply divided into three lobes. The upper leaves are smaller. The flowers vary from few to many and have five bright yellow petals and five green sepals (Figure 9.11). Buttercups are commonly found in wet areas throughout North America.

Some, but not all, species of buttercups contain ranunculin, a glycoside which forms the toxic blistering agent protoanemonin when the plant is chewed or crushed. When dried, buttercups lose their toxicity. Other plants that contain protoanemonins include hellebore (*Helleborus* spp.), marsh marigold (*Caltha palustris*), clematis (*Clematis* spp.), and anemone (*Ranunculus* spp.). Protoanemonins are irritants and cause stomatitis, excessive salivation, mild colic, and diarrhea, varying in severity depending on the amount the horse has eaten. In severe cases of colic, mineral oil (4 L/450 kg) or

activated charcoal should be given via nasogastric tube and the horse should be maintained on intravenous fluids as necessary.

9.2.7 Castor Oil Plant

Castor oil plants (*Ricinus communis*) are common perennial plants of tropical areas, growing 6–13 feet (2–4 m) high, with a hollow branching stem. The stem is often purplish with a waxy coating. Leaves are large, alternate, and usually eight lobed, each with a main vein that radiates from the off-centered attachment of the petiole (Figure 9.12). Yellowish flowers are produced in racemes at the end of the main stem and form fruits covered with soft spines that dry into sharp spines surrounding three characteristic seeds. Poisoning occurs from eating either the plants or grain contaminated with castor beans.

All parts of the plant and especially the seeds contain the toxalbumin ricin, a highly toxic lectin that inhibits protein synthesis. Similar toxic lectins are found in rosary peas, jequirity beans (*Abrus precatorius*) (Figure 9.13) and black locust (*Robinia pseudoacacia*) (Figure 9.14). Lectins

Figure 9.12 Castor oil plant (*Ricinus communis*) leaves and spiny fruit capsules.

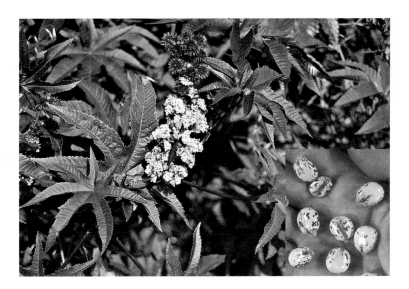

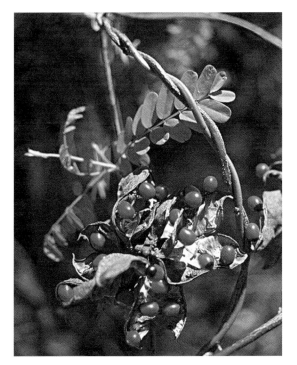

Figure 9.13 Rosary peas (*Abrus precatorius*) with characteristic black patch on the scarlet seeds.

are proteins that have the capability of binding to cells to cause agglutination and acute hypersensitivity reactions. Castor oil extracted from the seeds is not toxic, as ricin is insoluble in the oil. The oil contains predominantly ricinoleic acid that is an irritant and a potent cathartic.

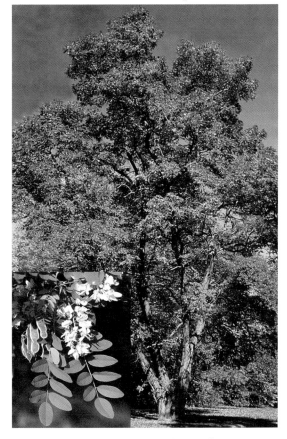

Figure 9.14 Black locust (*Robinia pseudoacacia*) flowers, compound leaves, and thorns on branches.

Horses are most likely to be poisoned by eating seeds (castor beans) in amounts as small as 0.01% of body weight (1–2% castor beans in the horse's grain).[12] The seeds need to be ground or well-chewed to expose the toxin. Early signs of castor bean poisoning in horses develop several days after the animal has eaten grain contaminated with castor beans and include trembling, sweating, and incoordination. Colic, diarrhea, and a rapid, weak pulse develop as the poisoning progresses.[12] Horses may also be poisoned by eating the bark from the black locust tree (*Robinia pseudoacacia*).[25] Therapy should include aggressive administration of intravenous fluids to counteract signs of shock. Mineral oil (4 L/450 kg) followed 4–6 h later by activated charcoal (0.5 kg/500 kg) in a saline solution cathartic should be given by nasogastric tube to reduce further absorption of ricin. Horses that develop clinical signs have a poor prognosis.

9.2.8 Jimson Weed, Potato, and Tomato

In the large diverse nightshade family (*Solanaceae*), horses have been poisoned by various genera that include nightshades (*Solanum* spp.),[26] jimson weed or thorn apple (*Datura stramonium*) (Figure 9.15),[14,27,28] tomato (*Lycopersicon* spp.), potato (*Solanum tuberos*um),[29] and jessamine (*Cestrum* spp.).[30] A variety of glycoalkaloids and tropane alkaloids are found in *Solanaceae* plants, especially in the green parts of the plant and the unripe fruits.

The glycoalkaloids common in the *Solanum* species are gastrointestinal irritants and neurotoxins. The tropane alkaloids, including scopolamine (hyoscine) and hyoscyamine, are similar to atropine in their effect on the autonomic nervous system, blocking the action of acetylcholine at muscarinic receptor sites. Dilated pupils, intestinal atony, decreased salivation, sweating, tachycardia, and tachypnea are typical signs of toxicity from the tropane alkaloids. Horses are most often poisoned by grain contaminated with jimson weed seeds (Figure 9.16), green or rotting potatoes,[15] or potato or tomato plants. Grain contaminated with as few as 595 seeds/kg will cause poisoning in horses. Compared to other livestock, horses may be more susceptible to the toxic effects of solanine alkaloids.[15] Initially, there may be central nervous system excitement, but depression follows with decreased heart and respiratory rates, muscle weakness, staggering, dilated pupils, colic, and watery diarrhea that may be hemorrhagic.[15] When large amounts of tropane alkaloids are ingested, death results

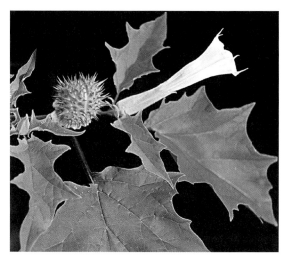

Figure 9.15 Jimson weed or thorn apple (*Datura stramonium*) showing characteristic trumpet-shaped flowers and spiny fruit (thorn apple).

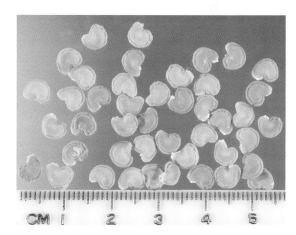

Figure 9.16 Jimson weed seeds (*Datura stramonium*).

from cardiac arrest. Interestingly, race horses eating bedding containing *Datura* species tested positive in their urine with the stimulant and illegal drug scopolamine.[31]

Therapy is symptomatic as there is no specific treatment. Oral administration of activated charcoal (0.5 kg/500 kg) as an absorbent, along with a saline cathartic may be effective if given soon after the plants have been eaten. Seizures should be managed with diazepam and not phenothiazine tranquilizers because of the anticholinergic effects of phenothiazines.

An interesting realtionship has been observed in horses that eat silverleaf nightshade (*Solanum elaeagnifolium*) and are treated with ivermectins. An increased permeabilty of the blood-brain barrier to ivermectin causes severe depression and death.[32]

Day and night blooming jessamines (*Cestrum* spp.) have a diferent effect causing excess calcification of the tissues, leading to weight loss, lameness, and debility (see Section 9.16 on Plant-induced calcinosis).

9.2.9 Kentucky Coffee Tree

Kentucky Coffee Tree (*Gymnocladus dioica*) is a deciduous, leguminous, tree native to eastern North America that produces numerous large dark brown seed pods

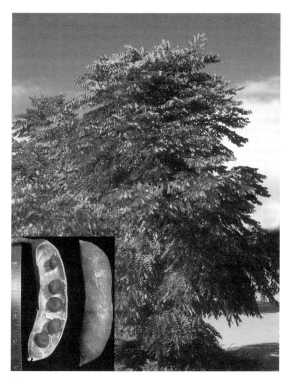

Figure 9.17 Kentucky coffee tree (*Gymnocladus dioica*).

containing 4–8 brown seeds (Figure 9.17). The specific toxin(s) in the plant and seeds have not been identified, but are possibly complex heat-labile saponins. Signs of poisoning include excessive salivation, diarrhea, colic, and excitement.[33]

9.3 Photodermatitis-Inducing Plants

Plant-induced dermatitis or photosensitization may be categorized into primary, secondary, or contact photosensitization. Primary photosensitization results when a horse eats plants that contain a photoreactive pigment; secondary photosensitization develops when plant alkaloids cause liver failure with photosensitization occurring secondarily to liver failure. Contact dermatitis as the name implies requires direct exposure of the skin to a substance, possibly a plant hapten that induces an immune reaction in the skin.

9.3.1 Primary Photosensitization

Primary photosensitizing plants (Table 9.3) contain photoreactive phenolic pigments that, once eaten and absorbed, accumulate in the skin. When these compounds are exposed to ultraviolet rays from sunlight, they fluoresce, releasing radiant energy that causes cellular necrosis. The mechanism of this reaction has been extensively reviewed.[34–36] Oxidation of amino acids in skin (histidine, tyrosine, tryptophan) provokes acute inflammation and necrosis. Horses fed a gluten concentrate may also develop primary photosensitization possibly from photoreactive metabolites. Non-pigmented skin is most severely affected (Figure 9.18). Horses with completely pigmented skin are fully protected even though the photodynamic pigments are present in the capillaries. In such animals, lacrimation and photophobia may be the only manifestations of photosensitivity.

Table 9.3 Primary photosensitizing plants.

Common Name	Scientific Name	Toxin
St. John's wort, Klamath weed	*Hypericum perforatum*	Hypericin
Buckwheat	*Fagopyrum esculentum*	Fagopyrin
Spring parsley	*Cymopterus watsonii*	Furanocoumarins
Bishop's weed	*Ammi majus*	Furanocoumarins

NB: See Figure 9.18 for clinical signs of photosensitization. All these plants may also cause excessive lacrimation and photophobia.

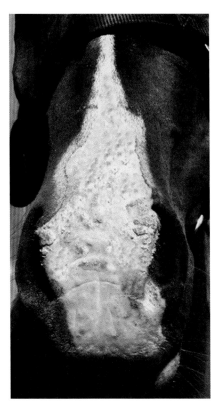

Figure 9.18 Photosensitization in a horse showing dermatitis affecting the nonpigmented skin only.

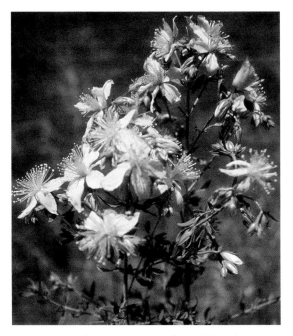

Figure 9.19 St. John's wort or Klamath weed (*Hypericum perforatum*).

Two plants historically associated with primary photosensitization in horses are buckwheat (*Fagopyrum esculentum*) and Saint John's wort (*Hypericum perforatum*).[37,38] Horses are also potentially at risk from plants such as spring parsley (*Cymopterus watsonii*) and bishop's weed (*Ammi majus*), which contain photoreactive furocoumarins that induce primary photosensitization in other livestock and poultry.[39]

9.3.1.1 Saint John's Wort or Klamath Weed
Saint John's wort (*Hypericum perforatum*) grows throughout North America. It is an erect perennial herb that grows up to 3 feet (1 m) tall with woody lower stems. The branches are opposite and sterile. Usually both stems and branches are two-edged or winged. The leaves are opposite, sessile, linear-oblong, 3/4 inch (2 cm) long, and dotted with glands that appear as tiny translucent dots when held against the light. The flowering part of the plant has a cyme arrangement with numerous flowers 0.5–0.75 inch (1–2 cm) in diameter with five bright yellow petals, five green sepals, many stamens in clusters of 3–5, and an ovary with three widely spreading styles (Figure 9.19). The petals have fimbriate margins and may have black glandular dots on the margins. These dots contain the toxin hypericin.[40] Hypericin is a photodynamic pigment that remains chemically intact through digestion and is readily absorbed into the blood. It has no effect on the liver or other organs unless it is exposed to ultraviolet light. This occurs especially in nonpigmented skin, causing primary photosensitization. Its presence in the glandular dots on the leaves suggests that all *Hypericum* spp. with similar glands are potentially capable of causing primary photosensitization. Young plants are as toxic as mature plants and are more palatable to livestock; thus they are more likely to cause poisoning in grazing animals. However, the toxin is not destroyed by drying and, therefore, hay may also cause poisoning.

9.3.1.2 Buckwheat
Buckwheat (*Fagopyrum esculentum*) is a glabrous herbaceous annual plant with erect stems and alternate hastate or cordate leaves. The stipules are united as a sheath

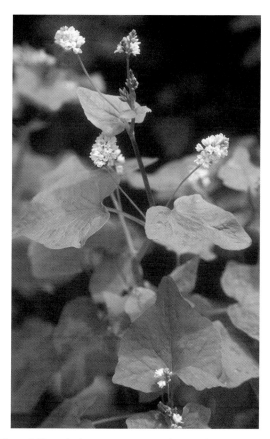

Figure 9.20 Buckwheat (*Fagopyrum esculentum*) showing the typical heart-shaped leaves and white flowers.

(ochrea) around the stem at the nodes. The greenish white flowers occur as terminal or axial panicles and have eight stamens and three-parted styles, which form three-angled brown-colored seeds from which buckwheat flour is made (Figure 9.20). Commonly grown as a cover crop to be plowed under for soil enrichment, it has escaped in many areas to become a weed of waste places.

Both the green and dried plant contain the pigment fagopyrin that, if ingested in sufficient quantities and then exposed to sunlight, is capable of producing primary photosensitization in all domestic livestock.

9.3.2 Secondary Photosensitization

Secondary, or hepatogenous, photosensitization occurs more commonly than primary photosensitization. Unlike primary photosensitization, liver disease is the underlying etiology of a secondary photosensitivity. The plant toxins themselves are not photoreactive, but cause liver damage. Once 80% or more of the liver is affected, it is unable to eliminate phylloerythrin, a normal breakdown byproduct of plant chlorophyll, which then accumulates in the blood. Phylloerythrin fluoresces when exposed to ultraviolet light, causing cellular damage resulting in photosensitization.[34,35,38] The prognosis for animals with secondary photosensitization is always far poorer than that for primary photosensitization because the underlying liver disease is frequently irreversible and eventually fatal in most affected animals. The plants that are most frequently associated with secondary photosensitization in horses in North America are discussed in the next Section 9.3.3 on liver disease-inducing plants and are listed in Table 9.4.

Treatment of photosensitization, whether it is primary or secondary, requires keeping the animal completely out of the sun and preferably stalled during the day. Sunlight through a glass window is not harmful, as ultraviolet rays are filtered out by glass. Gentle daily cleaning of the skin with a mild organic iodide solution will aid recovery. Appropriate systemic antibiotic therapy based on bacterial antibiotic sensitivity is indicated if there is secondary bacterial dermatitis. Recovery of the skin and hair regrowth may take 2–3 months.

9.3.3 Liver Disease-Inducing Plants

Few plant toxins cause liver disease because the liver has great capacity for detoxifying many compounds that are absorbed from the gastrointestinal tract. Furthermore, the liver has a large reserve capacity and will continue to function at near optimal levels until approximately 80% of it has been destroyed. Only then will clinical signs of liver failure such as weight loss, depression and abnormal behavior, icterus, hemoglobinuria, anemia, and photosensitization be observed. Photosensitization occurs because of the damaged liver's inability to eliminate phylloerythrin, the body's normal breakdown product of plant chlorophyll, which then accumulates in the blood. When this photoreactive compound is exposed to sunlight, it fluoresces, causing cellular damage in nonpigmented skin as seen in secondary or hepatogenous photosensitization (Figure 9.18–9.20). As described in the

Table 9.4 Hepatotoxic plants.

Common Name	Scientific Name	Toxin
Fiddleneck, tarweed	*Amsinckia* spp.	Pyrrolizidine alkaloids[a]
Rattlepod, rattlebox	*Crotolaria* spp.	Pyrrolizidine alkaloids[a]
Hound's tongue	*Cynoglossum officinale*	Pyrrolizidine alkaloids[a]
Salvation Jane[b]	*Echium plantagineum*	Pyrrolizidine alkaloids[a]
Heliotrope	*Heliotropium spp!*	Pyrrolizidine alkaloids[a]
Creeping indigo	*Indigofera spicata*	Indospicine[c]
Birdsville indigo	*Indigofera dominii*	Indospicine[c]
Alsike clover	*Trifolium hybridum*	Possible mycotoxin[d]
Kleingrass	*Panicum coloratum*	Possible mycotoxin[e]
Cocklebur	*Xanthium* spp.	Carboxyactractyloside[f]
	Senecio spp.	Pyrrolizidine alkaloids[a]

[a] In addition to signs of liver failure, often first noted by abnormal behavior followed by weight loss, icterus, hemoglobinuria, anemia, and photosensitization. Pyrrolizidine alkaloids are also carcinogenic, teratogenic, and abortifacients with effects often not occurring for months after ingestion.

[b] Salvation Jane has been introduced into California and may become an invasive toxic plant in North America.

[c] Several weeks of eating indigo may also result in ataxia, depression, corneal opacity, dyspnea, and abortion.

[d] Horses grazing alsike clover pastures during warm, humid weather may develop acute photosensitization of thin haired and white-skinned areas, especially around the lips, nose, and feet, which has been referred to as "dew poisoning."

[e] Predominantly Klein grass pasture or hay can cause hepatitis in horses and other livestock.

[f] Cocklebur seedlings in the coteledonary or two-leafed stage are hepatotoxic to all animals. The mature plant is not toxic.

previous section, photosensitization may also be caused by the ingestion of plants, such as buckwheat (*Fagopyrum esculentum*) or Saint John's wort (*Hypericum perforatum*), that contain photoreactive pigments but do not cause liver damage. Because signs of secondary or hepatogenous photosensitization or other clinical signs of liver disease appear only when a majority of liver function is destroyed, horses showing clinical signs as the result of any plant-induced liver disease have a guarded to poor prognosis.

9.3.3.1 Plants Causing Pyrrolizidine Alkaloid Hepatotoxicosis

The most important plant toxins responsible for causing secondary photosensitization, as well as other manifestations of liver damage, are pyrrolizidine alkaloids (PA). Pyrrolizidine alkaloids, the major plant hepatoxin, are present in many of the plants listed in Table 9.4.[16,41]

Senecio Species

There are some 1,200 different species of *Senecio* that are distributed throughout the world, with about 70 species occurring in North America.[41] Approximately 25 of these have been proven to be poisonous, but all species of *Senecio* should be considered toxic unless known

Table 9.5 Toxic *Senecio* species in North America.

Common Names	Scientific Name
Tansy ragwort, stinking Willie	*S. jacobaea*
Lambstongue groundsel	*S. integerrimus*
Woolly or threadleaf groundsel	*S. douglasii*
Riddell's ragwort	*S. riddellii*
Groundsel	*S. plattensis*
Broom groundsel	*S. spartioides*
Butterweed	*S. glabellus*
Common groundsel	*S. vulgaris*

otherwise. The most common species responsible for poisoning in horses in North America are listed in Table 9.5. *Senecio* species have a wide overlapping geographic range, but are selective in their habitats; some prefer high altitude, subalpine, moist conditions, while others prefer dry, rocky, sandy soils at lower elevations.

Identification of individual *Senecio* species is difficult. However, recognition of a plant as a member of the genus *Senecio* can be based on the presence of a single layer of touching, but not overlapping, greenish bracts surrounding the flower head (Figure 9.21). *Senecio* species have alternate leaves that are generally

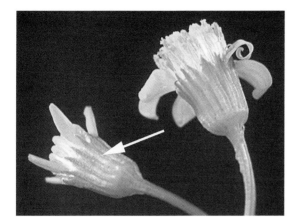

Figure 9.21 *Senecio* flower showing the characteristic single layer of bracts surrounding the petals.

lanceolate to ovate, dentate, and often irregularly and deeply pinnately divided. Some species are densely covered with white hairs. The composite heads are flattened terminal clusters with showy yellow ray and disk flowers. Seeds have a dense ring of white hairs (pappus) at one end to aid in wind distribution.

The PA concentration and thus toxicity of *Senecio* species varies considerably with the stage of growth and mature plants are the most toxic. Ridell's ragwort (*S. ridellii*) when near maturity has been reported to contain exceptionally high concentrations of PA (10–18% dry weight).[42] Acute poisoning and death in 1–2 days has been associated with a few days' consumption of green *Senecio* plants high in PA concentration equal to 1–5% of the animal's body weight. Chronic poisoning, however, is more common in horses and cattle and is usually associated with ingestion of smaller amounts of *Senecio* over a period of 3 weeks or longer.[43] Horses eating green tansy ragwort or stinking willie (*S. jacobaea*) (Figure 9.22) in amounts in excess of 1–2% of their body weight develop clinical signs 20 days to 5 months later.[12] This equates to a minimum cumulative exposure for 20 days or a total dose equal to 2% of body weight in plant dry matter.

Hound's Tongue

Hound's tongue (*Cynoglossum officinale*) is a PA-containing common biennial weed of cultivated and waste areas that grows up to 3 feet (1 m) tall with alternate tongue-shaped, hairy basal leaves up to 20 inches (0.5 m) long (Figure 9.23). The upper leaves are

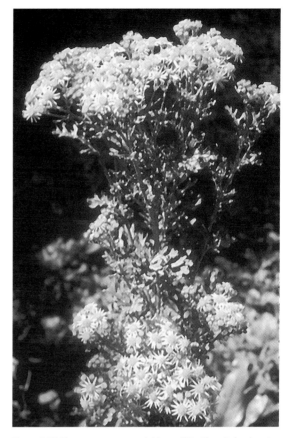

Figure 9.22 Tansy ragwort or stinking willie (*Senecio jacobaea*).

lanceolate and sessile. The flowers are small, regular, reddish purple, and produced on terminal racemes. The fruits separate into 4 brown nutlets at maturity which are covered with hooked barbs that readily attach to animal hair and aid in their dispersal. Hound's tongue contains the PA heliosupine and echinatine with the greatest concentration (2.1% dry weight) in the pre-flowering rosette stage.[44] Although reduced in quantity, the alkaloids remain in the dried plant.

Fiddleneck

Fiddleneck or tarweed (*Amsinckia intermedia*) is an erect, sparsely branched annual weed that grows up to 3 feet (1 m) tall and is covered with numerous, fine white hairs. Leaves are hairy, lanceolate, and alternate. The perfect five-parted, small, orange to yellow flowers are borne terminally on a characteristic fiddleneck-shaped raceme, with the flowers all inserted on one side of the

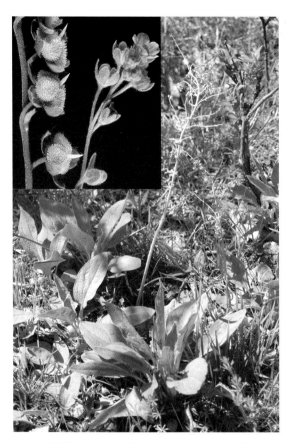

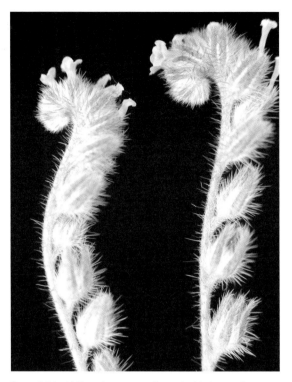

Figure 9.24 Fiddleneck or tarweed (*Amsinckia intermedia*) showing its characteristic fiddleneck shape of the inflorescence.

Figure 9.23 First-year growth or rosette stage of hound's tongue (*Cynoglossum officinale*). Inset shows flowers and fruits.

axis (Figure 9.24). Mature fruits separate into 2–4 black-ridged nutlets.

Horses, cattle, and pigs have been poisoned by eating fiddleneck plants, especially the seeds.[45] The symptoms and lesions in all species of animals poisoned consist of liver necrosis and fibrosis characteristic of PA toxicity. *Amsinckia* species have also been reported to accumulate levels of nitrate potentially toxic to ruminants but probably not to horses.

Rattlebox or rattlepod (*Crotalaria* spp.) are erect, herbaceous, variably hairy plants that may be annuals or perennials. The leaves are simple, alternate, lanceolate to obovate, with a finely haired undersurface. The flowers are yellow, with the leguminous calyx longer than the corolla (Figure 9.25). The fruit is a leguminous pod, inflated, hairless, becoming black with maturity, and containing 10–20 glossy, black, heart or boxing glove-shaped seeds, which often detach and rattle within the pod. Several species of *Crotalaria* have been associated with livestock poisoning, including *C. sagittalis*, *C. spectabilis*, and *C. retusa*.

Crotalaria species contain PA, the most notable of which is monocrotaline.[41] The alkaloid is present in greatest quantity in the seeds, lesser amounts being present in the leaves and stems. All livestock, including domestic fowl, are susceptible to poisoning.[46] Although acute deaths will occur from eating large quantities of *Crotalaria* seeds or plants, more often, as with other PA-containing plants, clinical signs develop from a few days to up to 6 months later.

Toxicity of Pyrrolizidine Alkaloids

Variations in the PA content of plants, the quantity eaten, and susceptibility of individual animal species result in a wide severity of PA poisoning in animals. Flowers tend to contain the greatest amount of the alkaloid, although seeds of rattlebox or rattlepod, fiddleneck, and tarweed contain high levels of PA.[16,47]

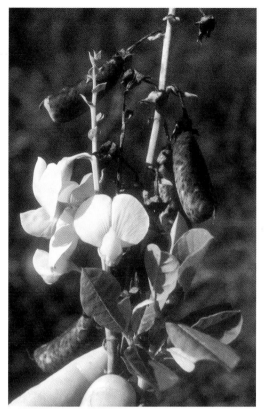

Figure 9.25 Rattlebox or rattlepod (*Crotalaria spectabilis*) showing the pea-like flowers and seed pods.

Pigs are most susceptible to PA, followed by poultry, cattle, horses, goats, and sheep.[41,47] Sheep can eat approximately 20 times the amount of *Senecio* it would take to poison a cow on an equivalent body weight basis. Horses show about the same susceptibility to pyrrolizidine toxicosis as do cattle.[41,48] The chronic lethal dose of dried tansy ragwort (*S. jacobaea*) in cattle is only 0.02–0.05 mg/kg body weight fed over several months.[41] This would equate to a 1000-lb (450-kg) horse eating about 5% of its body weight in green tansy ragwort over a period of 1–3 months.

Fortunately, herbivores will not readily eat plants containing PA unless they are forced to do so with lack of other feed. However, the dried plants which have only a minimal reduction in their alkaloid content are more palatable making them a particular risk when present in hay.[49] Although acute poisoning and death can occur after a few days' consumption of plants high in PA, chronic poisoning is more common. The effects of

PA are cumulative, so symptoms of liver disease and photosensitization may not appear for many months after animals have eaten toxic quantities of PA-containing plants. This makes identification of the suspected poisonous plants difficult, since the plants will often not be present in the pasture or hay when clinical signs become evident in the horse.

Pyrrolidizine alkaloids are readily absorbed from the digestive tract of horses and are converted in the liver to toxic pyrroles and possibly other reactive metabolites.[41,47,50,51] Large doses of pyrroles bind to cellular proteins, causing rapid cell death. Chronic low-level exposure to pyrroles allows binding to the endoplasmic reticulum, which inhibits mitosis and replication of hepatocytes. As a result, the liver typically responds with megalocytosis, bile duct hyperplasia, and fibrosis.[50] Similar cellular damage may also occur in the kidneys, intestinal tract, and lungs.[47,50] Pyrrolizidine alkaloids are also carcinogenic, teratogenic, and abortifacient.[16] Although secretion of PA in mare's milk has not been established, there is potential risk to the suckling foal, as PA has been shown to be present in small quantities in the milk of cows and goats fed tansy ragwort (*Senecio jacobaea*).[52,53]

Clinical Signs of Pyrrolizidine Alkaloid Hepatotoxicosis

Acute PA poisoning occurs occasionally in horses that ingest large amounts of alkaloid-containing plants over a few days. Affected animals may show only depression, coma, and death as a result of acute hemorrhagic necrosis of the liver.

Chronic PA poisoning, which is more common, is characterized by irreversible liver disease clinically manifested by one or more of the following clinical signs: weight loss, nervous system signs, icterus, anemia, hemoglobinuria, and photosensitization.[34,44,54–57] Nervous system signs with hepatic encephalopathy are often the first clinical indication of PA poisoning and may include drowsiness, head pressing, blindness, aimless wandering or "walking disease," frequent yawning, and incessant licking of objects.[54,58] The nervous system signs of PA poisoning are attributed to the liver's failure to detoxify various metabolic products such as ammonia and its failure to maintain a normal balance of branched chain and aromatic amino acids that affects brain neurotransmission.[48] A small percentage of horses with PA poisoning may present with inspiratory dyspnea with no obvious anatomic cause if eating *Crotolaria* species.[59,60] In such cases, the horse should be examined carefully for liver failure. Hemolysis with hemoglobinuria occurs occasionally in horses, possibly as the result of toxins accumulating in the blood as a consequence of liver failure.[52] Photosensitization may occur in some horses (Figures 9.18–9.20). In these horses, severe dermatitis develops when horses are exposed to sunlight from the liver's failure to metabolize phylloerythrin, a photoreactive byproduct of chlorophyll breakdown. The pathogenesis of photosensitization is described earlier in this chapter in the section on primary photodermatitis.

Diagnosis of Pyrrolizidine Alkaloid Hepatotoxicosis
Pyrrolizidine alkaloid poisoning is usually not suspected and, therefore, not detected until severe liver damage has occurred and clinical signs of liver failure are evident. Elevations in serum activities of gamma glutamyl transpeptidase (GGT) and sorbitol dehydrogenase are indicative of active liver necrosis.[61,62] Gamma glutamyl transpeptidase is an especially useful indicator of PA-induced liver disease because it remains elevated in the presence of active liver necrosis and biliary hyperplasia significantly longer than other liver enzymes.[61–63] The measurement of GGT activity is therefore beneficial for detecting asymptomatic liver disease that may or may not progress to fatal liver failure.[63] Elevated serum bile acid concentration may also be indicative of severe liver disease.[64] Liver function tests and activities of various liver enzymes can be measured, but they give no indication as to the cause of liver damage.[49]

Elevated blood ammonia concentrations are a consistent finding in horses exhibiting signs of hepatic encephalopathy.[48] Changes in the ratio of serum branched chain amino acids (leucine, isoleucine, valine) to aromatic amino acids (phenylalanine and tyrosine) correlate with the severity of liver disease and may be useful for the prognosis and treatment of PA poisoning in horses.[48,61] A decline in this ratio, measured at monthly intervals, is indicative of a progressive decrease in liver function. Ratios of 2.0 or less indicate a high probability of the horse developing liver failure and encephalopathy.[65] The ability to detect sulfur-bound pyrrolic metabolites on hemoglobin using thin layer chromatography or high pressure liquid chromatography offers a promising and specific means of detecting and monitoring exposed animals.[66]

At the present time, the only widely available and reliable means of confirming PA-induced liver failure is histopathologic examination of a liver biopsy or section of the liver obtained at necropsy. The presence of hepatomegalocytosis, biliary hyperplasia, and fibrosis are diagnostic for PA toxicosis. The only other disease to mimic this triad of histopathologic findings is aflatoxicosis, which occurs when horses eat moldy grains containing aflatoxins and it is uncommon in horse.[67]

Treatment of Pyrrolizidine Alkaloid Hepatotoxicosis
Intravenous administration of electrolyte-containing fluids with glucose may be necessary in severely affected animals. Dietary supplementation of branched chain amino acids (leucine, isoleucine, and valine) may result in clinical improvement by helping to restore the ratio of branched chain to aromatic amino acids and thus influencing the levels of false neurotransmitters.[61] However the use of vitamin B_{12}, cysteine, and hydroxyanisole in an attempt to increase liver sulfhydryl conjugation of PA in horses did not provide any protective effect.[68] A guarded to poor prognosis is warranted in all confirmed cases of PA poisoning.

Animals showing signs of photosensitization should be provided shelter from the sun and preferably kept stalled completely out of sunlight. Sunlight through glass will not induce photosensitization as it blocks ultraviolet rays. Gentle daily cleaning of the affected skin with a mild organic iodine antiseptic solution will aid in the healing process. Antibiotics may be indicated in cases where there is severe secondary bacterial dermatitis.

9.3.3.2 Non-Pyrrolizidine Alkaloid Hepatotoxic Plants
Indigo
Creeping indigo (*Indigofera spicata*) is a legume that was introduced into southern Florida where it has become well established. It causes a fatal neurologic disease resulting from liver failure.[69] "Grove poisoning," originally thought to be due to chemicals used in the citrus industry is now known to be due to horses' eating creeping indigo.[69] In Australia, a similar disease of horses and other livestock referred to as "Birdsville disease" is caused by Birdsville indigo (*Indigofera dominii*).[70]

Creeping indigo is a prostrate plant of tropical and subtropical areas with many branched runners fanning out from the crown of a white tapering taproot that may be up to 3 feet (1 m) in length. The stems are usually pale

Figure 9.26 Creeping indigo (*Indigofera spicata*) young flowering plant showing prostrate form.

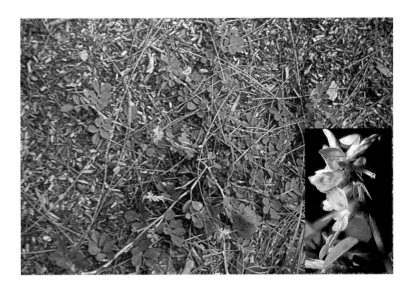

Table 9.6 Protein, sulfur-containing amino acid, and arginine content of horse feeds.[229]

	% Protein in Air Dried Feed	% Cysteine + Methionine in Air Dried Feed	% Cysteine + Methionine in Feed Protein[a]	% Arginine Air Dry Feed	% Arginine in Feed Protein[a]
Alfalfa	17	0.52	3.1	0.73	4.3
Corn	9	0.18	2.0	0.45	5.0
Cottonseed meal	41	1.5	3.7	4.25	10.4
Fish meal	61–66	2.7–3.2	4.5–4.8	4.0–4.5	6.5–6.8
Grain, small	11–13	0.3–0.45	3.0–3.5	0.5–0.8	4.6–6.6
Peanut meal	47	1.0	2.1	5.9	12.5
Rapeseed meal	41	1.5	3.7	1.9	4.7
Soybean meal	46	1.3	2.8	3.2	7.0
Sunflower seed meal	47	2.2	4.7	3.5	7.5
Wheat bran	16	0.4	2.5	1.0	6.2
Yeast, brewer's	45	1.2	2.7	2.2	4.9

[a] The percentage of cysteine and methionine content is most important value to consider in selecting a feed that is high in these two amino acids. It is calculated as [amino acids (%)/protein (%)] in the feed.

green with alternate pinnate leaves, and alternate ovate leaflets on a short petiole (Figure 9.26). The pink to dark red flowers are produced on short spikes from the leaf axils. The pointed seed pods are produced in downward-pointing clusters. The plant is a prolific seed producer and tends therefore to be capable of spreading readily.

The hepatotoxic amino acid indospicine is present in various *Indigofera* species.[71] Leaves may contain from 0.1–0.5% of this toxin in dry weight and the seeds contain as much as 2.0%.[72] Horses apparently find the plant highly palatable and seek it out. The toxin acts as a specific antagonist of the amino acid arginine and is therefore an inhibitor of protein synthesis.[71,73] Horses fed sufficient peanut meal or cottonseed meal, both of which are rich in arginine, are protected from the effects of indospicine.[74] Arginine constitutes 10–12% of the protein in these two protein supplements as compared to 4–7% in other horse feeds (Table 9.6).

After consuming creeping indigo for several weeks, affected horses develop incoordination, ataxia, difficulty in turning, and inability to walk in a straight line, eventually collapsing.[69] They become severely depressed, lose weight, and have been reported to develop corneal opacity and respiratory difficulty. Pregnant mares may abort. Death results from liver necrosis and nodular fibrosis. Animals eating meat from horses that have been poisoned by creeping indigo may also suffer similar fatal poisoning.[75]

Alsike Clover and Kleingrass

Occasionally, horses grazing alsike clover (*Trifolium hybridum*) during wet or humid weather develop a photosensitivity and hepatitis referred to as trifoliosis.[12,76,77] A similar condition may also occur in horses or sheep grazing kleingrass (*Panicum coloratum* and *P. dichotomiflorum*) pastures during wet or humid weather.[78–80] The toxin responsible for either trifoliosis or kleingrass poisoning has not been identified, but the sporadic nature of the diseases and their occurrence only during wet humid weather suggests that mycotoxins or plant metabolites produced under humid, high-moisture growth conditions may be responsible.[77,78,81,82]

Affected horses on alsike clover pasture characteristically develop an acute photosensitization involving thinly haired and white-skinned areas, especially around the lips, nose, and feet (see Figs 9.18–9.20). The condition has been referred to as "dew poisoning" because there is an association between the location of the dermatitis and contact with moisture on dew-laden clover pasture.[12] Affected horses may exhibit icterus and other signs of liver disease including elevations in serum liver enzymes. In such cases, there may be significant hepatomegaly and histopathologic evidence of liver degeneration. Horses generally recover rapidly from photosensitization if they are removed from the toxic pasture. Horses may graze the pasture again without problem under different growing conditions in subsequent years or after the pasture dries out.

Lantana

Although rarely reported as a problem in horses, Lantana (*Lantana camara*) or red sage are commonly planted as ornamentals and escape readily to become invasive weeds. Prostrate or upright, branching shrubs with pungent, opposite or whorled leaves, *Lantana* species are grown for their showy, flat-topped heads of variably colored flowers (Figure 9.27). The round fruits turn shiny black when ripe. The toxins have been identified as triterpenoid lantadenes. If *Lantana* foliage is consumed by horses and other livestock over a period of weeks, the lantadenes cause cumulative damage to bile canaliculi that results in obstruction of the bile ducts and cholestasis. The chronic hepatitis ultimately causes icterus, weight loss, and secondary photosensitization.[83,84]

9.4 Neurologic Disease-Inducing Plants

Behavioral alterations, blindness, inability to prehend and chew food, ataxia, depression, convulsions, and other physical abnormalities are all indicators of

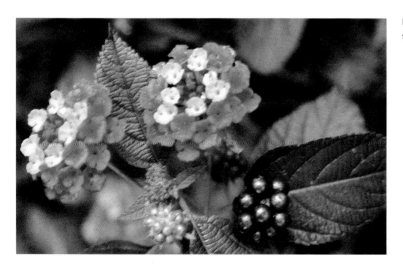

Figure 9.27 Lantana (*Lantana camara*) showing the flowers and ripe fruits.

Table 9.7 Protein, sulfur-containing amino acid, and arginine content of horse feeds.[229]

	% Protein in Air Dried Feed	% Cysteine + Methionine in Air Dried Feed	% Cysteine + Methionine in Feed Protein[a]	% Arginine Air Dry Feed	% Arginine in Feed Protein[a]
Alfalfa	17	0.52	3.1	0.73	4.3
Corn	9	0.18	2.0	0.45	5.0
Cottonseed meal	41	1.5	3.7	4.25	10.4
Fish meal	61–66	2.7–3.2	4.5–4.8	4.0–4.5	6.5–6.8
Grain, small	11–13	0.3–0.45	3.0–3.5	0.5–0.8	4.6–6.6
Peanut meal	47	1.0	2.1	5.9	12.5
Rapeseed meal	41	1.5	3.7	1.9	4.7
Soybean meal	46	1.3	2.8	3.2	7.0
Sunflower seed meal	47	2.2	4.7	3.5	7.5
Wheat bran	16	0.4	2.5	1.0	6.2
Yeast, brewer's	45	1.2	2.7	2.2	4.9

[a] The percentage of cysteine and methionine content is most important value to consider in selecting a feed that is high in these two amino acids. It is calculated as [amino acids (%)/protein (%)] in the feed.

nervous system disorders. The brain, spinal cord, and peripheral nervous systems are susceptible to a variety of infectious, toxic, and congenital diseases that are often indistinguishable clinically. A variety of plants that grow throughout North America are known to produce neurologic abnormalities in horses and, therefore, should be considered in the differential diagnosis of nervous system disorders. These plants, along with the major clinical signs that they cause in horses, are listed in Table 9.7.

9.4.1 Sagebrush

The sagebrushes (*Artemisia* spp.) of the western United States are perennials ranging from the woody stemmed 3–10 feet (1–3 m) tall big sagebrush (*A. tridentata*) to the smaller sand sage (*A. filifolia*) (Figure 9.28) and the low-growing fringed sage (*A. frigida*) (Figure 9.29). Considerable variation exists in the 200 or more species of sagebrush. Leaves are usually alternate, covered with very fine hairs that give the leaves a silvery green appearance, and when crushed give the characteristic smell of sage. Flowers are usually inconspicuous and born on panicles from the leaf axils.

The toxins in sagebrush are volatile terpenoid oils, which vary considerably in quantity depending on growing conditions and season and are highest in the fall and winter months.[8,85,86] Sand sage (*A. fiifolia*),

common in the sandy soils along the eastern side of the Rocky Mountains and south into Mexico, has been associated with a syndrome in horses called "sage sickness."[87] Budsage (*A. spinescens*) has been reported to cause similar problems in California and Nevada.[82,89] The author has encountered a neurologic syndrome of horses that were wintered on an overgrazed range in Colorado where fringed sage (*A. frigida*) was the predominant forage available.[89]

Although the actual toxin that causes sage sickness has not been defined, some monoterpenes present in *Artemisia* species are known to be neurotoxins. Thujone, a monoterpene present in wormwood (*A. absinthium*), has been associated with a neurologic syndrome in people who chronically consume absinthe, an alcoholic beverage produced from wormwood.[90] A similar toxicosis is presumed to develop in horses that consume a sufficient quantity of sage.

Horses develop neurologic signs after they are forced to eat sagebrush because other forages are depleted or unavailable either as a result of deep snow cover or pasture overgrazing. After eating sage for several days, horses suddenly exhibit abnormal behavior characterized by ataxia and a tendency to fall down or react abnormally to stimuli that would not normally have elicited such a response. Tying an affected horse to a fence, for example, will cause the animal to pull back

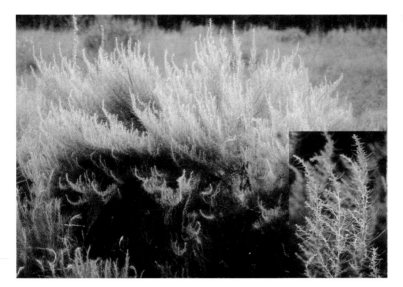

Figure 9.28 Sand sage (*Artemisia filifolia*).

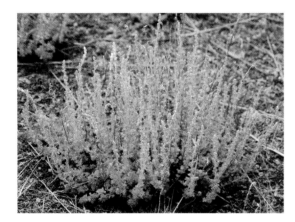

Figure 9.29 Fringed sage (*Artemisia frigida*).

violently, eventually throwing itself to the ground in panic. If left undisturbed, the animal will recover and act relatively normal. Ataxia is particularly noticeable in the forequarters, with the hindquarters seemingly normal. Some animals may circle incessantly; others may become excitable and unpredictable. The characteristic smell of sage is often noticeable on the breath and in the feces. Sage-poisoned horses maintain appetite and have normal temperature, pulse, and respiration. It is the author's observation that the clinical signs closely resemble those of a horse that has been poisoned by locoweed.[89] However, unlike "locoed" horses that have a poor prognosis for recovery, "saged" horses tend to recover in 1–2 weeks after they stop eating sage and

are fed a nutritious diet. Supportive therapy, including protection from extreme climatic conditions will aid in recovery. Affected horses should not be ridden until fully recovered and evaluated for normal behavior and neurologic function.

Histopathologic lesions in sage-sick horses are a nonspecific degenerative toxic encephalopathy evident in severely affected cases as intraneuronal pigment accumulation and degeneration, especially in the medulla, brain stem, and cerebellum.[89]

9.4.2 Locoweeds and Milkvetches

At least 375 species of locoweed and milkvetch (*Astragalus* and *Oxytropis* spp.) occur in North America, many of which are known to cause severe poisoning of livestock.[45,87] Taxonomically it is difficult to identify individual species, even by an experienced botanist. The genus *Oxytropis*, which like many *Astragalus* spp. is also commonly called locoweed, is a closely related genus and produces identical locoism in horses, cattle, sheep, and elk.[91–93] However, not all species of *Astragalus* and *Oxytropis* are toxic and some are useful forage plants.

Astragalus spp. are perennial legumes growing to a height of 3 feet (1 m) with branching stems from a stout crown and extensive taproot. The leaves are alternate and pinnately compound, with each leaflet being elliptical or oval and minutely hairy. The white to purple pea-like flowers are produced in racemes at the ends of the branches depending on the species. The leguminous

Figure 9.30 Locoweed (*Astragalus molissimus*) showing the typical flowers, leaves, and pea-like seed pods.

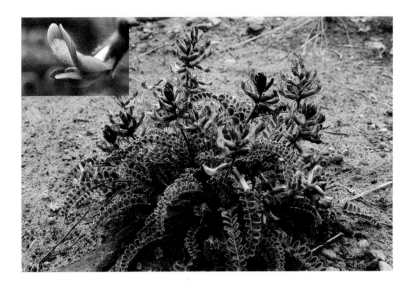

seed pods vary considerably in shape and contain many bean-shaped seeds (Figure 9.30).

Oxytropis species differ from *Astragalus* in that their hairy leaves and flower stems arise directly from the taproot crown. The leaves are pinnately compound with each having a single apical elliptical leaflet. The flowers are either white (*O. sericea*) or purple (*O. lambertii*) and have a characteristic pointed keel (Figures 9.31 and 9.32).

Locoism, blind staggers, alkali disease, and a syndrome characterized by respiratory difficulty and ataxia have all been attributed to species of *Astragalus* and *Oxytropis*.[80,94–97] Three distinct syndromes are recognized by virtue of the different toxins that various species of these plants may accumulate.[91,98] *Astragalus* species can be categorized into the locoweeds that contain indolizidine alkaloids (swainsonine), milkvetches that contain nitroglycosides (miserotoxin) and milkvetches that, as discussed in the section in this chapter on lameness, accumulate toxic amounts of selenium.[91,98] Some species may contain more than one toxin and consequently can cause a combination of clinical signs in affected animals.[89,99]

9.4.2.1 Locoweed Neurotoxicosis

Locoism results from the cumulative effects of the indolizidine alkaloid swainsonine, named after its isolation from various species of *Swainsona* (Darling pea) in Australia. It has subsequently been demonstrated in *Astragalus lentiginosus*, *A. mollisimus*, and *A. bisulcatus* amongst others, and *Oxytropis lambertii* and *O. sericea* in North America.[98,100–103] Current research has shown that swainsonine is not produced by the plants directly and it is a product of an endophytic fungus (*Embellisia* spp.) that grows in the locoweed.[6,104] This symbiotic relationship between the plant and the endophyte causes no apparent harm to the plant and may assist in its adaptation to adverse conditions.

Signs of poisoning do not become evident until animals have consumed significant quantities of locoweed over many weeks and the toxic threshold is reached.[105] Some horses develop a preference for locoweed, especially when it is blooming. Young animals are most severely affected, as maturing neurons are more vulnerable to the effects of the toxin. Swainsonine inhibits the action of two lysosomal enzymes that aid in the metabolism of saccharides. The inhibition of alpha-mannosidase causes cells to accumulate oligosaccharides, which interferes with normal cell function. The second enzyme, golgi mannosidase II, when inhibited, affects the normal structure of oligosaccharide components of glycoproteins.[100,106] In effect, swainsonine causes a generalized lysosomal storage disease, eventually causing irreversible neuronal damage similar to mannosidosis.[100]

Clinical Signs of Locoism

Horses with locoism will show a variety of signs including changes in behavior, ataxia, high stepping gait, head bobbing, marked excitement, and overreaction to various stimuli. Some horses become totally unpredictable in their response to normal handling and may fall down when being haltered or ridden.[74,91,92]

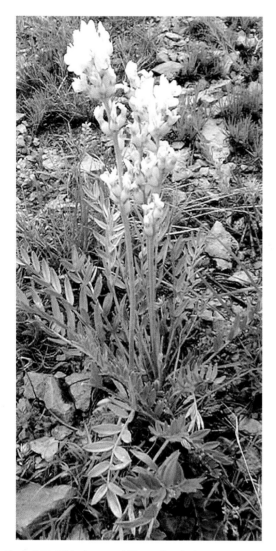

Figure 9.31 White locoweed (*Oxytropis sericea*).

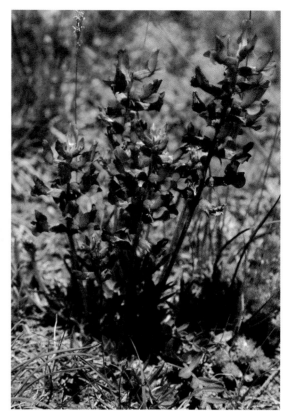

Figure 9.32 Purple locoweed (*Oxytropis lambertii*).

When left undisturbed, horses are depressed and may appear asleep. Weight loss is progressive due to the animal's impaired ability to prehend food. If removed from locoweed and fed a nutritious diet, horses will show some improvement and appear relatively normal after several months. However, if the horse has been chronically affected by locoism, then the animal will only partially recover and will remain a liability for human safety. The prognosis for locoed horses therefore is always poor. Pregnant mares that consume quantities of wooly loco (*A. mollisimus*) (Figs 9.20–9.30) in early gestation may produce foals with various limb deformities.[24] The teratogenic effects of locoweeds are discussed further in Section 9.19 on teratogenic plants.

Diagnosis of Locoism

Locoweed poisoning should be suspected when horses exhibit abnormal behavior and there is evidence that they have been eating locoweed. Horses that have been recently eating locoweed may have peripheral blood lymphocytes with cytoplasmic vacuoles that are diagnostic.[8,107,108] At postmortem examination, there are no gross pathognomonic lesions. Emaciation, occasional stomach ulcers, thyroid hypertrophy, and pale color of the liver and kidneys have been reported.[92] In acute poisoning of horses exhibiting neurologic signs, severe cytoplasmic vacuolation of neurons in the brain is characteristic. Similar vacuolation is often present in the pituitary gland, thyroid, pancreas, kidneys, liver, and other exocrine glands.[92] In horses that are chronically affected and have not eaten locoweed for more than a month, vacuolation is restricted to hepatocytes and neurons of the brain. Purkinje cells of the cerebellum retain vacuoles for over a year and there is noticeable loss of these cells with time, which would account for the residual neurologic abnormalities typical of locoweed poisoning in horses.[92]

Treatment of Locoism

There is no proven effective treatment for locoweed poisoning in horses. Further access to the plants should be prevented immediately and thereafter, as horses may retain a preference for the plants in subsequent years. Early recommendations of treatment with Fowler's solution and reserpine are unwarranted in light of the current knowledge of locoweed poisoning.[45]

9.4.3 Milkvetch Neurotoxicosis

Nitroglycosides or nitrotoxins have been demonstrated in some 263 species of milkvetch (*Astragalus* spp.). These plants are found growing in vast areas of rangelands in the western United States, Canada, and northern Mexico,[109] and have been associated with severe livestock losses.[110–112] Horses, although not frequently affected, are susceptible to poisoning by nitrotoxins.[111]

Nitrotoxin-containing *Astragalus* contains at least two toxic compounds: 3-nitro-1-propanol (miserotoxin) and 3-nitro-propionic acid.[112] These toxins, once absorbed from the digestive tract, act primarily on the respiratory and central nervous systems, initially causing depression, incoordination, and hindleg weakness. Difficulty breathing, weight loss, and paralysis of the hindquarters develop as the animal continues to eat milkvetch. Animals appear to recover if they are removed from the source of the plants before neurologic signs become severe.

9.4.4 Yellow Star Thistle and Russian Knapweed

Horses that eat yellow star thistle (*Centaurea solstitialis*) or Russian knapweed (*Acroptilon repens*) for prolonged periods develop an irreversible brain disease characterized by weight loss caused by the inability of the horse to prehend and chew its food.[113–116] It is characterized by necrosis of the globus pallidus and substantia nigra (nigropallidal encephalomalacia). This irreversible brain damage destroys the horse's ability to prehend and masticate food. The disease is unique to the horse and has been reported in only those areas of the western United States, Australia, and Argentina where these plants are abundant.[117,118] Cattle and sheep appear to be able to eat both yellow star thistle and Russian knapweed without problem.

Yellow star thistle originated in the Mediterranean region. It has become extensively established in California and has spread through the southern states to the Atlantic coast. It is an annual weed, with multiple branching stems growing to 3 feet (1 m) in height. The stems have longitudinal wings or ridges formed by the downward extension of the leaf bases. The basal leaves are markedly lobed with linear stem leaves covered with fine white hairs. The characteristic, star-like yellow flowers are produced at the ends of branches and protected by bracts with long spines (Figure 9.33). The seeds have a terminal tuft of whitish hairs.

Russian knapweed was introduced from Russia and has become a noxious weed in many Rocky Mountain states. It is a perennial with woody stems up to 3 feet (1 m) tall and invasive, branching underground stems. The name knapweed is derived from the grey hairs, or knap, that cover the leaves and stems, giving the plant a gray-green appearance. The stems branch terminally and end in a purple thistle-like flower (Figure 9.34). The bracts are papery white and lack the stiff long spines seen in yellow star thistle. The seed heads tend to remain closed and do not shed the seeds readily.

The specific toxin that causes localized destruction of the globus pallidus and substantia nigra of the brain has not been identified in either yellow star thistle or Russian knapweed. However, a sesquiterpene lactone, repin, found in Russian knapweed has been shown to have specific toxicity toward chick embryo neurons. Repin may therefore be the toxin that is responsible for the effects found in the brain of horses poisoned by Russian knapweed and yellow star thistle. In addition, yellow star thistle has also been shown to contain the potent neurotoxins aspartic and glutamic acid that may contribute to the pathogenesis.[119]

Horses must consume large quantities of green or dried plants for extended periods of time before the toxic threshold is reached and clinical signs abruptly appear. Horses have to consume an amount of green Russian knapweed or yellow star thistle equal to 59–71% and 86–200% of their body weight, respectively, before clinical signs develop. This indicates that Russian knapweed is apparently the more toxic of the two species. Horses can develop a preference for the plants and will eat them even in the mature spiny state. In California, there are two times of the year, from June–July and

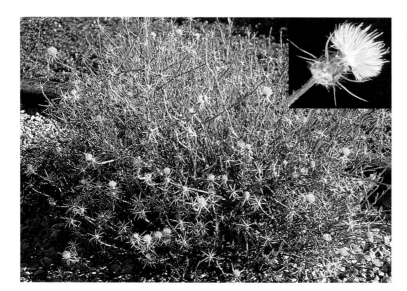

Figure 9.33 Yellow star thistle (*Centaurea solstitialis*) showing the long spiny bracts surrounding the flowers.

October–November, when yellow star thistle poisoning is most prevalent, suggesting some seasonal variation in palatability or toxin content of the plants.[117]

The pathogenesis of the disease apparently involves the initial release of the neurotransmitter dopamine from the substantia nigra and its subsequent depletion once the nigrostriatal cells are destroyed.[117] The resulting dopamine deficiency causes hypertonicity of the muscles innervated by the trigeminal, facial, and hypoglossal cranial nerves producing the clinical signs.

Clinical signs are not apparent until a toxic threshold is reached, at which time signs occur suddenly in association with the development of lesions in the brain. Initially, affected horses exhibit hypertonicity of muzzle and lip muscles so that the mouth is held open with the incisors exposed and the tongue hanging out. Continuous movements of the tongue and hypertonicity of the lips may cause frothing of saliva as the horse tries to eat. Some horses may wander about with their lips brushing through the grass, which to the unobservant, could be mistaken for normal grazing. If offered hay, the horse will attempt to scoop up hay and hold it in its mouth but normal prehension and mastication are severely impaired. Swallowing, however, is unaffected and some less severely affected horses may learn to submerge their heads far enough into a deep trough of water to allow water to reach the pharyngeal area and be swallowed. Some affected horses appear depressed and, if the lesions in the brain affect one side more than the other, the lips may be pulled to one side and they

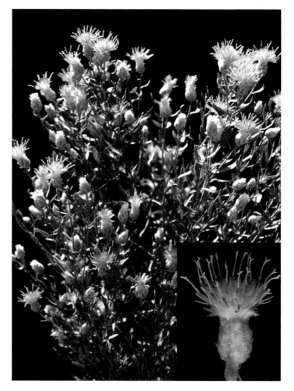

Figure 9.34 Russian knapweed (*Acroptilon repens*) with spineless papery bracts surrounding the purple thistle-like flowers.

may circle in one direction. Other abnormal behaviors may include violent head tossing and excessive yawning. Weight loss becomes severe as the horse is unable to eat. If not euthanized, affected horses eventually die from starvation and/or aspiration pneumonia.

There is no effective treatment as the affected areas in the brain undergo liquefactive necrosis and do not regenerate. Affected horses may be kept alive by administering water, electrolytes, and a high-energy liquid diet through a nasogastric tube or an esophagostomy as described in Chapter 3. Euthanasia of affected horses is eventually necessary because of the debilitating and irreversible effects of the brain lesions.

9.4.5 Horsetail

Horsetail, marestail, horserush, or snake grass are common names given to members of the genus *Equisetum*, of which *E. arvense* is the most common. Horses are rarely poisoned by horsetail today, but reports 30–40 years ago indicate that plants in hay were a problem.[12] Hay containing 20% horsetail fed to horses for over 2 weeks caused neurologic signs.[120] Successful treatment of the affected horses with thiamin hydrochloride (vitamin B1) indicated that the primary toxin in horsetail was a thiaminase.[120] Although a variety of other substances have been identified including silica, various alkaloids, and organic acids, the primary toxin effects appear to be related to horsetail's antithiamin properties.[12]

Horsetails are perennial rush-like plants with characteristic jointed hollow stems arising from an extensive underground root system. The plant appears leafless but has small scale-like leaves with black tips that surround the stem at each node. The plants reproduce by spores produced in a cone-like structure at the ends of the stems. Horsetails also produce sterile much-branched stems (Figure 9.35). Found throughout North America, the plants prefer wet soils and tend to form dense stands.

Affected horses show signs of weakness, depression, and ataxia, especially of the hindquarters. Other signs that have been associated with horsetail poisoning include diarrhea, constipation, muscle tremors, and corneal opacity.[12] A diagnosis of horsetail poisoning is generally based upon the presence of significant quantities of the plant (20% or more) in the hay being fed and the animal's response to the administration of large doses of thiamin hydrochloride (5–10 mg/kg).[38] Thiamin should be diluted in a liter of isotonic saline and given slowly intravenously to avoid adverse reactions. Intravenous 5% glucose may also be beneficial. Thiamin

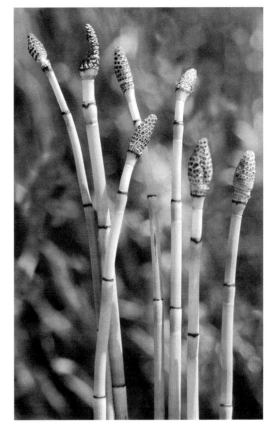

Figure 9.35 Horsetail, marestail, horserush, or snake grass (*Equisetum hymale*) with spore-producing heads.

should be administered intramuscularly once daily for an additional 5–7 days.

9.4.6 White Snakeroot and Crofton, Jimmy, or Burrow Weeds

White snakeroot or richweed (*Eupatorium rugosum*) has been known for many years to cause "trembles" in horses and other livestock and milk sickness in people who drink the milk from cows that have eaten white snakeroot.[59,121–123] Sporadic cases of white snakeroot poisoning occur in horses allowed access to the plant or when it is present in their hay. "Trembles" is also encountered in horses and other livestock that eat Jimmyweed or rayless goldenrod (*Haplopappus heterophyllus*) and burrow weed (*H. tenuisectus*), which grows in the southwestern United States and northern Mexico.[124,125]

White snakeroot is an erect perennial growing about 5 feet (1.5 m) tall and having opposite ovate leaves with

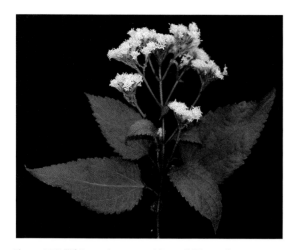

Figure 9.36 White snakeroot or richweed (*Eupatorium rugosum*).

markedly toothed edges (Figure 9.36). Flowers are white and produced terminally in clusters of 20–30 small 5-petaled flowers (3–5 mm) across. The seeds contain white hairs at one end that aid in wind distribution. The plant prefers to grow in moist wooded areas from Minnesota south to eastern Texas and all of the eastern states.

The principal toxin in white snakeroot is tremetol, a fat-soluble higher alcohol.[121,125,126] Jimmyweed, burrow weed, and Crofton weed (*Eupatorium adenophorum*) also contain tremetol and cause poisoning in horses.[123,125] The toxin is present in greatest quantity in the mature plant, particularly the leaves, and persists in frozen and dried leaves.[127] Tremetol is a cumulative toxin in animals; consequently, the amount consumed at any one time is not critical.[127] Small doses over a period of time will produce poisoning. An amount of green plant equal to 1–10% of body weight is potentially lethal to horses and other animals. Tremetol is readily soluble in fat and excreted in milk, which is the primary means that nursing animals and infants are poisoned. Nonlactating animals tend to show more severe signs of poisoning since tremetol cannot be excreted except by lactation.

When sufficient tremetol accumulates in the body, muscle tremors occur as the name "trembles" implies. In addition, horses may present with difficulty swallowing, excessive salivation, and the appearance of being choked. Depression, patchy sweating, ataxia, greenish discharge from the nostrils, and death within a few days after the onset of clinical signs have been reported in horses poisoned with white snakeroot.[127,128] Other diseases that can resemble white snakeroot poisoning include botulism, rabies, lead poisoning, and esophageal obstruction. The most significant necropsy finding is patchy myocarditis and fibrosis that may be severe enough to be the cause of death.

There is no specific antidote to tremetol. Affected horses should be removed immediately from pastures or hay that contain white snakeroot or other tremetol-containing plants. Laxatives, including mineral oil (1 gallon/1000 lb or 4 L/450 kg horse) or activated charcoal (1 lb/1000 lb or 0.5 kg/500 kg horse) with a saline cathartic, should be given orally to help prevent further absorption of the toxin. Mares should be hand milked frequently to help remove the toxin from the body. Foals should be removed immediately from affected mares to prevent further intake of toxic milk.

9.4.7 Bracken Fern

Bracken fern (*Pteridium aquilinum*) is found throughout the world and has been associated with poisoning in cattle, sheep, and horses whenever they are deprived of adequate normal forage. Poisoning has been reported most frequently in cattle in England and Europe and is relatively uncommon in horses. In North America, bracken fern poisoning is most common in the northwest.[12,129] Sensitive fern (*Onoclea sensiblis*) has also occasionally been reported to cause poisoning in horses.

Bracken fern is a common perennial fern of woodlands and grows from an underground, dark brown, branching rhizome. Fronds emerge directly from the rhizome and may be up to 6.5 feet (2 m) in height. The overall leaf shape is triangular with each leaflet having curved-under edges (Figure 9.37). Spores are produced on the underside of the leaflets and appear as brown dots lining the leaf edge.

The toxic principle in bracken fern that causes disease in horses is a thiaminase enzyme that destroys thiamin and thus causes a thiamin (vitamin B1) deficiency.[129,130] Horses have to consume a diet containing 30–50% bracken fern for at least 30 days before clinical signs appear.[131] The rhizome is most toxic and the leaves are poisonous whether green or dried.

Bracken fern poisoning in cattle differs from that in horses in that cattle develop a fatal aplastic anemia with bone marrow depression, thrombocytopenia, and clinically evident as a hemorrhagic syndrome, hematuria, and anemia. Neoplasia of the upper digestive tract and urinary bladder are often encountered.[132] The carcinogenic compound in bracken fern has been identified as ptaquiloside that causes urinary bladder and intestinal tumors in cattle, other animals, and humans.[133,134] Sheep develop retinal degeneration and blindness due to bracken fern poisoning. Retinal degeneration and carcinogenesis have not been found in bracken fern-poisoned horses. Weight loss due to poor appetite, incoordination of the hindquarters, and bradycardia are the principal clinical signs seen in horses.[135,136] If horses continue eating bracken fern, progressive depression and posterior weakness develop that may result in recumbency, coma, and eventual death.[12]

Diagnosis of bracken fern poisoning is aided by the determination of low serum thiamin and increased pyruvate concentrations, absence of viral encephalomyelitis and hepatic encephalopathy, and evidence that the horse has eaten large quantities of bracken fern. Alleviation of clinical signs in 12–24 h following thiamin administration is also helpful to confirm the diagnosis.[136]

Affected horses should be removed from bracken fern and treated with large doses of thiamin hydrochloride (5–10 mg/kg, IV slowly). Dilution of thiamin in isotonic fluids will reduce the chances of adverse reactions. Daily intramuscular doses of thiamin should be given for 5–7 days. Recovery usually occurs in 2–3 days.

9.4.8 Johnsongrass and Sudangrass

Johnsongrass (*Sorghum halepense*) and sudangrass (*Sorghum sudanense*) and their hybrid varieties are annuals in northern states and perennials in southern states. Johnson grass is an invasive weedy coarse grass that spreads readily from its creeping rhizomes. The glabrous leaves are up to 1.5 feet (0.5 m) in length and form a sheath around the stem, which may reach 3–8 feet (1–2 m) in height. Many individual small flowers are produced in a loose terminal panicle (Figure 9.38).

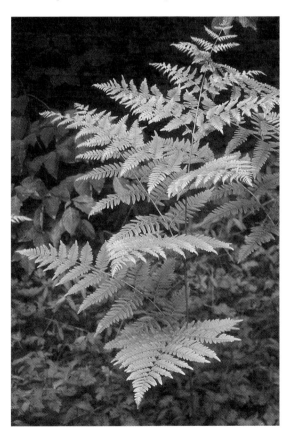

Figure 9.37 Bracken fern (*Pteridium aquilinum*).

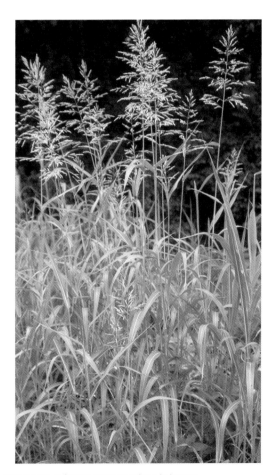

Figure 9.38 Johnson grass (*Sorghum halepense*).

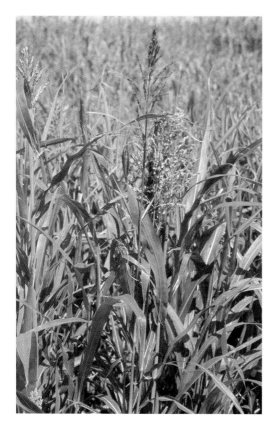

Figure 9.39 Sudan grass hybrid (*Sorghum sudanense*).

Sudan grass (Figure 9.39) and other grain sorghums such as milo are cultivated corn-like annuals that do not become invasive weeds like Johnson grass.

Sorghums have primarily been associated with poisoning due to the accumulation of toxic levels of cyanogenic glycosides and nitrates. Not all varieties of sorghum grasses are poisonous. It is possible to select varieties that are safe to feed animals.[137,1398] Sudan and Johnson grasses that are capable of accumulating high levels of cyanogenic glycosides and nitrates can cause acute fatalities in ruminants. Sorghum poisoning in horses, however, is due to low concentrations of cyanoalanine that causes chronic neurotoxicosis.

Horses, sheep, and cattle that consume cyanogenic varieties of these grasses for prolonged periods develop a syndrome of posterior ataxia, urinary incontinence, cystitis, and weight loss.[139-142] The disease results from degeneration of the lower spinal cord induced by cyanoalanine in the plants that causes demyelinization of peripheral nerves. It has been hypothesized that

T-glutamyl-B-cyanoalanine, a known lathyrogen, interferes with the neurotransmitter activity of glutamate. Lathyrogens affect the normal development of nervous tissue, causing signs of ataxia, urinary incontinence, and musculoskeletal deformities similar to those seen in mares grazing sudan grass in early pregnancy.[143]

Ataxia resulting from consumption of toxic sorghum grasses is most noticeable when the horse is backed or turned, which may cause it to sit on its hindquarters or fall over. Paralysis of the urinary bladder results in continual dribbling of urine which causes skin scalding and hair loss of the lower hind legs in males and of the perineal area in mares. Affected mares may have paralysis of the perineum so that the lips of the vulva stay open, causing vaginitis. Loss of tone to the rectum may occur, causing fecal impaction and constipation. Flaccid paralysis of the tail develops in some cases. Affected horses generally retain a good appetite and physical parameters remain normal until cystitis and ascending nephritis develop secondary to incontinence. As this occurs, the urine becomes thick and opaque and contains large amounts of amorphous sediment. On rectal palpation, the bladder is characteristically enlarged and flaccid and contains putty-like uroliths adhered to the dependent portion of the bladder (sabulous urolithiasis).[139]

Clinical signs of ataxia and posterior flaccid paralysis are similar to those caused by equine herpes virus-1 myeloencephalitis, equine protozoal encephalomyelitis, and the equine viral encephalitides. However, a history of feeding sorghum grasses over a period of weeks and the presence of cystitis, which is not usually a feature of the previously mentioned diseases, should confirm the diagnosis of chronic sorghum grass poisoning.

Postmortem examination of sorghum grass-poisoned horses generally reveals a severe ulcerative necrotizing urethritis and cystitis extending to pyelonephritis. Degeneration and demyelination of axons throughout the length of the spinal cord are evident histologically.[139]

Animals may slowly recover if they are removed from toxic sorghum grasses before cystitis and ataxia become complicated by secondary problems, such as ascending pyelonephritis. Complete recovery seldom occurs once horses have developed severe signs of ataxia and cystitis. Improvement can be accomplished by not feeding toxic sorghum grasses and treating urinary infections with appropriate antibiotics.

9.5 Lameness and Muscle Weakness-Inducing Plants

When lameness or muscle weakness are the predominant clinical signs in horses, plant poisonings that should be considered include: (1) contact with black walnut shavings; (2) ingestion of coffee weed or other *Cassia* species; (3) ingestion of plants that cause vitamin D toxicosis-like calcinosis; (4) chronic selenium toxicosis; or (5) oxalate-induced calcium deficiency. Excess oxalate intake decreases calcium absorption, causing hyperparathyroidism. If nutritional secondary hyperparathyroidism occurs for more than a few months, it results in shifting leg lameness, bone and joint tenderness, and a gradual reluctance to move. Emaciation, loose teeth, upper respiratory noise due to collapse of the nasal passages, enlarged facial bones, and sudden death during exercise may occur. The most common geographic locations where plant poisonings can cause lameness and muscle weakness are summarized in Table 9.8.

9.5.1 Black Walnut

Black walnut (*Juglans nigra*) is a widely distributed large native tree of North America growing 30–65 feet (10–20 m) in height. It is extensively used for its wood, aromatic oils, and edible nuts (Figure 9.40). Black walnut is a rich, dark, closed-grain hardwood commonly used for furniture and gun stocks. Horses are poisoned by contact with black walnut wood shavings or sawdust that may be present in bedding. The shavings range in color from purplish black to coffee-brown when freshly cut and have a distinctly sweet or acrid odor (Figure 9.41). In contrast, pine, fir, ash, oak, and most softwoods commonly used for bedding are all light colored. Bedding containing as little as 5–20% black walnut shavings can cause poisoning in horses.[144]

The toxin responsible is not known. Juglone, a naphthoquinone present in the roots, bark, nuts, and pollen of a variety of the walnut tree family has been proposed as the toxin. However, purified juglone applied topically to the feet of horses causes mild dermatitis but not laminitis. The variable severity of signs associated with black walnut shavings is poorly understood, but is apparently not related simply to contact of the horse's skin with the walnut shavings. Horses administered aqueous extracts of the heartwood of black walnut by nasogastric tube consistently develop acute laminitis, indicating that toxicosis is due in part to ingestion or inhalation of a toxic substance present in black walnut.[130,145–147] It has also been postulated that juglone and/or other possible substances cause the toxic reaction directly or by acting as an antigenic hapten.[148] Experimental evidence further

Table 9.8 Lameness and muscle weakness-inducing plants.

Common Name	Scientific Name	Toxin	Geographic Location	Predominant Clinical Effects
Black walnut	*Juglans nigra*	In shavings & sawdust	Widely distributed	Laminitis, leg edema, colic, anorexia, depression, and sometimes dyspnea
Hoary alyssum	*Berteroa incana*	Unknown	Central, northeast USA and Canada	Limb edema, fever, laminitis
Coffee weed or coffee senna	*Cassia occidentalis*	High in seeds	Southeast USA to Texas	Ataxia and sudden death
Day-blooming jessamine	*Cestrum diurnum*	Vitamin D-like	Florida, Texas, & California	Chronic weight loss, generalized stiffness to severe lameness, and recumbency; hypercalcemia and calcinosis
Golden oat grass	*Trisetum flavescens*	Vitamin D-like	England & Wales	
	Solanum malacoxylon	Vitamin D-like		
Selenium	See Table 9.9	Selenium accumulator plants	See Fig. 9.47	Mane and tail hairs break off, stiff and tender gait, hoof rings and cracks, sometimes emaciation, anemia, and cirrhosis
Many cultivated crops, alfalfa, and grasses grown on high-selenium soils				
		Oxalate-induced calcium deficiency		Shifting leg lameness, bone tenderness & possible emaciation, loose teeth, respiratory noise & "big head"

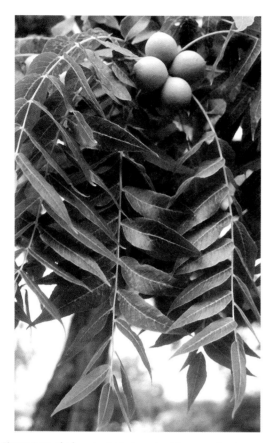

Figure 9.40 Black walnut (*Juglans nigra*) leaves and nuts.

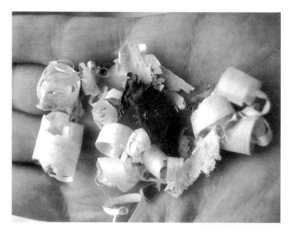

Figure 9.41 Walnut wood shavings.

anti-inflammatory agent, cold therapy, and keeping the horse on a soft pasture or sand for 1–2 weeks may be beneficial. If colic is present, mineral oil (4L/450kg horse) administered by nasogastric tube and other symptomatic treatments are indicated.

Although not all dark wood shavings are black walnut, it is safest to not use any wood shavings that contain dark wood unless it is known for certain that it is not black walnut. Poisoning of horses in pastures containing black walnut trees is also a concern, particularly during pollen shedding in the spring, and in the fall when the leaflets are shed from the walnut leaves. Reports of other species of walnut causing laminitis in horses are lacking but juglone and other phenolic compounds have been found in English walnuts (*Juglans regia*).[150]

9.5.2 Hoary Alyssum

Hoary alyssum (*Berteroa incana*) is an invasive weed of the northeastern and north central United States and Canada (Figure 9.42). A syndrome of limb edema, fever, colic, intravascular hemolysis, and laminitis has been recognized in horses eating hoary alyssum (*Berteroa incana*).[56] Hoary alyssum is toxic when incorporated into hay. The symptoms resemble those of black walnut poisoning.[56,63,151] A specific toxin has not been identified. Affected horses generally recover once they are removed from the plant source.

9.5.3 Coffee Weed or Coffee Senna

Occasionally horses, but more commonly cattle, in the southeastern United States to Texas have been poisoned by the ingestion of coffee weed (*Cassia*

indicates that the effects of the toxin do not directly cause contraction of the digital blood vessels, but enhance vasoconstriction in conjunction with the combined effects of catecholamines and corticosteroids.[107,145] Increases in laminar intravascular pressure may contribute to the collapse of capillary beds and lead to tissue necrosis.[149]

Clinical signs begin 8–24h after contact with black walnut shavings or sawdust. They are characterized by anorexia, lethargy, depression, and/or edema of the lower legs, which in severe cases may extend up to the ventral thorax. Colic, respiratory distress, and rarely death may occur. The most common symptom is varying degrees of lameness due to laminitis.[46] The laminitis results in foot pain, foot warmth, and increased digital pulse pressure. If affected horses are removed from the source of the black walnut shavings early enough and treated for laminitis, then they recover without the severe consequences of hoof deformity and third phalanx rotation. Administration of a nonsteroidal

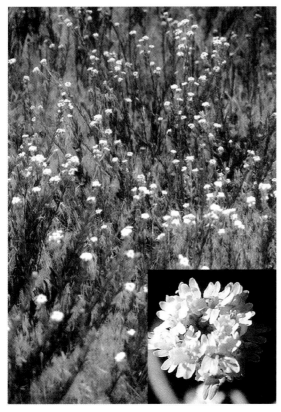

Figure 9.42 Hoary Alyssum (*Berteroa incana*).

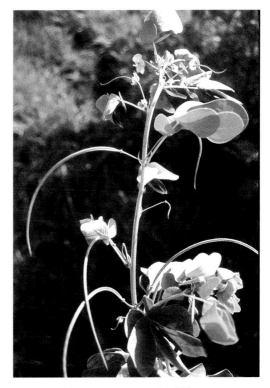

Figure 9.43 Sicklepod cassia (*Cassia obtusifolia*).

occidentalis).[88,152–154] Affected animals develop an acute myodegeneration that can be rapidly fatal.[69,75,124,154] Other species of *Cassia* are similarly toxic.[249]

Coffee weeds, like other *Cassia* species, are erect annual legumes growing to 6.5 feet (2 m) in height with pinnately compound leaves, each with 4–6 pairs of leaflets (Figure 9.43). The foliage has a strong distasteful odor. The yellow flowers are produced in axillary racemes and form long linear pods that are laterally compressed to show numerous seeds. The seeds appear to contain significant quantities of the toxin. The toxin's mode of action has not been determined, although it appears to be a water-soluble proteinaceous compound that binds tightly to cell membranes.[155]

Horses consuming sufficient quantities of *Cassia* plants are generally afebrile and severely ataxic and may die without showing other clinical signs. Serum liver enzyme activities may indicate acute liver degeneration. Unlike the disease in cattle, myoglobinuria and hemoglobinuria rarely occur in affected horses.

On postmortem examination, gross lesions are infrequently found, but skeletal muscle necrosis and renal tubular and hepatic centrilobular necrosis are detectable histologically.[154] Confirmation of the diagnosis is based upon knowing that the animal had access to and consumed *Cassia*, along with the presence of histologic lesions.

9.6 Plant-Induced Calcinosis

A generalized stiffness progressing to lameness occurs in horses from eating plants containing a vitamin D-like toxin that results in excessive calcium absorption and deposition in tissues.[156,157] Plants that have been incriminated to cause calcinosis in animals include *Solanum malacoxylon*,[30] golden oat grass (*Trisetum flavescens*),[158] and day-blooming jessamine (*Cestrum diurnum*).[84,159] The only one of these known to cause calcinosis in horses in North America is day-blooming jessamine.[30] Golden oat grass is common in England and Wales, particularly on calcareous soils. It grows well under adverse conditions and on poor soils and is quite palatable.

9.6.1 Day-Blooming Jessamine

Introduced from the West Indies as an ornamental tree, day-blooming jessamine or wild jasmine (*Cestrum diurnum*) has become widely distributed in Florida, Texas, and California. It is a shrub or small tree that grows up to 16 feet (5 m) high, with alternate elliptic leaves that have a dark green, glossy upper surface. Its fragrant white tubular flowers are borne in small clusters on axillary peduncles. Multiple green berries that turn black when ripe are produced after flowering (Figure 9.44).

The toxin in day-blooming jessamine is similar to 1,25-dihydroxy-cholecalciferol, the active metabolite of vitamin D.[30,160] Consequently, horses eating it absorb excessive amounts of calcium, resulting in hypercalcemia and tissue calcinosis. Prolonged ingestion of the plant results in calcification of the elastic tissues of the arteries, tendons, and ligaments.[30,83] Hypercalcemia causes hypoparathyroidism and hypercalcitoninism, which inhibit normal bone resorption and result in osteopetrosis.[30] Other members of this genus, such as night-blooming jessamine (*Cestrum nocturnum*) (Figure 9.45) and green cestrum or willow-leafed jessamine (*C. parqui*) are also poisonous, but not due to a vitamin D-like toxin. Their toxicity is instead due to atropine-like glycoalkaloids that are common in the family *Solanaceae*.

Characteristic clinical signs of plant-induced calcinosis in horses are chronic weight loss despite normal appetite and generalized stiffness leading to severe lameness and prolonged periods of recumbency. Lameness is due to pain in calcified ligaments and tendons. Plasma calcium concentration in affected horses is elevated from a normal of 11–13 mg/dl (2.75–3.25 mM/L) to 12–16 mg/dl (3–4 mM/L).[30] Other blood parameters, including phosphorus concentration, are generally normal.

Radiographically, horses show marked osteopetrosis as increased bone density and decreased size of the medullary cavity. Calcification of cartilage and increased metaphyseal and epiphyseal trabeculae are also evident radiographically.[30] Postmortem examination of affected horses shows severe calcification of the tendons, ligaments, and elastic arteries. Mineralization of tissues is confined to those containing elastic tissue.

Recovery from plant-induced calcinosis is rarely reported, as animals are usually chronically affected. Recovery is likely in less severely affected horses if they

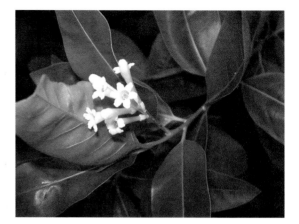

Figure 9.44 Day-blooming jessamine (*Cestrum diurnum*) (Courtesy of Forest & Kim Starr).

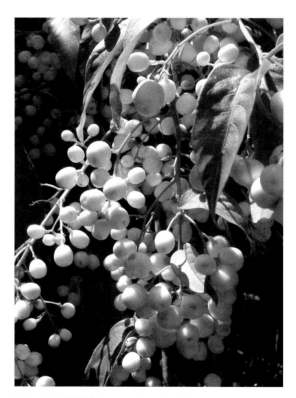

Figure 9.45 Night-blooming jessamine (*Cestrum nocturnum*) (Courtesy of Forest & Kim Starr).

are denied further access to toxic plants and fed a balanced diet. Care should be taken to ensure that horses are not placed in pastures or pens that contain *Cestrum* species or other calcinosis-inducing plants.

9.6.2 Flatweed

A plant that has recently been implicated in a stringhalt-like lameness is flatweed, cat's ear, or false dandelion (*Hypochoeris radicata*).[63,68] This perennial native plant of most of North America, Australia, and New Zealand has become a nuisance weed in some areas. Resembling the common dandelion, *Hypochoeris radicata* has a rosette of basal, hairy leaves and multiple branching flower stems. The flowering stalks are up to 2 feet tall with each branch terminating in a single yellow flower head with up to 30 yellow rays, each with 5 small teeth at the outer edge. The leaves have a milky sap and the seeds are wind dispersed (Figure 9.46).

Horses grazing the plants over time develop a spasmodic hyperflexion of one or both hind legs similar to classic stringhalt. Experimentally, horses fed 9.8 kg of the green plant daily for 50 days develop hyperflexion of one or both hock joints.[161] When both hindlegs are involved, a characteristic hopping gait devlops. In severe cases, the foot is lifted sharply up to the abdomen and then slapped to the ground.

Turning, backing, or other stimulation exacerbates signs. The specific toxin in flatweed has not been determined, but it induces increased electromyographic activity in the long digital extensor muscles and affects conduction in the long nerves of the body. Atrophy of the lateral thigh muscles may occur in chronic cases. Laryngeal hemiplegia resulting in "roaring" may occur in some affected horses.

Other plants that have been associated with stringhalt include sweet peas (*Lathyrus* species), dandelion (*Taraxacum officinale*), and mallow (*Malva parviflora*). "Australian stringhalt" referes to a similar condition in horses in Australia associated with grazing *Hypochoeris radicata*.

Treatment involves removing the horse from the pasture containing the plants and, in more severe cases, administering phenytoin (15 mg/kg, PO, for 2 weeks). Thiamine has been reported to aid in the recovery of Australian stringhalt. Recovery may take a few weeks and up to 18 months after horses are removed from flatweed. Horses with persistent signs may benefit from tenectomy of the lateral digital extensor tendon(s).

9.7 Selenium Toxicosis

Selenium is an essential micronutrient of a horse's diet with numerous impacts on cellular functions. A number of detrimental effects including generalized myopathy occur if the diet contains less than 0.1 ppm (mg/kg) of selenium. However, selenium in excess of 5 ppm in the total diet is harmful and causes chronic selenium poisoning of livestock.[162,163] Levels of selenium greater than 25–50 ppm may cause acute selenium poisoning and sudden death due to pulmonary congestion and edema. In excess, selenium profoundly inhibits cellular enzyme oxidation reduction reactions, especially those involving sulfate or sulfur-containing amino acids.[164,165] This antagonistic effect of selenium on sulfate alters the metabolism of the sulfur-containing amino acids methionine and cystine, which affects cell division and growth. These effects are greatest on hoof and hair which contain the highest concentrations of sulfur-containing amino acids. With chronic selenium poisoning, this is seen clinically as abnormal hoof and hair growth. Selenium will also cross the placenta, causing fetal abnormalities through its effects on fetal cellular metabolism.[164]

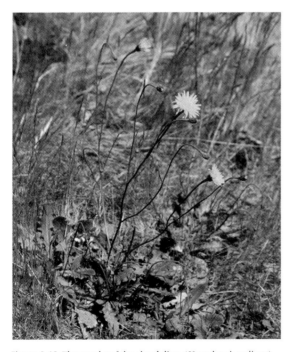

Figure 9.46 Flatweed or false dandelion (*Hypochoeris radicata*).

9.7.1 Causes of Selenium Toxicosis

Selenium poisoning of herbivores occurs when excess selenium has inadvertently been administered or added to the animal's diet, is present at toxic concentrations in drinking water, or when plants high in selenium content are consumed. There are three types of plants that may accumulate sufficient selenium to cause selenium poisoning. These are: (1) obligate selenium accumulator or indicator plants, (2) secondary or facultative selenium accumulator plants, and (3) crops, alfalfa, and grasses, that are normally good horse feeds but may contain 1–30 ppm selenium if grown on selenium-rich soils.

Selenium-rich soils occur in areas of low rainfall where minimal leaching of selenium from the soil is likely to occur. In North America, this occurs primarily in the Rocky Mountain and Great Plains regions (Figure 9.47). In a recent survey, selenium toxicosis attributed to native plants was reported in only eight states (California, Colorado, Idaho, Montana, Oregon, South Dakota, Utah, and Wyoming).[163] In contrast, in all states except four (Delaware, Rhode Island, West Virginia, and Wyoming), selenium deficiency was reported to be a problem.

Even in high selenium-containing soils, plant uptake of selenium is variable according to the species, depending on the chemical form of selenium in the soil, soil acidity, climate, and is highest during plant growth.[166] Selenium is taken up more readily by plants in alkaline soils. Selenium toxicosis is unlikely from plants grown on acidic soils. Soils high in readily available selenium for plants can be determined. Therefore, the potential for selenium poisoning in herbivores is recognized by the presence of obligate selenium accumulator plants that are growing in the area (Table 9.9). These plants are referred to as selenium indicator plants. The high selenium content gives these plants an unpleasant garlic-sulfur odor, which makes them relatively unpalatable and assists in identifying them. The odor is increased by rubbing their leaves together. Horses will avoid eating these plants if sufficient other feed is available. Referred to as obligate selenium accumulator plants, they grow only on soils high in available selenium because they require a high amount of selenium for their normal growth. Selenium accumulator plants are capable of accumulating up to 10 times the amount of selenium present in the soil. Some may contain up to 10,000 ppm selenium, or 2,000 times the total dietary concentration of selenium that is toxic and thus may cause acute selenium poisoning. It is important to recognize that other plants and grasses growing in the same area as selenium indicator plants will have increased levels of selenium that may also be toxic to animals grazing them. In such pastures, it is important to ensure that horses receive adequate sulfur and copper in their diet to counter the absorption of toxic levels of selenium.

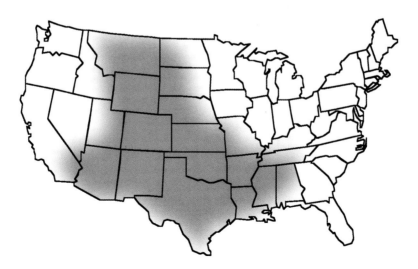

Figure 9.47 Approximate geographic distribution of selenium-rich soils in the continental United States.

Table 9.9 Selenium accumulator plants.

Obligate selenium accumulator or indicator plants	
Milkvetches	Astragalus (24 spp.)
False golden weeds	Oonopsis spp.
Woody asters	Xylorrhiza glabriuscula
Prince's plume	Stanleya pinnata
Secondary or facultative selenium accumulator plants	
Asters	Aster and Machaeranthera spp.
Saltbrush	Atriplex spp.
Indian paintbrush	Castllleja spp.
Broomweed, snakeweed, Turpentine, or matchweed	Gutierrezia spp.
Beard tongue	Penstemon spp.
Gumweed, resinweed	Grindelia squarrosa
Ironweed	Sideranthus grindelioides
Bastard toadflax	Comandra pallida

Selenium poisoning is most often caused by secondary, or facultative, selenium accumulator plants (also listed in Table 9.9) and common forages grown on selenium-rich soils.[26,104,168] Secondary selenium accumulator plants may cause either acute or chronic selenium poisoning. In contrast to the obligate selenium accumulator plants, secondary accumulator plants do not require selenium for growth, but may accumulate up to several hundred ppm of selenium when grown on soils high in available selenium. The toxic effects of selenium in animals varies, depending on the amount and rate of its absorption, individual susceptibility, type of selenium in the plant, and the interaction of selenium with other dietary minerals, such as sulfur, arsenic, or copper.[168] These minerals and possibly others competitively interfere with selenium absorption and therefore adequate amounts of these minerals in the diet may help prevent selenium toxicity.

9.7.2 Two-Grooved Milkvetch (*Astragalus bisulcatus*)

Two-grooved milk vetch is an obligate selenium accumulator capable of containing very high concentrations of selenium. It also contains the neurotoxic indolizidine alkaloid swainsonine and nitroglycosides that cause neurologic disease. Two-grooved milkvetch is a perennial plant forming large clumps that reach 3 feet (1 m) in height. Stems are purple in mature plants. The leaves are pinnate with numerous paired hairy leaflets. Flowers are in dense spike-like racemes, generally purple but varying from pink to white (Figure 9.48). The fruit is a leguminous, heavily textured pod about 0.5 inch (11–15 mm) in length. The pod has two characteristic longitudinal grooves on the upper surface, which gives this milkvetch its name. It typifies the 24 or more species of *Astragalus* that grow on the alkaline seleniferous soils of the western states.

9.7.3 False Golden Weed (*Oonopsis species*)

False golden weed is an obligate selenium accumulator that is a perennial subshrub with a woody root stock. The stems are from 4–12 inches (10–30 cm) tall with brown bark below and are hairless. The leaves are 1–3 inches (3–7 cm) long and less than 1/8 inch (1–3 mm) wide, narrowly linear, rigidly erect, and glabrous. The heads range from one to several per stem. The flowers are few to many with bracts in three or more lengths. The disk flowers are yellowish and the pappus is brown. There are no ray flowers.

9.7.4 Woody Aster (*Xylorhiza glabriuscula*)

Woody aster is an obligate selenium accumulator that prefers rocky and clay soils at higher altitudes. It is a perennial arising from a thick woody crown with roots. Numerous unbranched hairy stems reaching a height of 1 foot (30 cm) have entire leaves 0.75–2.0 inches (2–5 cm) long and about to 0.25 inch (2–6 mm) wide tipped with a callus point. The daisy-like flowers have stiff white ray flowers and yellow disk flowers (Figure 9.49).

9.7.5 Prince's Plume (*Stanleya pinnata*)

Prince's plume is a common obligate selenium accumulator that is a coarse herbaceous perennial ranging from 1.5–5.0 feet (0.5–1.5 m) in height. The stems are stout and mostly unbranched. The leaves are entire to pinnately compound, 1.5–6.0 inches (4–15 cm) long. The petals are yellow with long claws and are arranged in plume-like inflorescences (Figure 9.50). The fruit is slender and nearly round in cross section with a stripe from 0.4–1.2 inches (1–3 cm) long.

9.7.6 White Prairie Aster (*Aster falcatus*)

White prairie aster is a secondary selenium accumulator. It is a branched perennial plant of the dry plains with extensive spreading roots and stalks. The leaves are 0.4–1.2 inches (1–3 cm) long, linear, and densely hairy,

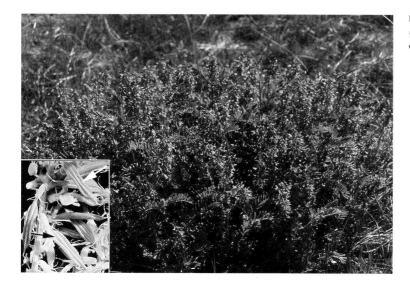

Figure 9.48 Two-grooved milkvetch (*Astragalus bisulcatus*) showing the two characteristic grooves on the seed pods.

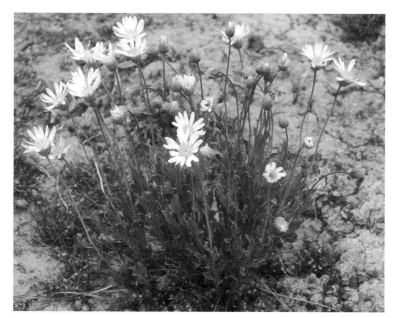

Figure 9.49 Woody aster (*Xyorrhiza glabriuscula*).

giving the plant a rough feeling. The flowers are small and daisy-like with white ray flowers about 1/8 inch (3–4 mm) long that produce many tawny pappus bristles in a head in late summer and fall (Figure 9.51).

9.7.7 Broom, Turpentine, Snake, or Match Weed (*Gutierrezia sarothrae*)

Broom, turpentine, snake, or match weed is a secondary selenium accumulator. It is a native perennial invasive plant with a woody base from which the closely grouped

branching stems arise each spring. Often it is an evergreen shrub in the milder climates of the southwestern states. The leaves are alternate, linear, and glabrous. It has many yellow flower heads, usually located in clusters at the ends of the branches (Figure 9.52). A given head will have no more than 3–8 yellow ray flowers and 3–8 disk flowers. The pappus is composed of several to many oblong scales. *Gutierrezia* spp. have been associated with abortion in cattle and sheep, but not horses.

Figure 9.50 Prince's plume (*Stanleya pinnata*).

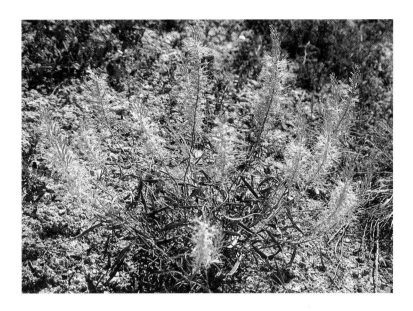

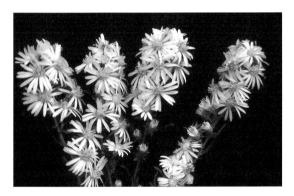

Figure 9.51 White prairie aster (*Aster falcatus*).

9.7.8 Gumweed or resinweed (*Grindelia* spp.)

Gumweed or resinweed are secondary selenium accumulators. They are common biennial or perennial herbaceous plants with leafy stems that grow up to 3 feet (1 m) tall. The leaves are alternate, simple with serrated edges, and have scattered glands that produce a sticky, gum-like substance. The yellow flowers are solitary and surrounded by several rows of curved bracts that produce a white gummy resinous material. The ray flowers, when present, are about 0.5 inch (8–10 mm) long and lemon-yellow to bright yellow (Figure 9.53). The pappus awns are about 2–3 mm long.

9.7.9 Saltbush (*Atriplex* spp.)

Saltbush is a secondary selenium accumulator that grows on dry soils. It is a perennial woody shrub that is more or less scaly and scurfy. The leaves are mostly alternate. The plants are dioecious with staminate flowers in terminal panicles without bracts. The characteristic fruits have four wings that are entire or deeply cut, giving rise to the common name "four-wing saltbush" (Figure 9.54).

9.7.10 Indian Paintbrush (*Castilleja* spp.)

Indian paintbrush is a secondary selenium accumulator. It is an annual or perennial plant that is herbaceous, but many are woody at the base only. It is a partial root parasite of various other plants. The leaves are alternate and sessile. The flowers are arranged in terminal bracted spikes that are usually petaloid and ranging from scarlet to yellow (Figure 9.55). The Indian paintbrush is common throughout the northern Rocky Mountain states, particularly at higher elevations.

9.7.11 Beard Tongue (*Penstemon* spp.)

Beard tongue is a secondary selenium accumulator. It is an herbaceous perennial plant, usually erect, but many are low and creeping. The leaves are opposite with the upper ones sessile and often clasping. The inflorescence is a panicle of flowers ranging from blue to red. The flowers are showy with a tubular corolla whose

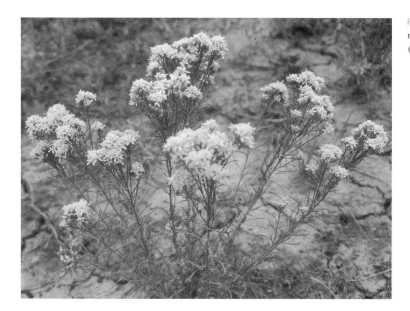

Figure 9.52 Snakeweed, broomweed, matchweed, or turpentine weed (*Gutierrezia sarothrae*).

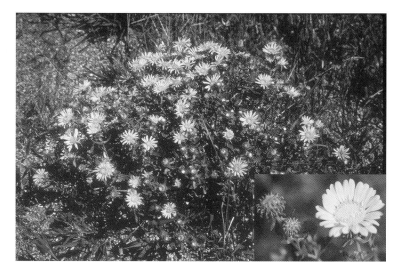

Figure 9.53 Gumweed or resinweed (*Grindelia* spp.) showing the whitish gummy resin in the tops of the flower buds.

upper lip is two-lobed and the lower lip is three-lobed (Figure 9.56). There are four fertile stamens in two pairs with arched filaments. A fifth stamen, called a staminode, is represented by a conspicuous sterile filament attached to the upper side of the corolla. It is widened and bearded at the apex.

9.7.12 Effects of Acute Selenium Toxicosis

Acute selenium poisoning from plant ingestion is rare since animals rarely eat plants containing levels of selenium over 50 ppm, as they generally are not palatable. Acute selenium toxicosis most commonly occurs as a result of the inadvertent addition of excess selenium to the diet or by administration of an overdose of selenium. However, when livestock are forced to graze plants high in selenium content or consume a diet containing high levels of selenium, they can rapidly accumulate levels of selenium in their tissues that will result in death.[26,169] Blood serum selenium levels greater than 72 ppm cause severe capillary damage in the lungs, liver, and kidneys. As a result of this, affected animals frequently die before clinical signs are evident. Death results from respiratory failure attributable to pulmonary congestion and edema. Congestion, edema, and necrosis of the lungs, liver, and kidneys are the major lesions

seen at postmortem examination of animals that have died of acute selenium poisoning.

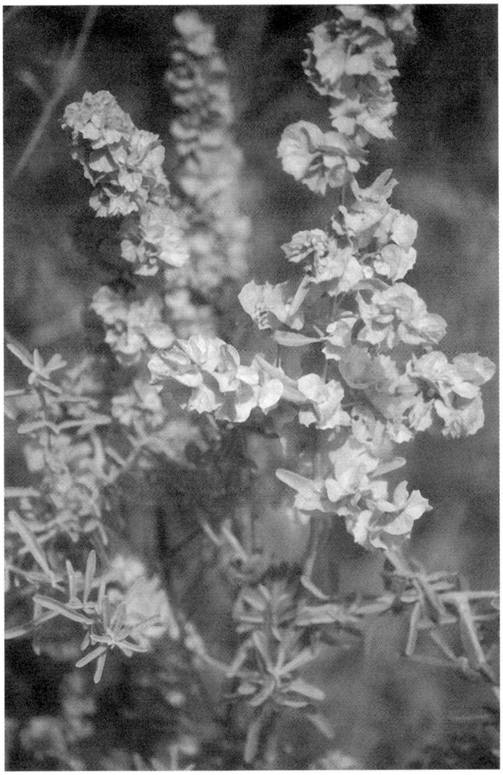

9.7.13 Effects of Chronic Selenium Toxicosis

Traditionally, chronic selenium poisoning has been divided into two syndromes referred to as blind staggers or alkali disease.[27] Both syndromes are associated with chronic ingestion of forage and crop plants that have accumulated 5–50 ppm selenium.[26]

Blind staggers is primarily a problem of cattle and sheep from the ingestion of selenium accumulator plants. Affected animals characteristically exhibit aimless wandering, circling, disregard for objects in their way, loss of appetite, and apparent blindness.[26,164] The disease progresses to foreleg weakness and inability to stand. Weight loss accompanies inappetence. Teeth grinding, indicating abdominal pain or colic, is common. Death results from respiratory failure, which usually occurs if the plants causing the disease are not removed from the animal's diet early in the course of disease. Recent evidence suggests that blind staggers syndrome is rarely due to selenium toxicity, as originally thought. Sheep fed the obligate selenium accumulator and neurotoxin-containing plant two-grooved milkvetch (*Astragalus bisulcatus*) developed classic signs of blind staggers but did not develop lesions typical of selenium toxicosis.[164] Instead, microscopic lesions in the brain (cytoplasmic vacuolation) typical of those from locoweed poisoning, were present. This suggests that blind staggers may be due to chronic locoweed poisoning and

Figure 9.54 Saltbush (*Atriplex* spp.) showing four-winged fruits.

Figure 9.55 Indian paintbrush (*Castilleja* spp.).

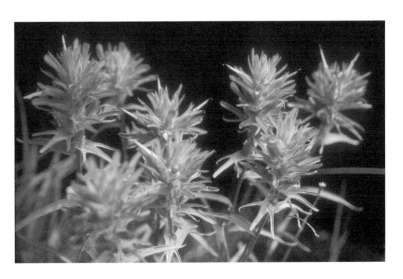

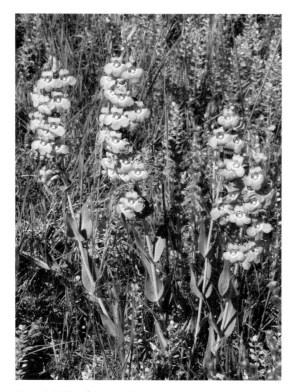

Figure 9.56 Beard tongue (*Penstemon* spp.).

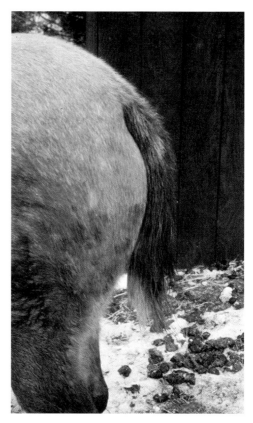

Figure 9.57 Horse with "bob-tail" due to hair loss from chronic excess selenium consumption.

not selenium toxicity.[91,99] Further evidence suggests that blind staggers may also be related to high sulfate in plants and therefore in the diet of animals grazing the plants.[170,171]

Alkali disease is the name given to chronic selenium toxicity by the early Great Plains and Rocky Mountain settlers because they noted it occurred only in livestock grazing semiarid regions with high alkali soil. These areas are now known to be soils high in readily available selenium. Chronic selenium toxicosis affecting horses, cattle, pigs, sheep, and poultry is associated with the consumption of forages or cereal crops grown in seleniferous soils or diets to which excess selenium had been inadvertently added.[27,74,142,171] Poisoning occurs after high selenium-containing plants or a diet high in selenium has been consumed for several months. Excess selenium consumption results in the substitution of selenium for sulfur in keratin. This results in defective formation of keratin, the principal protein present in the hoof and hair. Initially, affected horses lose the long hair from the mane and tail and it breaks off at the site where excess selenium was incorporated into the hair shaft. This gives the horse a "clipped" mane and bobtailed

appearance and is the reason that the syndrome has been referred to as "bobtail disease" (Figure 9.57). Lameness develops as a result of coronitis and abnormal hoof wall formation and affects all feet. Initially, affected horses walk stiff-legged with tenderness followed by pronounced lameness. Horizontal hoof wall rings or ridges that may progress to full-thickness cracks causing severe lameness are characteristic (Figure 9.58). Some horses may slough the hoof entirely. Chronic selenium poisoning has also been associated with anemia, liver cirrhosis, emaciation, heart atrophy, and bone and joint degeneration in horses and cattle.[169,172]

9.7.14 Diagnosis of Selenium Toxicosis

A diagnosis of selenium poisoning is best confirmed by submitting samples of feeds and forages for analysis and then determining the selenium concentration in the total diet. Selenium levels greater than 5 ppm of total dietary dry matter should be considered potentially toxic.[162]

Normal serum selenium levels are in the range of 0.09–0.3 ppm. Levels of selenium from 1–4 ppm are suggestive of chronic selenium poisoning. Serum levels up to 25 ppm have been reported in acute selenium poisoning. Greater than 4 ppm dry matter in liver or kidney or 1.2 ppm wet weight is indicative of selenium toxicosis.[162]

Generally, the more chronic that selenium toxicosis becomes, the lower the levels in tissues. However, hair and hoof samples retain high concentrations and are useful in the diagnosis of chronic selenium poisoning. It is important to collect hoof and hair samples from areas where the hoof is cracked or the hair is broken off, because this is where selenium is incorporated in the keratin. Hoof wall or hair selenium concentration in excess of 5–10 ppm indicates excessive selenium

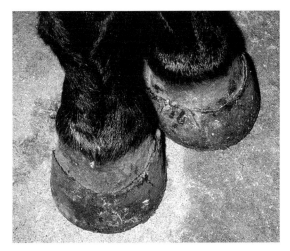

Figure 9.58 Circular horizontal cracks in the hoof wall of all feet characteristic of chronic excess selenium consumption.

intake.[169] However, hair selenium content is affected by intake of other minerals and external or surface selenium contamination.

Successful treatment of selenium poisoning depends on its early recognition and removal of horses from the source of excess selenium. Feeding a low selenium and high protein diet rich in the sulfur-containing amino acids cysteine and methionine will help counteract selenium's toxic effect (Table 9.6). Good-quality alfalfa hay, provided it does not contain high levels of selenium from being grown on selenium-rich soils, is a good source of cysteine and methionine. Any cereal grain except corn may be fed with 15–20% cottonseed, rapeseed, or fish meal, which will increase the protein content of the grain mix to 15–20%. Corn, soybean meal, and bran are low in sulfur-containing amino acids and, therefore, are not preferred. In addition, ensure that the total diet contains at least 10 ppm and preferably 25 ppm of copper, as copper is necessary to reduce the toxic effects of selenium. Recovery from chronic selenium poisoning will occur gradually as the affected horse's hooves grow out if the horse is fed a diet low in selenium and attention is given to regular trimming of cracked and overgrown hooves. Grain or hay, known (tested) to be low in selenium should be fed to horses grazing pastures with plants high in selenium to prevent chronic selenium toxicosis.

9.8 Anemia-Inducing Plants

Anemia due to hemolysis or hemorrhage may occur in animals ingesting plants such as onions (*Allium* spp.), red maple (*Acer rubrum*), and moldy sweet clover (*Melilotus officinalis*), or phenothiazine toxicosis (Table 9.10).

Table 9.10 Anemia-inducing plants.

Common Name	Scientific Name	Toxin	Major Effects
Onions, wild and cultivated	*Allium* spp.	N-propyl disulfide in plants and bulbs	Onion odor to breath; anemia (Hct 10–15%); hemoglobinuria, icterus, Heinz bodies, tachycardia, and tachypnea
Red maple	*Acer rubrum*	Bark and dry or wilted, but not green leaves	Develop rapidly; increased AST, SDH, and bilirubin
Moldy sweet clover	*Melilotus* spp.	Dicoumarol anticoagulant in moldy hay or haylage	Hematomas; normal appetite, temperature, pulse and respiratory rate until terminal; hemorrhaging; increased prothrombin and partial thromboplastin times

All these effects may also be caused by phenothiazine toxicity or babesiosis (both rare in USA), equine infectious anemia, and immune-mediated hemolytic anemia. Heinz bodies may also occur with equine lymphosarcoma.

Hemolysis is accompanied by hemoglobinuria and icterus. Anemia due to hemorrhage may be caused by the ingestion of spoiled or moldy sweet clover hay or haylage. Horses infected with the protozoan parasite *Babesia caballi* or *Theileria equi* may exhibit similar signs. Since phenothiazine is rarely used in horses today and babesiosis is uncommon in North America, poisoning by these plants should be of prime consideration when horses develop signs of anemia and hemoglobinuria. Other causes of similar clinical signs include immune-mediated hemolytic anemia and equine infectious anemia.

9.8.1 Onions

Poisoning from wild onions (*Allium* spp.) and domestic onions (*A. cepa*) will occur in horses that have eaten large quantities of the plants or the bulbs.[60] Cattle are the most susceptible, with horses and dogs being less so. Sheep and goats can tolerate eating considerably more onions than other animals.[173,174] Although species of wild onion are found in moist areas of most states, onion poisoning is most often caused by feeding culled domestic onions.

Onions contain the alkaloid n-propyl disulfide, which inhibits 6-phosphate dehydrogenase in red blood cells, causing hemoglobin denaturation and precipitation. This is recognized as Heinz bodies in red blood cells. Reticuloendothelial cells remove these altered red blood cells from circulation, causing anemia and the clinical signs.

Depending on the quantity and rate at which onions are eaten by the horse, effects vary from mild anemia without clinical signs to severe hemolytic anemia-induced icterus, increased heart and respiratory rates, weakness, hemoglobinuria, and death. The odor of onions is often detectable on the breath. The presence of Heinz bodies in red blood cells is highly suggestive of onion poisoning. However, Heinz body anemia also occurs from red maple leaf ingestion and may occur in equine lymphosarcoma.[136] Hematocrit is often as low as 10–15%. Horses with onion poisoning should not be stressed. They should be removed from the source of onions and fed a balanced diet. Severely anemic animals may require blood transfusion.

9.8.2 Red Maple

Red maple (*Acer rubrum*) trees are common throughout most of eastern North America and south to Florida and Texas. They adapt to moist or dry areas and may reach a height of 100 feet (30 m) at maturity. The characteristic leaves are three-lobed and shiny green above and they turn a brilliant red in the fall (Figure 9.59). Flowers are red, grow in clusters, and appear before the leaves. Fruits are red with two smooth wings.

Poisoning occurs when horses eat wilted or dried red maple leaves.[51,78,171,175,208,231] Fresh green leaves are not toxic, but once dried, they remain toxic for up to 30 days.[178] The bark from red maple trees is also apparently toxic.[171] Fatal poisoning from feeding ponies 1.5 g/lb (3.0 g/kg) body weight of dried red maple leaves

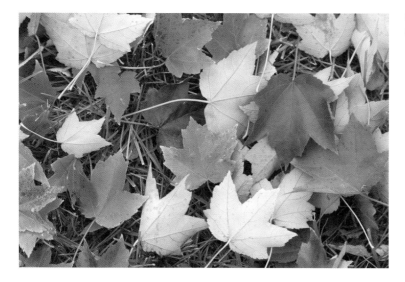

Figure 9.59 Red maple leaves (*Acer rubrum*).

occurred in 1–5 days.[176] Half of this amount will induce hemolytic anemia with the formation of Heinz bodies. The precise oxidant that forms in wilted maple leaves has not been determined. The toxicity of other maple species has not been fully investigated but oxidants similar to those in red maples have been identified in sugar maples (*Acer saccharum*).[104] Red maple hybrids (Crimson king) should also be considered toxic.

After eating even relatively small amounts of wilted maple leaves, horses exhibit clinical signs within 1–2 days. Poisoning is characterized by an acute hemolytic anemia that causes weakness, increased respiratory and heart rates, cyanosis, icterus, and hemoglobinuria.[177] Pregnant mares may abort without showing typical signs of hemolytic anemia. Some horses may present with colic, laminitis, and signs of renal failure. Blood changes include a marked reduction in hematocrit, methemoglobinemia, Heinz bodies in erythrocytes, and depletion of reduced glutathione in erythrocytes.[132,178] Serum aspartate amino transferase and sorbitol dehydrogenase activity and total protein and bilirubin concentrations are elevated.[177]

A diagnosis of red maple poisoning can generally be made when horses develop an acute hemolytic anemia with Heinz body formation and there is evidence that they have had access to and eaten wilted or dried red maple leaves or bark. Other conditions that should be considered include onion, moldy sweet clover, and phenothiazine poisoning, and diseases such as equine infectious anemia, anaplasmosis, and babesiosis. The prognosis is always guarded to poor for horses with red maple poisoning because of rapid intravascular hemolysis, coagulopathy, hemoglobin nephropathy, and vascular thrombosis that may occur.[176,179]

Successful treatment of horses with red maple poisoning must be initiated as early as possible in order to counteract the hemolytic crisis and secondary effects. Appropriate intravenous fluid therapy to maintain cardiac output and renal function and transfusions with packed erythrocytes may be effective.[1830] Large doses of vitamin C (ascorbic acid; 30 mg/kg, IV, q 12 h) as an antioxidant along with blood transfusions and other supportive therapy has proven beneficial if administered early in the course of toxicity.[181] It is important to note that the use of corticosteroids in treating red maple toxicity greatly decreased the chance a horse surviving the toxicity.[177] Although methylene blue is advocated as a treatment for oxidant toxicities of erythrocytes, it should be used with considerable caution in the horse,

as it will induce a Heinz body hemolytic anemia in excess. It is recommended that a no greater than 1% methylene blue solution be administered intravenously to give a total dose of no more than 8.8 mg/kg. This amount is provided using 1% methylene blue at a dose of 0.88 ml/kg. Administration may be repeated every 6–8 hours if necessary.

9.8.3 Spoiled Sweet Clover

Yellow sweet clover (*Melilotus officinalis*) and white sweet clover (*M. officinalis* var. *alba*) are legumes commonly grown in the northwestern United States and western Canada as livestock forage. Yellow sweet clover has become a self-sustaining weed in most of North America.[163] As biennials, both species grow to 5 feet (1.5 m) in height and have compound leaves with three leaflets that have serrated edges with the terminal leaflet on a stalk. The leguminous flowers are produced in axillary racemes up to 5 inches (12–13 cm) in length. The flowers are yellow or white, depending on the species (Figure 9.60).

Neither yellow nor white sweet clover is toxic, unless they are improperly cured as hay or haylage and become moldy. Molds, such as *Penicillium* spp., convert the non-toxic glycoside coumarin in the plant to dicoumarol. Dicoumarol has strong anticoagulant properties that interfere with the vitamin K-dependent coagulation factors VII, IX, X, and prothrombin. The rate of depletion of these factors is directly related to the duration and amount of dicoumarol ingested.

Moldy and improperly cured sweet clover hay or haylage, although not always toxic, should be used for animal feed only after it has been tested for dicoumarol. In one survey of 272 cured sweet clover hay samples, over one third contained more than 4.5 mg/lb (10 mg/kg) of dicoumarol (range 0–75 mg/lb or 0–165 mg/kg).[182] The concentration of dicoumarol tends to be higher in large round bales where the hay is more likely to have a higher moisture content. Moldy dicoumarol-containing sweet clover may be fed to livestock as long as it does not constitute more than 25% of the animal's total diet, although feeding any moldy feed is not recommended. There are varieties of sweet clover that contain very low levels of coumarin. Hay or haylage from these varieties will not interfere with coagulation, even if moldy.[182] However, to prevent the risk of moldy sweet clover poisoning, sweet clover hay or haylage should not be fed for at least 2–3 weeks before foaling or any elective surgery.

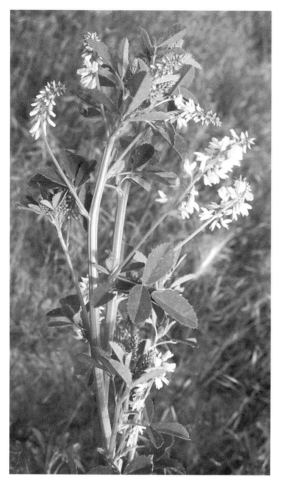

Figure 9.60 Yellow sweet clover (*Melilotus officinalis*).

Dicoumarol-containing sweet clover hay or haylage must be ingested for several weeks before clinical signs occur. The problem occurs most commonly in cattle, but horses and sheep may also be affected.[183,184] Generally, only a few animals in a herd will be affected, but mortality is high if untreated. Signs of poisoning include hemorrhage from the nose, intestinal tract, or into body cavities and soft tissues. Hematomas may develop over areas that are prone to trauma. Excessive hemorrhaging after any laceration is likely and can be life threatening. The degree of anemia depends upon the amount of blood loss and is reflected by tachycardia, pale mucous membranes, weakness, and other signs of hypovolemic shock. Blood prothrombin, activated partial thromboplastin, and clotting times are markedly prolonged from normal.

Affected horses should be treated with whole blood transfusions as necessary (10 ml blood/kg). Ideally, vitamin K_1 (2.0 mg/kg) should be injected to restore prothrombin time to normal within 24 hours. However, the cost may be prohibitive and vitamin K3 is often administered. Vitamin K_3 may cause a toxic reaction in horses and, in contrast to vitamin K_1, has been found to be ineffective in treating moldy sweet clover poisoning in calves.

Intravenous vitamin K_1 administration controls hemorrhage in 3–6 h and returns prothrombin time to normal in 12–24 h. If vitamin K_3 is given, therapeutic benefits are reported to occur within 1–2 days and the dosage should be less than 1 mg/kg and probably not more than 1–2 mg/kg. Parenteral doses of vitamin K_3 greater than 2 mg/kg greatly increase the risk of toxicosis.

9.9 Teratogenic Plants

Certain plants are known to be teratogenic and produce physical defects in the developing fetus, particularly if the plants are eaten by the dam during the first trimester of pregnancy. Plant teratogens are complex chemical compounds that cross the placenta and cause fetal resorption, abortion, stillbirths, or deformed newborns.[93,185–187] Teratogens have specific effects during precise stages of fetal organ development and are therefore most dangerous during the first trimester when fetal organ development is at its most critical stages. For example, western false hellebore or skunk cabbage (*Veratrum californicum*) is a classic teratogen that only induces the cyclops deformity in lambs if the pregnant ewe eats a sufficient quantity of the plant during the fourteenth day of gestation (Figure 9.61).[188] A teratogen must therefore be present in the developing conceptus at a specific stage of gestation and in sufficient quantity to exert its effect. In general, the fetus is most susceptible to teratogens during the first trimester of pregnancy. It is important to recognize, however, that plant teratogens are but a single entity in the spectrum of teratogens that include viruses, chemicals, and radiation.

Many plants have been suspected of causing infertility, fetal deformity, and abortion in livestock, and theoretically could cause similar effects in pregnant mares (Table 9.11). Relatively few cases of plant teratogenicity have been documented in horses. Mares consuming sudan grass (*Sorghum sudanense*) hay and sorghum hybrids (Figs 9.20–9.38 and 9.20–9.39) between the

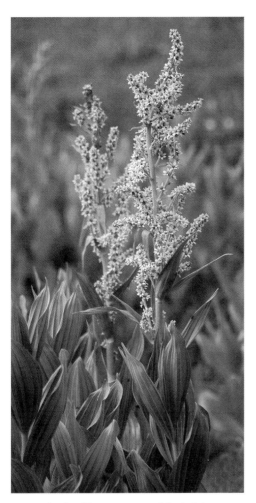

Figure 9.61 Skunk cabbage or western false hellebore (*Veratrum californicum*).

Table 9.11 Teratogenic plants for horses.

Known teratogenic plants for horses	
Milkvetch, locoweed	*Astragalus, Oxytropis* spp.
European or spotted hemlock	*Conium maculatum*
Lupine	*Lupinus* spp.
Wild tree tobacco	*Nicotiana glauca*
Tobacco	*Nicotiana tabacum*
Hellebore	*Veratrum viride*
Sudan grass	*Sorghum sudanense*
Suspected teratogenic plants for horses	
Akee	*Blighia sapida*
Autumn crocus	*Colchicum autumnale*
Cycad fern	*Cycas* spp.
Jimson weed	*Datura stramonium*
Creeping indigo	*Indigofera spicata*
Wild pea	*Lathyrus* spp.
Mimosa	*Leucaena leucocephala*
Poppies	*Papaver* spp.
Wild black cherry	*Prunus serotina*
Groundsel	*Senecio* spp.
Periwinkle	*Vinca rosea*

twentieth and fiftieth day of gestation have been reported to produce foals with a variety of skeletal deformities.[143] Sorghums are known to accumulate cyanogenic glycosides that can be converted to β-cyanolanine, a known precursor to the lathyrogen T-glutamyl-β-cyanoalanine, which is teratogenic.

Pregnant mares, cows, and ewes will abort or produce malformed offspring if they consume locoweed (*Astragalus* spp.) during early pregnancy.[73] Locoweed may also be neurotoxic to the dam. Wooly locoweed (*Astragalus mollissimus*) (Fig. 9.30) will cause mares to abort or produce foals with various limb deformities, including contracted flexor tendons, lateral rotation of the forelimbs, carpal flexural deformities, and laxity of the

hock joints.[24] Some foals with minor limb deformities recover spontaneously and more severely affected foals require surgical correction or euthanasia. Several other species of locoweed (*A. lentiginosus* and *A. pubentisimus*) are also known to cause congenital malformations and abortion in sheep, cattle, and horses.[168,189] The teratogenic components of *Astragalus* spp are nitroglycosides and not the toxic indolizidine alkaloid swainsonine that causes locoism; nor their high selenium content. A description of sorghum and *Astragalus* plants is given in the section on neurologic disease and in the section on sudden death-inducing plants for poison hemlock.

Poison, European, or spotted hemlock (*Conium maculatum*) contains the alkaloid coniine, which is a potent neurotoxin and a teratogen.[190] Cattle and pigs seem to be the most susceptible to its teratogenic effects, whereas in horses and ewes, it is neurotoxic and does not detectably harm the fetus.[191,192]

9.10 Sudden Death-Inducing Plants

Sudden death of horses due to plant poisoning with few or no previously occurring clinical signs is relatively uncommon. When it occurs, it is important to determine the cause as quickly as possible so that further losses can be avoided. Sudden death due to plants most often occurs when horses have been placed in situations where they have been compelled to eat unusual plants in hay or over-grazed pastures. Unintentional poisoning may occur when garden clippings or prunings are fed to horses or when horses are tied or placed in pens adjacent to plants to which they are unaccustomed and they would otherwise leave alone. Potential causes of plant-induced sudden death in horses are listed in Table 9.12 along with their predominant clinical effects.

9.10.1 Cyanide-Induced Sudden Death

All animals, including horses are susceptible to hydrogen cyanide (Prussic acid or HCN) poisoning.[192] Interestingly, horses and other monogastric animals are more susceptible to preformed cyanide salts (sodium or potassium cyanide) than ruminants, yet ruminants are highly susceptible to plant-induced cyanide poisoning. Horses are very rarely affected by cyanogenic plants. Some of the more common plants with a potential for cyanide poisoning in ruminants are listed in Table 9.12.

Table 9.12 Plants causing acute death.

Common Name	Scientific Name	Toxin	Predominant Clinical Effects
Serviceberry, Saskatoon berry	Amelanchier alnifolia	Cyanogenic glycosides throughout plant, especially high during growth	Bright red venous blood, dark red to cyanotic membranes, rapid labored breathing, frothing at mouth and dilated pupils Muscle tremors, ataxia, convulsions and death within minutes of eating plant Cyanide test kit positive on stomach contents, liver, or muscle.
Wild blue flax	Linum spp.		
Chockecherry	Prunus virginiana		
Elderberry	Sambucus spp.		
Johnson grass	Sorghum halepense		
Sudan grass, broom, kafir corn	Sorghum sudanense		
Arrow grass, goose grass	Triglochin spp.		
Milkweed	See Table 9.13		
Foxglove	Digitalis purpurea	Cardiac glycosides highest in green plant, but dry leaves more palatable and are toxic	Colic, diarrhea (may be bloody), chewing, dyspnea, cardiac arrhythmia, and shock Tetany and death less than 24 hours after eating small amounts of the plant
Oleander	Nerium oleander		
Yellow oleander	Thevetia peruviana		
Be-Still or lucky nut tree	T. thevetioides		
Lily of the valley	Convallaria majalis		
Dogbane or Indian hemp	Apocynum cannabinum		
Larkspur	Delphinium spp.	Diterpenoid alkaloids high in green leaves and flowers	Excitable, stiff, base-wide stance, cannot stand and may have colic; death occurs within a few hours of eating plants
Monkshood	Aconitum spp.		
Poison, European, spotted hemlock	Conium maculatum	Piperidine alkaloids high in leaves and stems before fruit	Salivation, colic, tremors, ataxia, dyspnea, cyanosis, coma, and death within 2–3 h of eating small amounts of plants
Water hemlock	Cicuta spp.	Cicutoxin alkaloid in whole plant, especially the root	Salivation, chewing, teeth grinding, dilated pupils, tremors, violent convulsions, respiratory paralysis, and death within hours of eating 0.5 lb of plant or 1 root.
Yew	Taxus spp.	Taxine alkaloid in the whole plant	Nervous, dyspnea, ataxia, diarrhea, bradycardia, convulsions, and death shortly after eating about 1 lb
Death Camas	Zigadenus spp.	Zigacine and zigadenine alkaloids in all of plant, especially the onion-like	Salivation, colic, weakness, ataxia, and death within several days of eating 8–10 lb of plant bulb
Avocado (Guatemalan, not Mexican smooth-skin variety)	Persea americana	Unknown toxin in plant but not in ripe fruit flesh	Diarrhea, colic, and ongestive heart failure-induced edema of abdomen, neck, head, and lungs causing dyspnea and death in <2 days after eating leaves.

9.10.2 Toxicity of Cyanogenic Glycosides

There are at least 2,500 plant species in many families including Asteraceae, Chenopodiaceae, Euphorbiaceae, Fabaceae, Juncaginaceae, Linaceae, Poaceae, and Rosaceae that contain cyanogenic glycosides in their stems and leaves.[12,172,193–197] These plants normally contain one or more complex cyanogenic glycosides that are biosynthesized from amino acids to nitriles before being hydroxylated and glycosylated to cyanogenic glycosides. The glycosides are compartmentalized in plant cells and protected from plant enzymes. Damage to plant cells liberates the enzymes (glycosidases) that start hydrolysis of cyanogenic glycosides to form hydrogen cyanide.[193,195,196] Optimally this occurs at a pH greater than 4 or when plants are damaged as a result of drought, wilting, freezing, or being chewed. Application of herbicides and nitrate fertilizers may increase the cyanogenic glycoside content of plants. Generally, all parts of the plant are toxic with young rapidly growing plants and new growth being the most toxic. Maturation of the plant and drying reduces its cyanogenic glycoside content.

Plant-induced acute cyanide poisoning in horses is a rarity and is poorly documented.[96] In contrast, cyanide poisoning in ruminants is well documented. This species difference is related to the low pH of the horse's stomach in contrast to the more alkaline rumen (pH 6–7) that optimizes hydrolysis of glycosides. Rumen microflora play an important role in the rapid hydrolysis of plant glycosides. Animals that drink water immediately after eating cyanogenic plants enhance the hydrolysis of glycosides to cyanide. Acute cyanide poisoning depends on the rapid ingestion of large quantities of plant material high in cyanogenic glycosides and their conversion to cyanide faster than the animal's ability to detoxify the cyanide.

The cyanide ion (CN-) is highly toxic to all animals when it is inhaled as gaseous hydrogen cyanide or it is ingested as sodium or potassium cyanide.[198] Once absorbed, it binds with trivalent iron of cytochrome oxidase and other enzyme systems in hemoglobin, inhibiting electron transport, which results in decreased oxidative metabolism and oxygen utilization by the cells.[194] This produces the characteristic cherry-red color of venous blood and mucous membranes that is typical of acute cyanide poisoning. This cherry red coloration of blood disappears as anoxia becomes severe and cyanosis predominates. Normally, small quantities of cyanide are detoxified by cellular enzymes and endogenous thiosulfate to thiocyanates that are excreted in urine. The lethal dose of preformed cyanide salts (NaCN and KCN) for most species is 2.0–2.5 mg/kg.[195] Plant material containing more than 200 ppm of cyanide (200 mg/kg) in dry matter is potentially lethal to all animals.[199]

However, if there is plenty of other plant material and carbohydrates present in the stomach, formation and absorption of cyanide may be slowed, thus allowing the animal to tolerate a higher dose of cyanide.

9.10.3 Serviceberry or Saskatoon berry (*Amelanchier alnifolia*)

Serviceberry or Saskatoon berry is a native shrub or small tree that grows up to 13 feet (4 m) tall, primarily on rocky slopes, canyons, and stream sides at altitudes from 5,000–9,500 feet (1,500–2,900 m). Its leaves are simple, alternate, petioled, oval to suborbicular with margins coarsely serrate or dentate. The inflorescence is a raceme with perfect regular flowers (Figure 9.62). The five petals are white and 0.25–0.5 inches (6–10 mm) long. The ovary has five styles, developing into a purple fruit when ripe.

9.10.4 Wild Blue Flax (*Linum* spp.)

Wild blue flax is widely distributed throughout North America. It is an herbaceous perennial with tough slender stems and alternate slender leaves. Its bright blue flowers have five petals that drop off by midday (Figure 9.63). New flowers open each day. The young succulent plants are particularly toxic.

9.10.5 Western Chokecherry (*Prunus virginiana*)

Western chokecherry commonly grows in thickets, especially along waterways, mountainsides below about 8,000 feet (2,500 m) elevation, and occasionally in the drier plains. It grows to about 8–15 feet (2.5–5.0 m) high as a shrub or small tree with gray bark marked by lenticels running around the stems. The leaves are simple, glossy, and alternate with serrated margins and a few glands on the petiole or base of the blade. The inflorescence is a cylindrical raceme of showy white fragrant flowers appearing in early spring after the leaves have appeared (Figure 9.64). The fruit changes from a red to a dark purple drupe when ripe. It is the only edible part of the plant, having an astringent but sweet taste when ripe. Other common members of the genus known to be

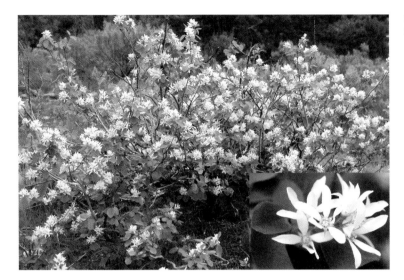

Figure 9.62 Serviceberry or Saskatoon berry (*Amelanchier alnifolia*) flowers.

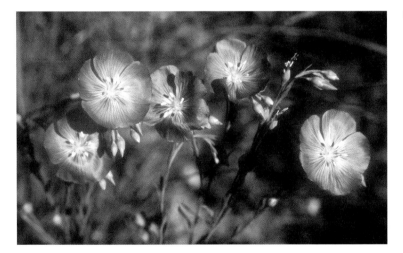

Figure 9.63 Wild blue flax (*Linum* spp.).

toxic include pin cherry (*P. pensylvanica*) and wild black cherry (*P. serotina*). All members of the cherry family should be considered toxic until proven otherwise.

9.10.6 Elderberry (*Sambuccus* spp.)

Elderberry is a woody shrub growing 6–10 feet (2–3 m) high and forming colonies from underground runners. Generally, elderberry bushes prefer open areas in rich moist soils surrounding ponds and along ditches and streams. The stems are thick and are filled with white pith. The leaves are opposite and pinnately compound with lanceolate serrated leaflets. It has conspicuous, terminal, round or flat-topped clusters of white five-petaled flowers

about 0.25 inch (4–6 mm) in diameter (Figure 9.65). Drooping clusters of dark purple (*S. canadensis*) or red (*S. racemosa*), juicy edible berries with several seeds form from July to September.

9.10.7 Sorghum Grasses

Johnson grass (*S. halepense*) is a coarse, drought-resistant perennial in the southern states and an annual in the northern states. It has scaly root stalks and relatively broad leaves and grows 6–8 feet (1–2 m) tall (Figure 9.38) as described previously in the section on neurologic disease-inducing plants. Sudan grass (*S. vulgare* var. *sudanense*) and its hybrids are corn-like in appearance

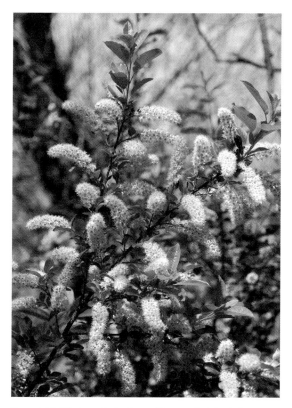

Figure 9.64 Western chokecherry (*Prunus virginiana*) flowers.

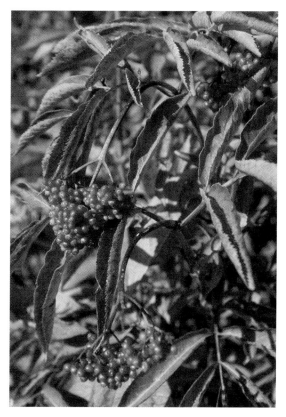

Figure 9.65 Elderberry (*Sambuccus* spp.) flowers and fruits.

(Figure 9.39) and are often grown as a forage crop. Cyanide-free varieties are available and are useful as forage crops.

9.10.8 Arrow grass or goose grass (*Triglochin* spp.)

Arrow grass or goose grass grows at most elevations throughout North America, preferring wet alkaline soils. It flourishes in marshy ground and irrigated pastures, often growing in native meadows cut for hay. It is a perennial grass-like plant with fleshy, half-rounded, dark green leaves clumped at the base of the plant. Leaves are 5–7 inches (12–18 cm) long, linear, unjointed, and sheathed at the base. The inflorescence is a pedicled raceme from 1.6–5.0 feet (0.5–1.5 m) in length that appears as an unbranched, unjoined flower spike (Figure 9.66). The flowers are inconspicuous and numerous with a greenish, 6-parted perianth. The fruits consist of three- to six-celled capsules that turn a golden brown before splitting.

9.10.9 Clinical Effects and Diagnosis of Acute Cyanide Poisoning

Animals poisoned by cyanogenic plants usually develop clinical signs and die within hours of consuming a lethal amount. Those that survive longer probably did not absorb a lethal dose and will recover. Sudden death is generally the presenting sign of cyanide poisoning. If observed early, poisoned animals show rapid labored breathing, frothing at the mouth, dilated pupils, ataxia, muscle tremors, and convulsions. Animals dying from acute cyanide poisoning may have characteristic cherry-red venous blood if examined immediately after death. The mucous membranes are often dark red to cyanotic because the animal is severely dyspneic and near death even though hemoglobin is saturated with oxygen. Generalized congestion and cyanosis is often seen at necropsy. Hemorrhages may be seen in the heart, lungs, and various other organs.

Acute cyanide poisoning can be confirmed by demonstrating the presence of either cyanide or cyanide-containing plants in the stomach of affected animals by

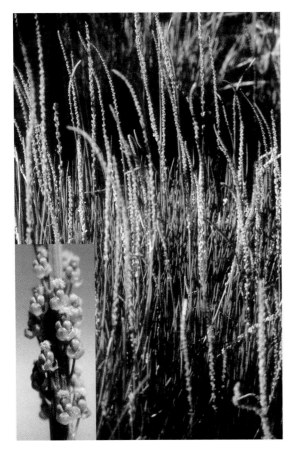

Figure 9.66 Arrow or goose grass (*Triglochin* spp.).

using the sodium picrate paper test.[200] Filter paper strips soaked in sodium picrate and dried will turn brick red if significant cyanide is present when they are suspended over suspect plant material in an airtight container.[199] A commercially available rapid test kit is also available and gives a blue reaction in the presence of cyanide.[201] Since cyanide is rapidly lost from animal tissues, specimens should be collected rapidly after death. If not analyzed immediately, they should be frozen in airtight containers for future analysis. Blood, spleen, liver, muscle, and stomach contents should be collected for analysis.

9.10.10 Treatment of Acute Cyanide Poisoning

Successful treatment of acute cyanide poisoning depends on rapid detoxification and excretion of the cyanide radical. Traditionally, this has been accomplished by intravenous sodium nitrite and sodium thiosulfate solution. Sodium nitrite converts hemoglobin to methemoglobin, to which cyanide binds to form relatively nontoxic cyanmethemoglobin. Sodium thiosulfate enhances cellular rhodonase biotransformation of cyanide to thiocynate which is excreted in urine. The recommended treatment for acute cyanide poisoning is a mixture of 1 ml of 20% sodium nitrite and 3 ml of 20% sodium thiosulfate/45 kg given intravenously.[19] This dose can be repeated in a few minutes if the desired response does not occur. Any stress to the animal should be avoided to avoid acute collapse.

Although not tested in horses, in sheep experimentally poisoned with cyanide, better results have been obtained by administering a 30–40% solution of sodium thiosulfate intravenously at 25–50 gm/100 kg.[202] Treatments tried in other animals with some benefit have not been validated in horses. These include the use of cobaltous chloride and α-ketoglutaric acid.[202,203] Sodium thiosulfate solution (30 g/450 kg) has been administered to cattle by orogastric tube to detoxify and remove toxic plant material still in the digestive tract. A similar treatment would seem logical for affected horses that have been observed eating new growth choke cherry leaves in the past few hours.

9.10.11 Cardiac Glycoside-Induced Sudden Death
9.10.11.1 Plant Causes of Cardiac Glycoside Poisoning
At least 34 plant genera contain cardiac glycosides that are potentially toxic to man and animals, but relatively few have attained importance as causes of animal poisoning.[2,12,97,204,205] The most important cardiac glycoside-containing plants in North America are listed in Table 9.12. These include milkweeds (*Asclepias* spp.), foxglove (*Digitalis* spp.), oleander (*Nerium oleander*), and lily of the valley (*Convallaria majalis*), which are widely grown as ornamental plants and have escaped to become established in the wild. Dogbane or Indian hemp (*Apocynum cannabinum*) is an indigenous plant containing cardiac glycosides but it is rarely a problem to livestock.

9.10.11.2 Milkweeds (*Asclepias* spp.)
Milkweeds are common cardiac glycoside-containing plants that are widely distributed throughout much of North America and are toxic either green or dried.

Table 9.13 Common toxic milkweeds.

Common Name	Scientific Name	Toxicity*
Labriform milkweed	*Asclepias labriformis*	0.05
Horsetail or whorled milkweed	*A. subverticillata*	0.2
Eastern whorled milkweed	*A. verticillata*	0.2
Woolypod milkweed	*A. eriocarpa*	0.25
Spider, antelopehorn milkweed	*A. asperula*	1–2
Plains or dwarf milkweed	*A. pumila*	1–2
Swamp milkweed	*A. incarnata*	1–2
Mexican whorled milkweed	*A. mexicana*	2.0
Showy milkweed	*A. speciosa*	2–5
Broad-leaf milkweed	*A. latifolia*	1.0
Slim-leafed milkweed	*A. stenophylla*	?
Butterfly milkweed	*A. tuberosa*	?
Green milkweed	*A. hirtella*	?
Green antelopehorn milkweed	*A. viridis*	?
Blood flower	*A. curassavica*	?

* Amount of green plant ingested as percent of body weight that is lethal (adapted from Kingsbury[240] and Ogden[217]).

Milkweed species identified to cause cardiac glycoside poisoning in sheep, goats, cattle, horses, and domestic fowl are listed in Table 9.13, as are their relative toxicities.[12,159,206–208] Greatest losses have occurred in sheep on western rangelands, but all animals are susceptible to poisoning, especially when other forages are scarce or milkweed is incorporated into hay.[159,209]

Milkweeds are perennial native plants with erect stems that have either broad-veined 2.5–5.0 inches (6–12 cm) leaves or narrow linear leaves seldom more than 1.0–1.5 inches (2–4 cm) wide, arranged either alternately or in whorls. Most species of milkweed (except butterfly weed, *A. tuberosa*) contain a milky sap. The flowers are produced in terminal or axillary umbels consisting of two five-parted whorls of petals, the inner one modified into a characteristic horn-like projection (Figure 9.67). The color of the flowers varies from greenish white to orange/red. The characteristic pod contains many seeds, each with a tuft of silky white hairs (Figure 9.68). The narrow-leafed species (Figure 9.69) generally tend to be the most toxic. A toxic dose of narrow leafed milkweed is 0.2% of body weight in green plant material.[210] Milkweeds grow in open areas along roadsides, waterways, and disturbed areas,

preferring the sandy soils of plains and foothills. Overgrazing will enhance the encroachment of milkweed.

9.10.11.3 Foxglove (*Digitalis purpurea*)
Foxglove is a native plant of Europe that was introduced to North America and escaped cultivation to become widespread in the northwest. It prefers disturbed rich soils along roadsides, fences, and unused areas. It is a perennial herb growing 3–5 feet (1–2 m) tall with alternate toothed, hairy basal leaves. The characteristic purple or white tubular pendant flowers have conspicuous spots on the inside bottom surface of the tube (Figure 9.70).

9.10.11.4 Oleander
Oleander (*Nerium oleander*) was introduced from the Mediterranean. It is an evergreen, showy, flowering shrub found in southern states from California to Florida. It is also grown as a potted house plant. Oleander is a perennial shrub or small tree up to 25 feet (8 m) tall with whorled, simple, narrow leathery leaves. All parts of the plant contain a sticky white sap. The showy white, pink, or red flowers (Figure 9.71) with five or more petals are produced in the spring and summer. Fruit pods contain many seeds, each with a tuft of brown hairs.

Yellow oleander, be-still or lucky nut tree (*Thevetia peruviana*) is a perennial branched shrub or small tree growing 30 feet (9 m) tall with dark green, glossy, alternate linear leaves up to 6 inches (15 cm) long and 0.5 inch (1 cm) wide containing a milky sap. The yellow to orange, showy, five-petalled tubular flowers are produced in clusters at the ends of branches (Figure 9.72).

Thevetia thevetioides is similar but tends to be much larger and has larger yellow flowers. Fruits are fleshy and triangular, turning yellow to black when ripe. Both species, native to tropical America, are widely cultivated in the southern United States and Hawaii and are a potential source of cardiac glycoside poisoning in all animals.

9.10.11.5 Pheasant's Eye (*Adonis aestivalis*)
Pheasant's eye is an introduced species from Europe that has become an invasive weed in some areas of North America. An annual, erect stemmed plant 8–40 inches (20–100 cm) tall with a taproot, basal leaves 1.2–2.0 inches (3–5 cm), pinnatifid, and 2–3 times divided.

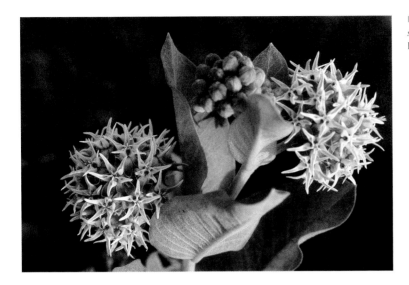

Figure 9.67 Milkweed flowers (*Asclepias speciosa*) showing the characteristic horn-like modified petal.

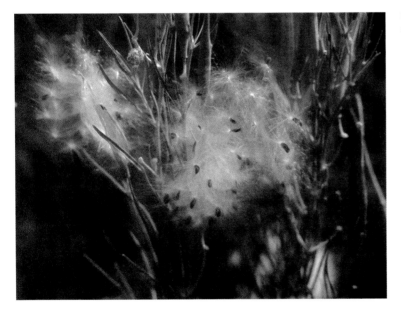

Figure 9.68 Milkweed pods and seeds (*Asclepias subverticillata*).

Flowers are showy, 0.6–1.4 inches (1.5–3.5 cm) in diameter with 6–8 petals; sepals appressed to petals, orange yellow, scarlet, or bright red-purple, usually with dark purple blotch at the base of the petals (Figure 9.73). Several cardenolides including adonitoxin, cymarin, and K-strophanthin are more potent than digitoxin and inhibit membrane–bound Na/K ATPase. Horses are most often poisoned by eating hay contaminated with the plant and exhibit gastrointestinal signs of colic, ileus, muscle tremors, tachycardia, and severe signs of shock.

9.10.11.6 Toxicity of Cardiac Glycosides

Cardiac glycosides are found in all plant parts and their concentrations are highest during rapid growth of the plant. Toxicity varies with the plant and growing conditions; however, all oleanders, foxglove, pheasant's eye, and narrow-leafed milkweeds should be considered potentially poisonous.[211] Only small amounts of these plants need to be eaten to invoke the potent effect of the toxins. In cattle and horses, as little as 0.005% of body weight or less than 1 oz for an 1100 lb horse (25 g/500 kg) of green

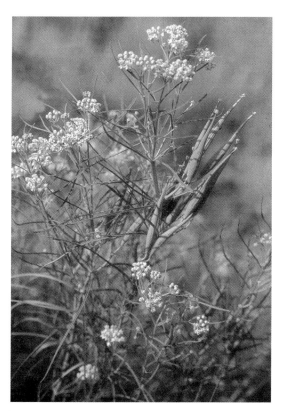

Figure 9.69 Narrow leafed or whorled milkweed (*Asclepias subverticillata*).

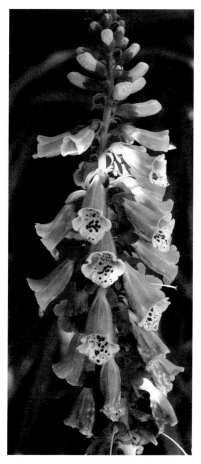

Figure 9.70 Foxglove (*Digitalis purpurea*).

oleander leaves is reportedly lethal.[28] About 2lb of green labriform milkweed is lethal to an 1100lb (500kg) horse. The relative toxicities of various species of milkweeds are given in Table 9.13. Horses, however, rarely eat green oleander or milkweed plants, apparently because of their taste, but seem to find the dried leaves more palatable. Because cardiac glycosides are retained in dried plants, although in reduced quantities, oleander, pheasant's eye, and milkweed pose the greatest threat if present in hay.

The most important of the cardiac glycosides are digoxin and digitoxin, present in *Digitalis* spp. and *Adonis* spp., oleandroside and nerioside in *Nerium oleander*, thevetin in yellow oleander (*T. peruviana*), and cardenolides in milkweed. Acute death from these plants results from their cardiac glycoside digitalis-like cardiotoxicity. This effect inhibits the cell membrane's sodium/potassium pump, resulting in irregular depolarization of myocardial cells.[159] This results in disorganized cardiac electrical activity that is manifested as a variety of arrhythmias and eventually cardiac arrest. The glycosides also act directly on the gastrointestinal tract, causing hemorrhagic enteritis that results in vomiting, colic, and diarrhea.[208] The cardiac glycosides, at least those in milkweed, also act on the respiratory and nervous systems, potentially causing dyspnea, muscle tremors, seizures, and head pressing.[212,213]

9.10.11.7 Clinical Signs of Cardiac Glycoside Poisoning

Animals consuming cardiac glycoside-containing plants are often found dead 8–10h later due to the profound effects of the toxins on the heart. Colic, vomiting, and diarrhea are also commonly encountered in animals poisoned with cardiac glycosides. If observed early in the course of poisoning, animals will exhibit labored breathing that may be rapid, although it is slow in sheep poisoned by milkweed. They also exhibit muscular

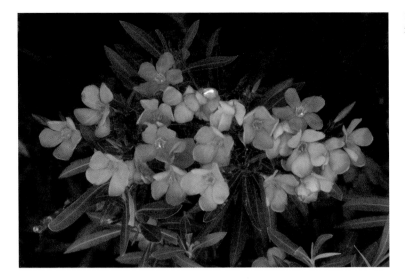

Figure 9.71 Oleander (*Nerium oleander*) flower with seed pod.

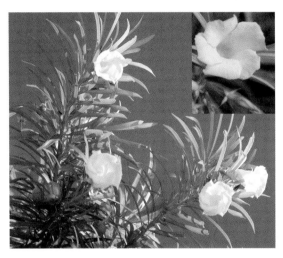

Figure 9.72 Yellow oleander (*Thevetia peruviana*) flower and fruit.

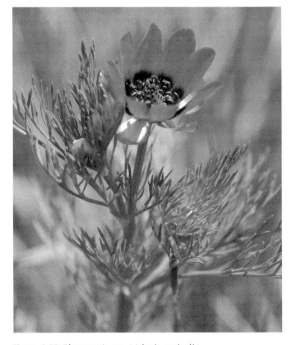

Figure 9.73 Pheasant's eye (*Adonis aestivalis*).

tremors, ataxia, inability to stand, bloating, and colic prior to death.[12,20,213] Horses, once recumbent, have periods of tetany and chewing movements.[12] The extremities are cold and there is a rapid, irregular and weak pulse due to the decreased cardiac output. All types of cardiac arrhythmias and heart blocks may be encountered at various stages of cardiac glycoside poisoning.[213] The duration of symptoms rarely exceeds 24 hours before death occurs. Convulsions prior to death are not common. There are no specific postmortem lesions in affected animals, but congestion of the lungs, stomach, and intestines is observed. Hemorrhages on the surfaces of the lungs, kidneys, and heart are commonly present.

9.10.11.8 Treatment of Cardiac Glycoside Poisoning

There is no specific treatment for counteracting the effects of cardiac glycosides. Horses should be given adsorbents such as activated charcoal (2–5 g/kg) by nasogastric tube with a saline cathartic to prevent further toxin absorption. Cardiac irregularities may be treated by carefully administering antiarrhythmic drugs such as potassium chloride, procainamide, lidocaine, dipotassium EDTA, or atropine sulfate. Although potassium administration helps control the severity of signs, potassium containing fluids should be administered only if hyperkalemia is not present and serum potassium concentration can be monitored closely. Intravenous fluids containing calcium should not be given because calcium augments the effects of the cardiac glycosides. Poisoned animals should be removed from the source of the plants, given fresh water, good-quality hay, shade, and kept as quiet as possible to avoid further stress on the heart. Animals that have not consumed a lethal dose of the plants recover over several days.

9.11 Larkspur

Larkspur poisoning is of greatest concern for cattle, causing more cattle fatalities in the western United States than any other naturally occurring plant species.[214,215] Horses are not as susceptible as cattle to the alkaloids in larkspur and are rarely poisoned. However, consumption of larkspur has the potential for causing poisoning in horses.

There are at least 80 species of larkspur or poison weed (*Delphinium* spp.) in North America, most of which grow in the western United States.[215] Larkspurs are erect, perennial herbaceous plants with simple or branched hollow stems and alternate, palmate divided leaves. The flowers are perfect and irregular and are carried in terminal racemes. They vary in color from white to red to dark blue/purple. The flower has five sepals, the uppermost one having an obvious spur (Figure 9.74). The corolla comprises two sets of two petals each with the two lower ones forming a claw and the upper two extending into the spur.

Larkspur poisoning is related to the quantity of toxic alkaloids in the plant. This varies with the plant species, stage of growth, amount ingested, and duration that the plant is eaten. Young, rapidly growing plants are the most toxic and the highest concentration of toxic alkaloids is in the leaves and flowers. *Delphinium barbeyi* is the most toxic of the larkspurs.[169,215,216] As little as 0.5% of body weight of green *D. barbeyi* is lethal to cattle.[217] Sheep can tolerate 3–4 times as much larkspur as cattle

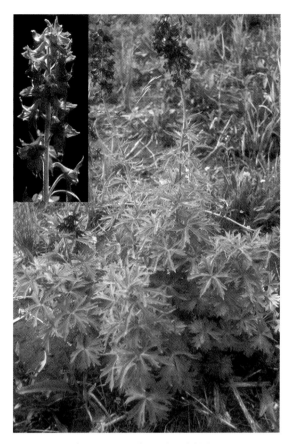

Figure 9.74 Larkspur or poison weed (*Delphinium* spp.) showing the characteristic spur of the flower.

and horses appear to be between cattle and sheep in susceptibility to larkspur poisoning.[215] A horse could therefore be poisoned by eating an amount equal to 1–2% of body weight in green larkspur, depending on the alkaloid content of the plant.

Larkspurs contain many diterpenoid alkaloids, 36 of which have been identified in the nine larkspur species that are most frequently associated with cattle poisoning.[175] To date, the most toxic of the alkaloids isolated from larkspur is methyllycaconitine.[175,218] The toxicity of the different larkspur species is, however, probably due to the combined effects of several alkaloids. The alkaloids act primarily at the neuromuscular junction (postsynaptic, nicotinic, and cholinergic receptors), causing a curare-like blockade with resulting muscle weakness and paralysis.[28,217]

Clinical signs of larkspur poisoning are best described in cattle but are similar in affected horses, sheep, and goats. Sudden death is often the first indication of lark-spur poisoning. Poisoned cattle initially show uneasiness, increased excitability, and muscle weakness that causes stiffness, staggering, and a base-wide stance. The front legs may be most severely affected, causing the animal to kneel before finally becoming recumbent. Frequent attempts to stand are uncoordinated and result in rapid exhaustion. Muscle twitching, abdominal pain, regurgitation, bloat, and constipation are common clinical findings. Aspiration of regurgitated rumen contents commonly leads to severe pneumonia and death. Cattle frequently die within 3–4 hours of consuming a lethal dose of larkspur.

Early diagnosis of larkspur poisoning through recognition of clinical signs and observation that horses have eaten larkspur is essential for successful treatment. Stress and excitement should be avoided as it will exacerbate respiratory distress and hasten death. Physostigmine (0.08 mg/kg, IV) has been shown to be effective in cattle about to collapse from larkspur poisoning.[169] Although not tested in horses, a similar dose may be used. Its administration may be repeated as needed over several hours until clinical signs have abated.

9.12 Monkshood

Monkshood or aconite (*Aconitum* spp.) frequently grows in the same habitat as larkspur and the alkaloids present in monkshood are similar in effects and toxicity to those of larkspur. The treatment for monkshood poisoning, therefore, is the same as for larkspur poisoning. Monkshood is a perennial herbaceous plant with tall leafy stems. The leaves are alternate, palmate lobed or parted, and similar to those of larkspur. The flowers are usually deep blue purple but occasionally white and carried on simple racemes or panicles. The flowers have five sepals that are petal-like with the upper sepal being larger and forming a characteristic helmet or hood (Figure 9.75). There are 2–5 petals, usually concealed within the hooded sepal.

9.13 Poison Hemlock

Poison, European, or spotted hemlock (*Conium maculatum*), although rarely eaten by horses or other livestock, will cause sudden death if consumed in even small

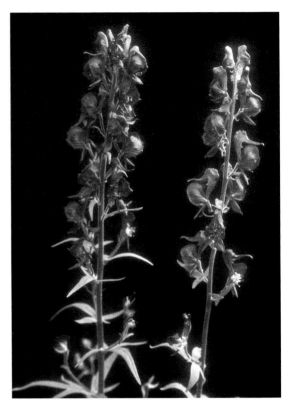

Figure 9.75 Monkshood or aconite (*Aconitum columbianum*)

amounts. Originally introduced from Europe, poison hemlock is found throughout North America growing along roadsides, ditches, cultivated fields, and waste areas, especially where the ground is moist. It is an erect, 3–6 foot (1–2 m) tall biennial or perennial plant. The branching stems are hollow and hairless, have purple spots especially near the base, and arise from a simple carrot-like tap root. Leaves are alternate, 3–4 times pinnately dissected, coarsely toothed, with a fern-like appearance. The terminal inflorescence is a compound, flat-topped, loose umbel with multiple, small, white five-petaled flowers (Figure 9.76). The fruits are gray-brown, ovoid, ridged, and easily separated into two parts.

At least five piperidine alkaloids, including coniine, are found in all parts of the plant, but especially in the leaves and stems prior to development of the fruit. Plants growing in the warmer southern states appear to be more toxic than those in the northern areas. Poison hemlock is toxic to all animals, including people.[12] Livestock seldom eat the plant because of its strong

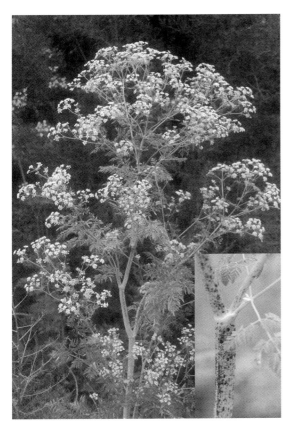

Figure 9.76 Poison, European, or spotted hemlock (*Conium maculatum*) showing the carrot-like leaves and spots on the stems.

pungent odor, but will do so if no other forage is available. Cattle have been fatally poisoned by eating as little as 1 lb (0.45 kg) of green poison hemlock plant. The mature or dried plant is less toxic.

Signs of poisoning develop within an hour of eating poison hemlock and, if a sufficient quantity has been consumed, death from respiratory failure occurs in 2–3 h. Salivation, colic, muscle tremors, and ataxia occur initially, followed by dyspnea, dilated pupils, weak pulse, cyanosis, coma, respiratory paralysis, and death.[219,220] Abortions may occur in pregnant animals that survive acute poisoning.[12]

Poison hemlock may cause abnormal fetal development if it is eaten early in gestation by ewes or sows,[220,221] but abortion has not been reported in mares.[191] Affected offspring may be born with crooked legs, deformed necks and spines, and cleft palates that are indistinguishable from similar deformities caused by the teratogenic effects of *Lupinus* and *Nicotiana* spp.[19,186,190,221–223] Although pregnant mares may exhibit the acute neurologic and gastrointestinal signs of poison hemlock poisoning, the fetus appears to be unaffected.[191]

Treatment should be directed at preventing further absorption of the toxin from the gastrointestinal tract and, if possible, providing positive pressure ventilation if respiratory paralysis is imminent. Respiratory stimulants are of questionable efficacy. Activated charcoal (0.5 kg/500 kg) in water with a saline cathartic should be given via nasogastric tube. Kaolin/pectin suspension (4 L) administered may also be used to prevent toxin absorption. Mineral oil may be administered (4 L/450 kg) as a laxative 4–6 h following the absorbents.

9.14 Water Hemlock

Water hemlock (*Cicuta* spp.) is extremely toxic, causing violent convulsions and sudden death within hours of consuming even a small amount. It is a stout, erect, hairless perennial growing to a height of 4–6 feet (1.2–1.8 m) from a close cluster of 2–8 thick tuberous roots. At the base of the hollow stem is a series of tightly grouped partitions containing an acrid yellow fluid (Figure 9.77). The leaves are alternate and 1–3 times pinnate; the lanceolate leaflets are 1–4 inches (3–10 cm) long, with toothed edges. The flowers are white and form a loose compound umbel (Figure 9.78). The fruits are oval and flattened laterally with prominent ribs. There are many species of water hemlock, with *C. maculata* found in the eastern half of North America and *C. douglasii* in the western half being the most common. Wet meadows, riverbanks, irrigation ditches, and water edges, are typical habitats.

The toxin in water hemlock is cicutoxin, a highly unsaturated alcohol and one of the most poisonous compounds known. All animals, including people, can be fatally poisoned by eating as little as 0.1–0.2 oz/100 lb (50–110 mg/kg) body weight of the plant. The lethal dose of fresh green *C. douglasii* for an adult horse is about 0.5 lb (250 g).[129] All parts of the plant, including the fluid found in the hollow stems are toxic. However, the toxin is concentrated in the roots. The roots are easily pulled up, as the ground is usually wet. Livestock consuming a single root are usually fatally poisoned.

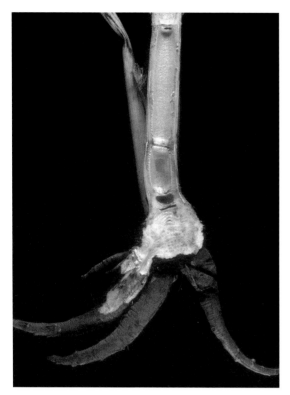

Figure 9.77 Water hemlock (*Cicuta douglasii*) tuberous roots and hollow partitioned stems.

The plant remains toxic when dry, although the mature leaves in late summer seem to have minimal toxicity to cattle. The roots, however, are highly poisonous at all times and 0.5% (wet weight) of body weight is fatal to horses.[12,220,224]

Cicutoxin is a potent neurotoxin causing rapid onset of muscle tremors and violent convulsions. Salivation, vigorous chewing movements, and teeth grinding are common. During the convulsions, animals have been known to bite off their tongues. Signs appear within a few hours of eating water hemlock and progress rapidly to convulsive seizures and lateral recumbency. Poisoned animals have dilated pupils and progress to a comatose state before dying from respiratory paralysis and asphyxia.

There is no specific antidote to cicutoxin. The animal should be heavily sedated or anesthetized to reduce the severity of the convulsions and laxatives should be given to hasten removal of the plant from the digestive system when possible.

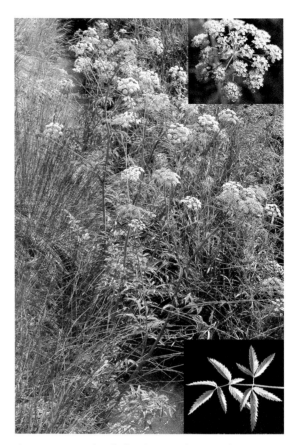

Figure 9.78 Water hemlock (*Cicuta maculatum*) umbel inflorescence and leaves with serrated edges.

9.15 Yew

Horses are highly susceptible to yews (*Taxus* spp.) with ingestion resulting in death following ataxia, nervousness, dyspnea, diarrhea, and convulsions.[225] Yews are evergreen shrubs or small trees with glossy, stiff, dark green, linear leaves 1.2–2.7 inches (3–7 cm) long with pointed ends, closely spaced on the branches. Inconspicuous axillary male and female flowers are produced on separate plants, forming showy red to yellow fruits containing a single seed (Figure 9.79). Several species of yew grow naturally or are grown as ornamental plants in North America. Yews generally prefer humid moist environments. Western yew (*Taxus brevifolia*) and Canada yew (*Taxus canadensis*) are two indigenous species. English yew (*Taxus baccata*) and Japanese yew (*Taxus cuspidata*) are commonly cultivated, non-native species in North America.

Figure 9.79 Yew (*Taxus* spp.) showing the fruits that resemble a pitted olive.

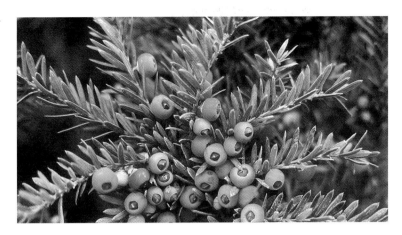

Yews contain the potent alkaloid taxine in all parts of the plant, green or dried, except the fleshy aril surrounding the seed.[12,236] Horses are highly susceptible to the cardiotoxic effects of the alkaloid, frequently dying shortly after eating small quantities of the plant (an amount equal to 0.05% of body weight in green leaves).[110] Livestock are often poisoned when fed yard trimmings from yews.

Sudden incoordination, nervousness, difficulty in breathing, slow heart rate, diarrhea, convulsions, and death are characteristic of yew poisoning in all animals.[12,237,238,239] Sudden death may be the only clinical sign observed in horses. There is no effective treatment for acute yew poisoning. A diagnosis of yew poisoning is usually made from the history of access to yew and sudden death, and pulmonary congestion, hemorrhage, and yew leaf fragments in the stomach at postmortem.[230,231] Taxine alkaloids in stomach contents can be detected using liquid chromatography and mass spectrometry.[232]

9.16 Death Camas

Horses that consume a sufficient amount of death camas (*Zigadenus* spp.) salivate and develop colic and ataxia and die within several days. There are approximately 15 species of death camas whose habitats range from moist mountain valleys to drier sandy hills and plains.[12] They appear in early spring, often growing amongst wild onion. They are herbaceous hairless perennials with grass-like, linear, V-shaped, parallel-veined leaves arising basally from an onion-like bulb

6–8 inches (15–20 cm) below the soil surface (Figure 9.80). However, death camas leaves are not hollow like those of onions, nor do they smell like onions when crushed. The bulb is covered with a membranous black outer coat. The inflorescence, a terminal raceme or panicle, has small, perfect, greenish white to yellow or pink flowers. The six-numbered perianth segments are separated, each with a gland at its base.

Several alkaloids, including zigacine and zigadenine are found in all parts of the plant, but especially the bulb.[12] Sheep are most frequently poisoned by death camas, but cattle, horses, and pigs may be affected.[13] Poisoning is most likely to occur in early spring when few other plants are available and the succulent shoots are especially enticing.

Sheep show signs of poisoning after eating as little as 0.5 lb (0.25 kg) of green plants. Convulsions, coma, and death occur if sheep eat 2–3% of body weight in green plants. Poisoning may occur in horses after they have eaten about 8–10 lb (4 kg) of plants. Salivation, colic, muscular weakness, and a staggering gait are reported in horses, with death occurring after several days. There are no specific lesions on postmortem examination.

In most cases of death camas poisoning, little can be done to reverse the toxicosis. Atropine sulfate (4 mg, SC) and picrotoxin (8 mg in 10 ml isotonic saline/100 kg) are reported to be effective in treating early poisoning in sheep.[57,166] The effectiveness in horses is not known. Horses may be given activated charcoal (0.5 kg/500 kg) or kaolin/pectin suspension (4 L) to decrease further alkaloid absorption. Supportive therapy, including intravenous fluid administration and analgesics is beneficial to manage signs of colic.

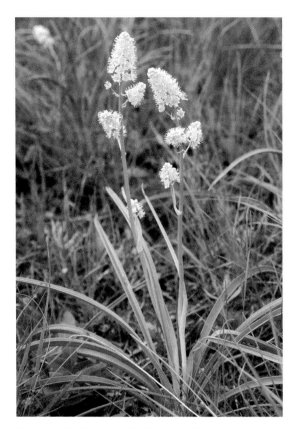

Figure 9.80 Death camas (*Zigadenus paniculatus*).

9.17 Avocado

Horses, cattle, goats, rabbits, and birds have been poisoned from eating leaves and other parts of the Guatemalan variety of avocado *Persea americana* var. *guatemalensis*.[29,171,232,233] The Mexican or smooth-skinned variety does not appear to be toxic.[90] The flesh of the ripe avocado fruit of neither variety is toxic. Horses are most likely to eat avocado plants if they are pastured in avocado orchards and normal forages are depleted. The toxin in the avocado plant is undefined. Horses develop a variety of clinical signs after eating the fruit, seeds, or leaves of avocado trees, including colic, diarrhea, and edema of the ventral abdomen, head, and neck.[29] In severely affected animals, there is marked edematous swelling of the head that is painful and causes upper respiratory dyspnea. Hydrothorax may develop, muffling heart sounds on auscultation. Elevation of serum creatinine phosphokinase and aspartate aminotransferase activity indicates muscle damage consistent with congestive heart failure.[29] Goats experimentally

poisoned with avocado leaves died within 48 hours and showed coagulative necrosis of the myocardium.[234] Birds also develop a cardiomyopathy.[235] In addition to the cardiotoxic effects of avocado, lactating mares and goats develop a noninfectious mastitis and agalactia due to necrosis of glandular epithelium of the mammary gland.[29,236] Horses should not be pastured in avocado orchards.

Glossary

Annual	A plant that lives only one growing season
Aril	A fleshy, usually colored, covering or attachment to a seed
Alternate	Singly along the stem, one leaf to a node
Awn	Bristle usually terminating a plant part
Axillary	Located at the junction of the leaf and the stem
Biennial	A plant that lives two growing seasons
Bract	A small leaf-like structure surrounding or below a flower
Calyx	An outer series or row of petals
Catkins	A scaly, spike-like inflorescence bearing unisexual flowers without petals, as in willows and cottonwoods
Chlorophyll	The green pigment of plants
Corolla	Collective term for petals
Cordate	Heart-shaped
Cyme	Flat-topped flower cluster, with the center flowers blooming first
Dentate	Tooth-like projections perpendicular to the leaf margin
Dioecious	Flowers that are unisexual; the staminate and pistillate are borne on separate plants
Diterpenoid	A compound with two hydrocarbon rings
Elliptic	A leaf that is tapered at both ends and widest in the middle
Fimbriate	Fringed
Flower, disk	A tubular flower in the central part of the floral head
Flower, ray	A single, petal-like symmetric flower around the edge of the floral head, as in sunflowers
Follicle	A dry, dehiscent fruit that splits down one side only, as in milkweeds
Frond	Leaf of a fern

Inflorescence The flowering part of the plant

Glabrous Smooth, without hairs

Hastate Shaped like an arrowhead, with the basal lobes turned outward

Involucre A circle of bracts under or at the base of a flower

Lanceolate Lance-shaped

Lectins A plant protein with carbohydrate-binding properties

Lenticels Wart-like spots on the bark

Monoecious Staminate and pistillate flowers on the same plant

Monoterpene A single-ringed hydrocarbon ($C_{10}H_{16}$)

Node The point of leaf attachment on the stem

Nutlet A small nut

Obovate Ovate leaf with the widest part near the apex and attached to the stem at its narrow end

Ocrea United appendages (stipules) surrounding the base of the petiole or leaf stock

Orbicular Circular in outline

Ovary Swollen base of the pistil (female reproductive organs of the flower) in which seeds form

Ovate Egg-shaped in outline, with attachment to the stem at its wide end

Opposite Two leaves per node or point of leaf attachment

Palmate Leaf lobes spreading like fingers on the palm of the hand

Panicle A compound raceme with the flowers on the terminal branchlets

Pappus Bristles at the tip of the single non-splitting fruit of the sunflower family

Pedicel Stalk of a single flower

Perennial A plant living more than two growing seasons

Perianth Collective term for flower structures

Petal One of the individual parts of the corolla or petals

Petaloid Having the form or appearance of a petal

Petiole The leaf stalk

Pinnate A compound leaf generally with pairs of leaflets along the rachis or the main stem bearing the leaves

Pistillate A flower with only female reproductive structures

Pome An apple-like fruit

Raceme An arrangement of flowers along a stem with one flower per node and the youngest flowers toward the apex

Rachis The main stem or axis bearing flowers or leaves

Rhizome An underground laterally growing stem that sends out shoots above ground and roots below

Saponins Plant glycosides capable of producing soap-like stable foam with water

Sepal Outer part of the flower or perianth, which is usually green

Serrate With pointed or sharp forward-pointing teeth

Sessile Without a stalk of any kind

Shrub Woody perennial, smaller than a tree, usually with several basal stems

Stamen Pollen-bearing structures of the flower

Staminate Having stamens only

Stipules Small leaf-like structure just below the leaf's attachment to the stem

Style The stalk attached to the tip of the ovary

Stylopodium A disk-like expansion of the style

Taproot The primary carrot-like root

Tuberous A thickened potato-like root, usually an underground stem with numerous eyes or nodes

Umbel A flat or rounded flower cluster in which the stalks radiate from a common point like an umbrella

Weed "A plant whose virtues have not yet been discovered" – Ralph Waldo Emerson

Whorled A circle of three or more leaves or branches at a node on the stem

Supplemental Reading

Poisonous Plants of the United States and Canada, John M. Kingsbury (Prentice-Hall Inc, Englewood Cliffs, NJ, 1964). This text provides historical information on poisonous plants in North America. It is particularly valuable when seeking information on early reports of plant poisoning, as it has an extensive bibliography covering plant poisoning reports from the beginning of the eighth century. Botanically, the book covers all groups of toxic plants. The limitation of the book is that it contains relatively few color photographs that would make plant identification easier for those that are not botanists. There has been no other edition of the book since 1964.

Toxic Plants of North America, George E. Burrows and Ronald J. Tyrl (Iowa State Press/Ames 2001). This is the most authoritative and comprehensive book on plant poisoning of animals in North America. It has an extensive bibliography and covers many new plant toxicities that are absent from Kingsbury's book. It is however relatively expensive and has relatively few photographs, relying on line-drawing illustrations

A Guide to Plant Poisoning of Animals in North America, Anthony P. Knight and Richard G. Walter (Teton New Media, Jackson, Wyoming 2001).

This book provides useful information to the horse owner while not being as expensive as the former. The book is organized by the major presenting clinical signs of poisoning with important poisonous plants illustrated with color photographs and their distribution, toxic principle, clinical signs, and treatments where possible.

Weeds of the West, Tom D. Whitson, published by the University of Wyoming in cooperation with the Western Society of Weed Science and the Western United States Land Grant Universities Cooperative Extension Services. (Pioneer of Jackson Hole, 132 West Gill Street, Jackson Hole, WY, 83001, 1991.) This book, although geographically limited to plants of the Rocky Mountain-Great Plains area of the United States and covering weeds that are not necessarily toxic, has outstanding color photographs of each plant that makes identification easy. It is written for livestock owners and is a useful book for weed identification important to pasture management. It does not, however, cover the toxicology of plants other than to mention those that are likely to be a problem to animals. With over 600 color pictures of the common important weeds, this book is well worth possessing.

References

1. Shupe JL, James LF. Teratogenic plants. Vet Hum Toxicol 1972;25:415–421.
2. Thompson GW, Barker IK. Japanese yew (Taxus cuspidata) poisoning in cattle. Can Vet J 1978;19:320–321.
3. James LF: Plant-induced congenital malformations in animals. World Rev Nutr Diet 1977;26:208–224.
4. Young S, Brown WW, Klinger B. Nigropallidal encephalomalacia in horses caused by the ingestion of weed of the genus Centaurea. J Am Vet Med Assoc 1970; 157:1602–1605.
5. James LF, Hartley WJ, Van Kampen KR. Syndromes of Astragalus poisoning in livestock. J Am Vet Med Assoc 1981;178:146–150.
6. Tehon LR, Morrill CC, Graham R. Illinois Plants Poisonous to Livestock. Univ Illinois, Coll Agr Ext Serv, Circular 1946; 599:55–57.
7. O'Sullivan BM. Crofton weed (Eupatorium adenophorom) toxicity in horses. Aust Vet J 1979;55: 19–21.
8. Cordy DR. Nigropallidal encephalomalacia in horses associated with the ingestion of yellow star thistle. J Neuropathol Exp Neurol 1954;13:330–342.
9. Keeler RF: Teratogens in plants. J Anim Sci 1984;58: 1029–1039.
10. True RG, Lowe JE, Heissen J. Black walnut shavings as a cause of laminitis. Proc Am Assoc Equine Pract 1978;24:511–515.
11. Couch JF. The toxic constituent of richweed or white snakeroot (Eupatorium urticaefolium). J Agr Res 1927;35: 547–576.
12. Giles CJ. Outbreak of ragwort (Senecio jacobaea) poisoning in horses. Equine Vet J 1983;15:248–250.
13. McDonald GK. Moldy sweet clover poisoning in a horse. Can Vet J 1980;121:250–251.
14. Way JL. Cyanide intoxication and its mechanism of antagonism. In: George R, Okun R, Cho AK, eds. Annual Review of Pharmacology and Toxicology. Volume 24. Annual Reviews, Palo Alto, CA, 1984;451–481.
15. Siegler DS. Plants of the northeastern United States that produce cyanogenic compounds. Economic Botany 1976;30:395–407.
16. Staley EE. An approach to the treatment of locoism in horses. Vet Med Small Anim Clin 1978;73:1205–1206.
17. Araya OS, Ford EJ. An investigation of the type of photosensitization caused by the ingestion of St. John's Wort (Hypericum perforatum) in calves. J Comp Pathol 1981;91: 135–141.
18. Gard GP, de Sarem WG, Ahrens PJ. Nigropallidal encephalomalacia in horses in New South Wales. Aust Vet J 1973;49:107–108.
19. Sockett DC, Baker JC, Stowe CM. Slaframine (Rhizoctonia legummicola) intoxication in horses. J Am Vet Med Assoc 1982;181:606.
20. White JL, Shivaprasad HL, Thompson U, et al. White snakeroot (Eupatorium rugosum) poisoning. Clinical effects associated with cardiac and skeletal muscle lesions in experimental equine toxicosis. In Seawright AA, ed. Plant toxicology. Proc Australia-USA Symp Poisonous Plants, Dominion Press-Hodges' & Bell, Melbourne, 1985;411–422.
21. Bull LB, Culvenor CCJ, Dick AT. The pyrrolizidine alkaloids: their chemistry, pathogenicity and other biological properties. North Holland Publishing Co, Amsterdam, 1968.

22. Clare NT. Photosensitization in animals. Adv Vet Sci Comp Med 1955;2:182–211.

23. James LF, Hartley WJ, Williams MC, et al. Field and experimental studies in cattle and sheep poisoned by nitro-bearing Astragalus and their toxins. Am J Vet Res 1980;41:377–382.

24. Panciera RJ. Oak poisoning in cattle. In: Keeler RF, Van Kampen KR, James LE, eds. Effects of poisonous plants on livestock. Academic Press, New York, 1978;499–506.

25. Molyneux RJ, James LF. Loco intoxication: indohizidine alkaloids of spotted locoweed (Astragalus lentigenosus). Science 1982;216:190–191.

26. Shrift A. Metabolism of selenium by plants and microorganisms. In: Kalyman DL, Gunther WHH, eds. Organic selenium compounds: their chemistry and biology. John Wiley & Sons, Inc., New York, 1973:763–773.

27. Rosenfeld I, Beath OA. Selenium. In: Geobotany, biochemistry, toxicity and nutrition. Academic Press, New York, 1964;141–213.

28. Williams MC, Barneby RC. The occurrence of nitro-toxins in North American Astragalus (Fabaceac). Brittonia 1977;29:310–326.

29. Panter KE, Bunch TD, Keeler RE. Maternal and fetal toxicity of poison hemlock (Conium maculatum) in sheep. Am J Vet Res 1988;49:281–283.

30. Minnick PD, Brown CM, Braselton WE, et al. The induction of equine laminitis with an aqueous extract of the heartwood of black walnut (Juglans nigra). Vet Hum Toxicol 1987;29:230–233.

31. Henderson JA, Evans EV, McIntosh RA. The antithiamine action of Equisetum. J Am Vet Med Assoc 1952;120:375–378.

32. Henson JB, Dollahite JW. Toxic myodegeneration in calves produced by experimental Cassia occidentalis intoxication. Am J Vet Res 1966;27:947–949.

33. Clarke ML. Cyanides. In Clarke ML, Harvey DG, eds. Veterinary toxicology. 2nd ed. Bailliere Tindall, Philadelphia, 1981;172–178.

34. Crinion RAP, O'Conner JP. Selenium intoxication in horses. Irish Vet 1978;J 32:81–86.

35. Kirk JH, Bulgin MS. Effects of feeding cull domestic onions (Allium cepa) to sheep. Am J Vet Res 1979;40:397–399.

36. Van Kampen KR. Sudan grass and sorghum poisoning of horses: a possible lathyrogenic disease. J Am Vet Med Assoc 1970;156:629–630.

37. Barneby RC. Atlas of North American astragalus. Memoirs

38. Lott DG. The use of thiamine in Mare's Tail poisoning in horses. Can J Comp Med 1951;15:274–278.

39. Garrett BJ, Holtman DW, Cheeke PR, et al. Effects of dietary supplementation with butylated hydroxyanisole, cysteine, and vitamin B on tansy ragwort (Senecio jacobaea) toxicosis in ponies. Am J Vet Res 1984;45:459–464.

40. Craigmill AL, Seawright AA, Mattilla T, et al. The toxicity of avocado (Persea americana) leaves for the lactating mammary gland of the goat. In: James LF, Keeler RF, Bailey EM, Cheeke PR, Hegarty MP, eds. Poisonous Plants Proceedings Third International Symposium. Iowa State University Press, Ames, 1992;623–625.

41. Cary CA. Poisonous action of red buckeye on horses, mules, cattle, hogs, and fish. Alabama Agr Exp Stat Bul 1922;218:1–40.

42. Pritchard JT, Voss JL. Fetal ankylosis in horses associated with hybrid pasture. J Am Vet Med Assoc 1967;150:871–873.

43. Young S, Brown WW, Klinger B. Nigropailidal encephalomalacia in horses fed Russian knapweed (Centaurea repens). Am J Vet Res 1970;31:1393–1404.

44. McKenzie RA, McMicking LI. Ataxia and urinary incontinence in cattle grazing sorghum. Aust Vet J 1977;53:496–497.

45. Olsen JD. Larkspur toxicosis: a review of current research. In: Keeler RE, Van Kampen KR, James LF, eds. Effects of poisonous plants on livestock. Academic Press, New York, 1978;535–543.

46. Cheeke PR, Shull LR. Natural toxicants in feeds and poisonous plants. AVI Publishing Co, Westport, CT, 1985;199–204.

47. Olsen JD, Manners GD. Toxicology of diterpenoid alkaloids in rangeland larkspur (Delphinium spp.). In: Cheeke PR, ed. Toxicants of plant origin. Vol 1. Alkaloids. CRC Press, Boca Raton, FL, 1989;291–326.

48. James LF. Suspected phytogenic selenium poisoning in sheep. J Am Vet Med Assoc 1982;180:1478–1481.

49. Morris KLM, Levack VM. Evidence for aqueous soluble vitamin D-like substances in the calcigenic plant, Trisetum flavescens. Life Sci 1982;30:1255–1266.

50. Keeler RF. Teratogenic effects of Conium maculatum and Conium alkaloids and analogs. Clin Toxicol 1978;12:49–64.

51. Olson OE: Selenium in plants as a cause of livestock poisoning. In: Keeler RE, Van Kampen KR, James LF, eds. Effects of poisonous plants on livestock. Academic Press, New York, 1978;121–133, 535–543.

52. Galey FD, Beasley VR, Twardock AR, et al. Pathophysiologic effects of an aqueous extract of black walnut (Juglans nigra) when administered via nasogastric tube to the horse. In: James LF, Keeler RF, Bailey EM, Cheeke PR, Hegarty MP, eds. Poisonous Plants Proc 3rd Intl Symp. Iowa State University Press, Ames, 1992;630–635.

53. Huxtable CR. Toxicity problems associated Swainsona spp., Stypandra imbricata, Isotropis spp. Vet Clin Toxicol Proc 103. University of Sydney, 1987;85–90.

54. Galey FD, Beasley VR, Schaeffer D, et al. Effect of an aqueous extract of black walnut (Juglans nigra) on isolated equine digital vessels. Am J Vet Res 1990;51:83–88.

55. Gulick BA, Liu 1K, Quails CW, et al. Effect of pyrrolizidine alkaloid-induced hepatic disease on plasma amino acid patterns in the horse. Am J Vet Res 1980;41:1894–1898.

56. Hooper PT, Hart B, Smith GW. The prevention and treatment of Birdsville disease of horses. Aust Vet J 1971;47:326–329.

57. Karns PA. Intoxication in horses due to ingestion of Japanese yew (Taxus cuspidata). Equine Pract 1983;5:12–15.

58. Humphreys DJ. Veterinary toxicology. 3rd Ed. Baillere Tindall, London, 1988;276–277.

59. Rowe LD. Photosensitization problems in livestock. Vet Clin North Am Food Anim Pract 1989;5:301–323.

60. Stair EL, Edwards WC, Burrows GE, et al. Suspected red maple (Acer rubrum) toxicosis with abortion in two Percheron mares. Vet Hum Toxicol 1993;35:229–230.

61. Duncan CS. Oak leaf poisoning in two horses. Cornell Vet 1961;51:159–162.

62. Traub-Dargatz JL, Knight AP, Hamar DW. Selenium toxicity in horses. Compend Contin Educ Pract Vet 1986;8:771–776.

63. Hooper PT. Epizootic cystitis in horses. Aust Vet J 1968;44:11–14.

64. Pierce KR, Joyce JR, England RB, et al. Acute hemolytic anemia caused by wild onion poisoning in horses. J Am Vet Med Assoc 1972;160:323–327.

65. Thorp F, Harshfield GS. Onion poisoning in horses. J Am Vet Med Assoc 1939;94:52–53.

66. Williams MC, Stermitz FR, Thomas RD. Nitrocompounds in Astragalus species. Phytochemistry 1975;14:2306–2308.

67. Keeler RF, Balls LD, Shupe JL, et al. Teratogenicity and toxicity of confine in cows, ewes and mares. Cornell Vet 1980;70:19–26.

68. Herbert CD, Flory W, Seger C, et al. Preliminary isolation of a myodegenerative toxic principle from Cassia occidentalis. Am J Vet Res 1983;44:1370–1374.

69. Rebhun WC, Georgi M, Georgi JR. Persistent corneal ulcers in horses caused by embedded burdock pappus bristles. Vet Med 1991;86:930–935.

70. Binns W, Keeler RE, Balls UD. Congenital deformities in lambs, calves and goats resulting from maternal ingestion of Veratrum californicum. Clin Toxicol 1972;5:245–261.

71. James LF, Van Kampen KR. Acute and residual lesions of locoweed poisoning in cattle and horses. J Am Vet Med Assoc 1971;158:614–618.

72. Morton JF. Creeping indigo (Indigofera spicata Forsk.) (Fabaccae)-A hazard to herbivores in Florida. Economic Botany 1989;43:314–327.

73. James LF, Shupe JL, Binns W, et al. Abortive and teratogenic effects of locoweed on cattle and sheep. Am J Vet Res 1967;28:1379–1386.

74. Keeler RF. Coniine, a teratogenic principle from Conium maculatum producing congenital malformations in calves. Clin Toxicol 1974;7:195–206.

75. McCulloch EC. Hepatic cirrhosis of horses, swine, and cattle due to ingestion of seeds of the tarweed, Amsinckia intermedia. J Am Vet Med Assoc 1940;96:5–18.

76. Rolins JB, Wigton DH, Clement TH. Heinz body anemia associated with lymphosarcoma in a horse. Equine Pract 1991;13:20–23.

77. Romane WM, Adams I.G, Bullard TL, et al. Cystitis syndrome in horses. Proc Am Assoc Equine Pract, 1965;65–69.

78. Divers TJ, George LW, George JW. Hemolytic anemia in horses after the ingestion of red maple leaves. J Am Vet Med Assoc 1982;180:300–302.

79. Rogers GR, Knight H, Gulick BA. Proposed method of diagnosis and treatment of pyrrolizidine alkaloid toxicity in horses.

In: Checke PR, ed. Symposium on pyrrolizidine (Senecio) alkaloids: toxicity, metabolism and poisonous plant control measures. Oregon State University, Corvallis, 1979;145–147.

80. Lowe JE, Hintz HF, Schryver HF, et al. Taxus cuspidata (Japanese yew) poisoning in horses. Cornell Vet 1970;60:36–39.

81. Burrows GE, Edwards WC, Tyrl RJ. Toxic plants of Oklahoma: groundsels and rattlebox. Oklahoma Vet Med Assoc J 1983;35:115–118.

82. Hagler WM, Croom WJ. Slaframine: occurrence, chemistry, and physiological activity. In: Cheeke PR, ed. Toxicants of plant origin. CRC Press, Boca Raton, FL, 1989;258–279.

83. Ralston SL, Rich VA. Black walnut toxicosis in horses. J Am Vet Med Assoc 1983;183:1095.

84. Wilson RB, Scruggs DW. Duodenal obstruction associated with persimmon fruit ingestion by two horses. Equine Vet Sci 1992;12:26–27.

85. Craig AM: Serum enzyme tests for pyrrolizidine alkaloid toxicosis in cattle and horses. In: Cheeke PR, ed. Symposium on Pyrrolizidine (Senecio) Alkaloids: Toxicity, Metabolism, and Poisonous Plant Control Measures. Nutrition Res Instit, Oregon State Univ, Corvallis, OR, 1979;135–143.

86. McDaniels LH. Perspective on the black walnut toxicity problem. Cornell Vet 1987;29:230–233.

87. Benson JM, Seiber JN, Bagley CV, et al. Effects on sheep of the milkweeds Asclepias eriocarpa and A. labriformis and of cardiac glycoside-containing derivative material. Toxicon 1979;17:155–165.

88. Warren CGB, Vaughan SM. Acorn poisoning. Vet Rec 1985;116:82.

89. McKenzie RA, Brown OP. Avocado (Persea americana) poisoning of horses. Aust Vet J 1991;68:77–78.

90. Barney GH, Wilson BJ. A rare toxicity syndrome in ponies. Vet Med 1963;58:419–421.

91. Krook L, Wasserman RH, Shively JN, et al. Hypercalcemia and calcinosis in Florida horses: implication of the shrub Cestrum diurnum as the causative agent. Cornell Vet 1975;65:26–56.

92. Lewis WIT, Elvin-Lewis MP. Contributions to herbology in modern medicine and dentistry. In: Keeler RF, Tu AT, eds. Plant and fungal toxins. Vol 1. Edited by Marcel Dekker, New York, 1983;802–810.

93. Mahin L, Marzou A, Huart A. A case of Nerium oleander poisoning in cattle. Vet Hum Toxicol 1986;26:303–304.

94. Benson JM, Seiber JN, Kceler RE, et al. Studies on the toxic principle of Asclepias eriocarpa and Aselepias labrtformis. In: Keeler RF, Van Kampen KR, James LF, eds. Effects of poisonous plants on livestock. Academic Press, New York, 1978;273–284.

95. Burrows GE, Way JL. Cyanide intoxication in sheep: enhancement of efficacy of sodium nitrite, sodium thiosulfate and cobaltous chloride. Am J Vet Res 1979;40:613–617.

96. Knight AP, Ingram JI, Traub-Dargatz J, et al. Personal communication, 1993.

97. Ogden L, Burrows GE, Tyrl RJ, et al. Experimental intoxication in sheep by Asclepias. In: James LF, Keeler RE, Bailey EM, Cheeke PR, Hegarty MP, eds. Poisonous Plants

Proceedings Third International Symposium. Iowa State University Press, Ames, 1992;495–499.

98. Craigmill AL, Eide RN, Schultz TA, et al. Toxicity of avocado (Persea americana var Guatemalan): Review and preliminary report. Vet Hum Toxicol 1984;26:381–383.

99. Lin TL Ramstad E, Heinstein P. In vivo biosynthesis of isopentyl-acetophenones in Eupatorium rugosum. Phyto Chem 1974;13:1809–1815.

100. George LW, Divers TJ, Mahaffey EA, et al. Heinz body anemia and methemoglobinemia in ponies given red maple (Acer rubrum L.) leaves. Vet Pathol 1982;19:521–533.

101. Kingsbury JM. Poisonous plants of the United States and Canada. Kingsbury JM, eds. Prentice-Hall, Englewood Cliffs, NJ, 1964;1–466.

102. Radostits OM, Searcy GP, Mitchall KG. Moldy sweet clover poisoning in cattle. Can Vet J 1980;21:155–158.

103. Sampson AW, Malmsten HE. Stock poisoning plants of California. Calif Agr Exp Sta Bull 1942;593:22–25.

104. Buck VT, Osweiler GD. Selenium. In: Van Gelder GA, eds. Clinical and diagnostic veterinary toxicology. 2nd Ed. Kendall Hunt, Dubuque, IA, 1976;345–354.

105. Stermitz FR, Lowry WT, Norris FA. Aliphatic nitro compounds from Astragalus species. Phytochemistry 1972; 11:1117–1124.

106. Geor RJ, Becker RL, Karnara EW, et al. Toxicosis in horses after ingestion of hoary alyssum. J Am Vet Med Assoc 1992;201:63–67.

107. Hegarty MP: Toxic amino acids of plant origin. In: Keeler RF, Van Kampen KR, James LE, eds. Effects of poisonous plants on livestock. Academic Press, New York, 1978;575–585.

108. Williams S Scott P. The toxicity of Datura stramonium (thorn apple) to horses. NZ Vet 1981;32:47.

109. Beath OA, Eppson HE, Gilbert CS, et al. Poisonous plants and livestock poisoning. University of Wyoming Agr Exp St. Bulletin 1939;231.

110. Fincher MG, Fuller HK. Photosensitization-trifoliosis-light sensitization. Cornell Vet 1942;32:95–98.

111. Kubota J, Allaway JH, Carter DL, et al. Selenium in crops in the United States in relation to selenium-responsive diseases in animals. J Agric Food Chem 1967; 15:448–453.

112. Oehme FW, Barbie WE, Hulbert LC. Astragalus mollissimus (locoweed) toxicosis of horses in western Kansas. J Am Vet Med Assoc 1968;152:271–278.

113. Dickinson JO, Cooke MP, King RR, et al. Milk transfer of pyrrolizidine alkaloids in cattle. J Am Vet Med Assoc 1986;169:1192–1196.

114. Hagler WM, Behlow RF. Salivary syndrome in horses: Identification of slaframine in red clover hay. Appl Environ Microbiol 1981;42:1067–1073.

115. Hargis AM, Stauber E, Casteel S, et al. Avocado (Persea americana) intoxication in caged birds. J Am Vet Med Assoc 1989;194:64–66.

116. Morris KLM. Plant-induced calcinosis: a review. Vet Hum Toxicol 1982;24:34–48.

117. Dewes HF, Lowe MD. Hemolytic crisis associated with ragwort poisoning and rail chewing in two Thoroughbred fillies. NZ Vet J 1985;33:159–160.

118. Henson JB, Dollahite JW, Bridges CH, et al. Myodegeneration in cattle grazing Cassia species. J Am Vet Med Assoc 1965;147:142–145.

119. Van Kampen KR, James LF. Manifestations of intoxication by selenium-accumulating plants. In: Keeler RF, Van Kampen KR, James LE, eds. Effects of poisonous plants on livestock. Academic Press, New York, 1978;135–145.

120. James LF, Van Kampen KR, Hartley WJ. Astragalus bisulcatus – a cause of selenium or locoweed poisoning. Vet Hum Toxicol 1983;26:86–89.

121. Dollahite JW, Younger RL, Hoffman GO. Photosensitization in cattle and sheep caused by feeding Ammi majus (Greater Ammi, bishop's weed). Am J Vet Res 1978;39:193–197.

122. Roberts HE, Evans ET, Evans WC. The production of "bracken staggers" in the horse, and its treatment with vitamin B1 therapy. Vet Rec 1949;61:549–550.

123. Siegler DS. Plants of Oklahoma and Texas capable of producing cyanogenic compounds. Proc Okla Acad Sci 1976;56:95–100.

124. Olsen JD. Tall larkspur poisoning in cattle and sheep. J Am Vet Med Assoc 1978;173:762–765.

125. Williams MC, Olsen JD. Toxicity of three Aesculus spp. to chicks and hamsters. Am J Vet Res 1984;45:539–541.

126. Benson ME, Casper HH, Johnson U. Occurrence and range of dicumarol concentrations in sweet clover. Am J Vet Res 1981;42:2014–2015.

127. Sharma RP, James LF, Molyneux RJ. Effect of repeated locoweed feeding on peripheral lymphocyte function and plasma proteins in sheep. Am J Vet Res 1984;45:2090–2093.

128. Welch BL, McArthur ED. Variation of monoterpenoid content among subspecies and accessions of Artemisia tridentata grown in a uniform garden. J Range Mgt 1981;34:380–384.

129. Mendel VE, Witt MR, Gitchell BS, et al. Pyrrolizidine alkaloid induced liver disease in horses: an early diagnosis. Am J Vet Res 1988;49:572–578.

130. Pigeon RE, Camp BJ, Dollahite JW. Oral toxicity and polyhydroxyphenol moiety of tannin isolated from Ouercus havardii (Shin oak). Am J Vet Res 1962;23: 1268–1270.

131. Couch JF. Trembles (or milk sickness). US Dept Agr, Washington, DC. Circular No. 306, 1933.

132. Hooper PT. Pyrrolizidine alkaloid poisoning: pathology with particular reference to differences in animal and plant species. In: Keeler RF, Van Kampen KR, James LE, eds. Effects of poisonous plants on livestock. Academic Press, New York, 1978;161–176.

133. Snyder SP. Livestock losses due to tansy ragwort poisoning. Oregon Agr Record 1972;255:2–4.

134. Stillman AE, Huxtable R, Consroe P, et al. Hepatic veno-occlusive diseases due to pyrrolizidine (Senecio) poisoning in Arizona. Gastroenterol 1977;73:349–352.

135. Richard JL. Mycotoxin photosensitivity. J Am Vet Med Assoc 1973;163:1298–1299.

136. Todd FG, Stermitz FR, Knight AP: Alkaloids of bindweed (Convolvulus arvensis). Unpublished data.

137. Ivie WG: Chemical and biochemical aspects of photosensitization in livestock and poultry. J Natl Cancer Inst 1982;69:259–262.

138. James LF, Ralphs MH. Water hemlock. Utah Sci 1980; 47:2–7.

139. Adams LG, Dollahite JW, Romane WM, et al. Cystitis and ataxia associated with sorghum ingestion in horses. J Am Vet Med Assoc 1969;155:518–524.

140. Keeler RF. Alkaloid teratogens from lupinus, conium, veratrum and related genera. In: Keeler RF, Van Kampen KR, James LE, eds. Effects of poisonous plants on livestock. Academic Press, New York, 1978;397–408.

141. Panter KE, Keeler RE, Baker DC. Toxicoses in livestock from the hemlocks (Conium and Cicuta spp.). J Anim Sci 1988;66:2407–2413.

142. True RG, Lowe JE. Induced juglone toxicosis in ponies and horses. Am J Vet Res 1980;41:944–945.

143. Stowe HD: Effects of copper pretreatment upon the toxicity of selenium in ponies. Am J Vet Res 1980;41:1925–1928.

144. Tennant B, Evans CD, Schwartz LW, et al. Equine hepatic insufficiency. Vet Clin North Am Eq Pract 1973;3: 279–289.

145. Haskins FA, Gorz HJ, Johnson BE. Seasonal variation in leaf hydrocyanic potential of low- and high-dhurrin sorghums. Crop Sci 1987;27:903–906.

146. Hatch RC: Poisons causing respiratory insufficiency. In: Jones ML, Booth NH, McDonald LE, eds. Veterinary pharmacology and therapeutics. 4th Ed. Iowa State University Press, Ames, 1977;1163–1166.

147. Hegarty MP, Pound AW. Indospicine, a new hepatotoxic amino acid from Indigofera spicata. Nature 1970;217:354–355.

148. Owen RR. Potato poisoning in a horse. Vet Rec 1985;117:246.

149. Glover GH, Newsom IF, Robbins WW. A new poisonous plant. Agric Exp Stat 1918;246:1–16.

150. Cronin EH, Williams MC, Van Kampen KR, et al. The poisonous timber milkvetches. US Dept Agr Handbook 1974;459.

151. Keeler RF. Known and suspected teratogenic hazards in range plants. Clin Toxicol 1972;5:529–565.

152. James LF, Van Kampen KR, Staker GR. Locoweed (Astragalus lentiginosus) poisoning in cattle and horses. J Am Vet Med Assoc 1969;155:525–530.

153. Johnson AE. Toxicologic aspects of photosensitization in livestock. J Natl Cancer Inst 1982;69:253–259.

154. Olsen JD. Rat bioassay for estimating toxicity of plant material from larkspur (Delphinium spp.). Am J Vet Res 1977;38:277–279.

155. Joubert JPJ. Cardiac glycosides. In: Cheeke PR, ed. Toxicants of plant origin. Vol 1. Alkaloids. CRC Press, Boca Raton, FL, 1899;63–92.

156. Moscley EL. The cause of trembles in cattle, sheep, and horses and of milk sickness in people. Med Rec 1909;75:699–715.

157. Peterson JE, Culvenor CCJ. Hepatoxic pyrrolizidine alkaloids. In: Keeler RE, Tu AT, eds. Handbook of natural toxins. Vol 1. Plant and fungal toxins. Marcel Dekker, New York and Basel, 1983;637–641.

158. Reagor JC. Increased oleander poisoning after extensive freezes in the South/Southeast Texas. Southwest Vet 1985;36:95.

159. Broquist HP. Livestock toxicosis, slobbers, locoism, and the indolizidine alkaloids. Nutr Rev 1986;44:317–323.

160. Keeler RF, Balls LD. Teratogenic effects in cattle of Conium maculatum and conium alkaloids and analogs. Gun Toxicol 1978;12:49–64.

161. Arnold WN. Vincent van Gogh and the thujone connection. J Am Med Assoc 1988;260:3042–3044.

162. Carpenter KJ, Phillipson AT, Thompson W. Experiments with dried bracken (Pteris aquilina). Br Vet J 1950;106:292-308.

163. Goplen BP. Sweet clover production and agronomy. Can Vet J 1980;21:149–151.

164. Uhlinger C: Black walnut toxicosis in ten horses. J Am Vet Med Assoc 1989;195:343–344.

165. Witte ST, Will LA, Olsen CR, et al. Chronic selenosis in horses fed locally produced alfalfa hay. J Am Vet Med Assoc 1993;202:406–409.

166. Kelsey RG, Stephens JF, Shafizadeh F. The chemical constituents of sagebrush foliage and their isolation. J Range Mgt 1982;35:617–622.

167. Knight AP, Kimberling CV, Stermitz FR, et al. Cynoglossum officinale (hound's tongue) – a cause of pyrrolizidine alkaloid poisoning in horses. J Am Vet Med Assoc 1984;185: 647–650.

168. Levander OA: Metabolic relationships between arsenic and selenium. Environ Health Perspect 1977;19:159–164.

169. Seiber JN, Nelson CJ, Lee SM. Cardenolides in the latex and leaves of seven Asciepias species and Calotropis procera. Phytochemistry 1982;21:2343–2348.

170. Smetzer DL, Coppack RW, Ely RW, et al. Cardiac effects of white snakeroot intoxication in horses. Equine Pract 1983;5:26–32.

171. Tennant B, Dill SG, Glickman LT, et al. Acute hemolytic anemia, methemoglobinemia, and Heinz body formation associated with ingestion of red maple leaves by horses. J Am Vet Med Assoc 1981;179:143–150.

172. Edwards WC, Burrows GE, Tyrl RJ. Toxic plants of Oklahoma: milkweeds. Oklahoma Vet Med Assoc 1984; 36:74–79.

173. Wolfe C, Lance WR. Locoweed poisoning in a northern New Mexico elk herd. J Range Mgt 1984;37:59–63.

174. Kelly WR, Young MP, Hegarty MP, et al. The hepatotoxicity of indospicine to dogs. In: James LF, Keeler RF, Bailey EM, Cheeke PR, Hegarty MP, eds. Poisonous Plants Proceedings Third International Symposium. Iowa State University Press, Ames, 1992;126–130.

175. Semrad SD. Acute hemolytic anemia from the ingestion of red maple leaves. Compend Contin Educ Pract Vet 1993;15: 261–264.

176. Hultine JD, Mount ME, Easley KJ, et al. Selenium toxicosis in the horse. Equine Pract 1979;1:57–60.

177. Anderson GA, Mount ME, Vrins AA, et al. Fatal acorn poisoning in a horse: Pathologic findings and diagnostic considerations. J Am Vet Med Assoc 1983;182:1105–1110.

178. Flemming CE. Poisonous range plants. Nevada Ag Exp Sta Ann Report 1920;1919:39.

179. Nation PN. Hepatic disease in Alberta horses; A retrospective study of "alsike clover poisoning" (1973–1988). Can Vet J 1991;32:602–607.

180. Williams MC, James LF. Livestock poisoning from nitrobearing Astragalus. In: Keeler RF, Van Kampen KR, James LE, eds. Effects of poisonous plants on livestock. Academic Press, New York, 1978;378–389.

181. Ormsby OB: A poisonous California plant. USDA Mo Rep, 1873;503–504.

182. Bruce EA. Astragalus campestris and other stock poisoning plants of British Columbia. Bulletin 88. Can Dept Agric, 1927.

183. Pamukcu AM, Price JM, Bryan GT. Naturally occurring and bracken fern-induced bovine urinary bladder tumors. Vet Pathol 1976;13:110–122.

184. Szabuniewicz M, Schwartz WL, McGrady JD, et al. Experimental oleander poisoning and treatment. Southwest Vet 1972;25:105–114.

185. Konishi K, Ichijo S. Experimentally induced equine bracken poisoning by thermostable antithiamine factor (SF factor) extracted from dried bracken. J Jpn Vet Med Assoc 1984;37:730–734.

186. Marsh CD, Roe GC. The "alkali disease" of livestock in the Pecos Valley. USDA Bulletin 1921;180:1–8.

187. Witzel DA, Dollahite JW, Jones LP. Photosensitization in sheep fed Ammi majus (bishop's weed) seed. Am J Vet Res 1978;39:320–321.

188. Buck WB, Osweiler GD. Cyanide. In: Van Gelder GA, ed. Clinical diagnostic veterinary toxicology. Kendall Hunt, Dubuque, IA, 1976;105–108.

189. Larson KA, Young S. Nigropallidal encephalomalacia in horses in Colorado. J Am Vet Med Assoc 1970;156:626–628.

190. Majak W, McDiarmid RE, Hall WJ. The cyanide potential of Saskatoon service berry (Amelanchier alnifolia) and choke cherry (Prunus virginiana). Can J Anim Sci 1981; 61:681.

191. Marsh CD, Clawson AB: The locoweed disease. USDA Bulletin 1919;1054:1–32.

192. Mattocks AR. Recent studies on mechanisms of cytotoxic action of pyrrolizidine alkaloids. In: Keeler RF, Van Kampen KR, James LE, eds. Effects of poisonous plants on livestock. Academic Press, New York, 1987;177–187.

193. Swick RA. Hepatic metabolism and bioactivation of mycotoxins and plant toxins. J Anim Sci 58: 1984; 1017–1028.

194. Dalvi RR, Sawant SG, Terse PS. Efficacy of alpha ketoglutaric acid as an effective antidote in cyanide poisoning in dogs. Vet Res Commun 1990;14:411–414.

195. Rainey DP, Smalley DB, Crump MH, et al. Isolation of salivation factor from Rhizoctonia leguminicola-infected red clover hay. Nature 1973;205:203–204.

196. Stevens KL, Riopelle RJ, Wong RY. Repin, a sesquiterpene lactone from Acroptilon repens possessing exceptional biological activity. J Nat Prod 1990;53:218–221.

197. Wolf FA, Curtis RS, Kaupp BF. A monograph on trembles or milk sickness and white snakeroot. N Carolina Agr Exp Stat, Bulletin 1918;15.

198. Watson WA, Terlecki S, Patterson SP, et al. Experimentally produced progressive retinal degeneration (bright blindness) in sheep. Br Vet J 1972;128:457–468.

199. Conn EE. Cyanogenesis, the production of hydrogen cyanide by plants. In: Keeler RF, Van Kampen KR, James LE, eds. Effects of poisonous plants on livestock. Academic Press, New York, 1978;301–310.

200. Campangnolo ER. USDA Animal and Plant Health Inspection Service, Springfield IL. Personal communication, June 1993.

201. Thompson U. Depression and choke in a horse: probable white snakeroot toxicosis. Vet Hum Toxicol 1989;31:321–322.

202. Cheeke PR, Shull LR. Glycosides. In: Cheeke PR, Shull LR, eds. Natural toxicants in feeds and poisonous plants. AVI Publishing Co, Westport, CT, 1985;190–192.

203. Fowler ME. Nigropallidal encephalomalacia in the horse. J Am Vet Med Assoc 1965;147:607–616.

204. Craig AM, Meyer C, Koller LD, et al. Serum enzyme tests for pyrrolizidine alkaloid toxicosis. Proc Am Assoc Vet Lab Diagnost, 1978;161–178.

205. MacDonald H. Hemlock poisoning in horses. Vet Rec 1937;49:1211–1212.

206. Bridges CH, Camp BJ, Livingston CW. Kleingrass (Panicum coloratum) poisoning in sheep. Vet Pathol 1987;24: 525–531.

207. Gorz HL Haskins FA, Vogel KP. Inheritance of dhurrin content in mature sorghum leaves. Crop Sci 1986;26:65–67.

208. Williams MC, James LE. Poisoning in sheep from emory milkvetch and nitro-compounds. J Range Mgt 1976;29:165–167.

209. O'Hara PL Pierce KR, Read WK. Degenerative myopathy associated with the ingestion of Cassia occidentalis L: clinical and pathologic features of the experimentally induced disease. Am J Vet Res 1969;30:2173–2180.

210. Cheeke PR, Shull LR. Hypericin. In: Cheeke PR, Shull LR, eds. Natural toxicants in feeds and poisonous plants. AVI Publishing Co, Westport, CT, 1985;348–350.

211. Moran EA. Cyanogenic compounds in plants and their significance in the animal industry. Am J Vet Res 1954;15:171–176.

212. Craigmill AL, Seawright AA, Mattilla T, et al. Pathological changes in the mammary gland and biochemical changes in the milk of the goat following oral dosing with leaf of the avocado (Persea americana). Aust Vet J 1989;66:206–211.

213. Sanders M. White snakeroot poisoning in a foal: a case report. Equine Vet Sci 1987;3:128–131.

214. Aiyar VN, Bern MH, Hanna T. The principle toxin of Delphinium brownii and its mode of action. Experientia 1979;35:1367–1368.

215. Farrel RK, Sande RD, Lincoln SD. Nigropallidal encephalomalacia in a horse. J Am Vet Med Assoc 1971;158:1201–1204.

216. Seawright AA, Hrdlicka J, Wright JD, et al. The identification of hepatotoxic pyrrolizidine alkaloid exposure in horses by the demonstration of sulphur-bound pyrrolic metabolites on their hemoglobin. Vet Hum Toxicol 1991;33:286–287.

217. Schmutz EM, Freeman BN, Reed RE. Jimmyweed (Haplopappus heterophylus). In: Schmutz EM, Freeman BN, Reed RE, eds. Livestock Poisoning plants of Arizona. University of Arizona Press, Tucson, 1974;42–45.

218. Rook JS, Marteniuk JV, Alden W, et al. An outbreak of impaction colic due to ingestion of cockspur hawthorn fruit. Equine Pract 1991;13:28–32.

219. O'Dell BL, Regan WO, Beach TJ. A study of the toxic principle in red clover. Missouri Univ Ag Exp St Res Bulletin 1959;702:3–12.

220. Sperry OE, Dollahite JW, Hoffman GO, et al. Isocoma wrightii (Aplopappus heterophylus). In: Sperry OE, Dollahite JW, Hoffman GO, Camp BJ, eds. Texas plants poisonous to livestock. Texas Agr Exp Stat and Texas A&M University, College Station, Texas B-1028: 1968;26–27.

221. Marsh CD. Poisonous properties of the whorled milk-weeds Asclepias pumila and A. verticillata var. Geyeri. USDA Bulletin 1921;942:1–14.

222. Goeger DE, Cheeke PR, Buhier DR, et al. Effect of tansy ragwort consumption on dairy goats and goat milk transfer of pyrrolizidine alkaloids. In: Cheeke PR, ed. Symposium on Pyrrolizidine (Senecio) Alkaloids: Toxicity, Metabolism and Poisonous Plants Control Measures. Oregon State University, Corvallis, 1979;77–83.

223. Martin BW, Terry MK, Bridges CH, et al. Toxicity of Cassia occidentalis in the horse. Vet Hum Toxicol 1981;23:416–417.

224. Spoerke DG, Spoerke SE: Three cases of Zigadenous poisoning. Vet Hum Toxicol 1979;25:346–347.

225. Cunha TJ, Chairman, and Subcommittee on Swine Nutrition: Nutrient Requirements of Swine. 7th Ed. National Academy of Sciences, Washington, DC, 1973.

226. Kelleway RA, Geovjian L. Acute bracken fern poisoning in a 14-month-old horse. Vet Med Sm Anim Clin 1978; 73:295–296.

227. Alden CL, Fosnaugh JF, Smith JB, et al. Japanese yew poisoning of large domestic animals in the midwest. J Am Vet Med Assoc 1977;70:314–316.

228. Nation PN, Bern MH, Roth SH, Wilkens JL. Clinical signs and studies of the site of action of purified larkspur alkaloid, methyllycaconitine, administered parenterally to calves. Can Vet J 1982;23:264–266.

229. MacDonald MA. Timber milkvetch poisoning in British Columbia ranges. J Range Mgt 1952;5:16–21.

230. McPherson A. In: Kinghorn AD, Pokeweed and other lymphocyte mitogens in toxic plants. Columbia University Press, New York, 1979;81–102.

231. Edmonds LD, Selby LA, Case AA. Poisoning and congenital malformations associated with consumption of poison hemlock by sows. J Am Vet Med Assoc 1972;160:1319–1324.

232. James LF, Keeler RF, Binns W. Sequence in the abortive and teratogenic effects of locoweed fed to sheep. Am J Vet Res 1967;30:377–383.

233. Williams MC, James LF. Effects of herbicides on the concentration of poisonous compounds in plants: a review. Am J Vet Res 1981;44:2420–2422.

234. Cedarleaf JD, Welch BL, Brotherson JD. Seasonal variation in monoterpenoids in big sagebrush (Artemisia tridentata). J Range Mgt 1983;36:492–494.

235. Edmondson AJ, Norman BB, Suther D. Survey of state veterinarians and state veterinary diagnostic laboratories for selenium deficiency and toxicosis in animals. J Am Vet Med Assoc 1993;202:865–872.

236. McClean EK. The toxic actions of pyrrolizidine (Senecio) alkaloids. Pharmacol Rev 1970;22:429–483.

Index

Nutritional Management of Equine Diseases and Special Cases, First Edition. Edited by Bryan M. Waldridge.
© 2017 John Wiley & Sons, Inc. Published 2017 by John Wiley & Sons, Inc.